BIOCHEMISTRY OF PARASITIC HELMINTHS

BIOCHEMISTRY OF PARASITIC HELMINTHS

JOHN BARRETT
Department of Zoology
The University College of Wales
Aberystwyth, Dyfed

UNIVERSITY PARK PRESS
Baltimore

595.1
B275b

LIBRARY
ATLANTIC CHRISTIAN COLLEGE
WILSON, N. C.

First published 1981 by
Macmillan Publishers Ltd
London and Basingstoke

Published in North America by
UNIVERSITY PARK PRESS
233 East Redwood Street
Baltimore, Maryland 21202

Printed in Hong Kong

British Library Cataloguing in Publication Data

Barrett, John, *b. 1943*
   Biochemistry of parasitic helminths.
   1. Worms, Intestinal and parasitic
   2. Biological chemistry
   I. Title
   595′.1′04524   QL392

   ISBN 0-8391-4141-6   LCCCN 80-50999

To Sara and Kate

Contents

Preface

It is the aim of this book to give a comparative account of the biochemistry of parasitic helminths and to relate the biochemistry of parasites not only to that of mammals but also to that of free-living invertebrates. The emphasis is on regulation and deals with metabolic control both at the cellular and at the developmental level.

A difficulty in parasite biochemistry is that the information is patchy, some aspects are known in great detail and others not at all. In the text, I have tried to indicate those areas of parasite biochemistry that have been neglected, in the past, since, in some ways, what is not known about helminths is almost as interesting as what is known.

The book does not deal with nerve–muscle physiology, nor with osmoregulation, and nor does it discuss, in detail, the mode of action of anthelmintics. However, a table of the possible biochemical modes of action of the more important anthelmintics is given in Appendix 7.1.

For the purpose of this book, I have taken helminths to include acanthocephalans, cestodes, trematodes, nematodes and nematomorphs. Throughout the text, *Ascaris lumbricoides* is used, rather than *A. suum* or var. *suis*. In almost all cases, it is the ascarid from pigs which has been investigated and not the human worm.

The literature has been covered up to December 1978, and the sheer number of references poses a severe problem. The compromise I have adopted is to have a general reading list composed of relevant reviews at the end of each chapter, as well as the specific references. Any reference that can easily be found from the general reading list is not included in the specific list; in particular, T. von Brand's book, *The Biochemistry of Parasites* (2nd edn, 1973), gives comprehensive references to all of the literature prior to 1973. In this way, it should be possible to find the reference to any particular point of interest, yet keep the reference lists to manageable proportions.

It is inevitable that some of the information in this book will rapidly become out of date or prove to be incorrect. What I hope the text will provide is a framework within which the reader can place new developments in context.

In conclusion, I should like to thank those colleagues who have sent me reprints or allowed me to quote from their unpublished work. Also, I am grateful to R. W. Walker, J. M. Paul and, in particular, G. M. Lloyd for reading and commenting on various aspects of the manuscript.

June, 1979   *J.B.*

1 Introduction to Parasite Biochemistry

Biochemistry consists of both variant and invariant elements. The invariant aspects of biochemistry are features like the use of DNA and RNA and the major metabolic pathways that are common to all living organisms. The variant part of biochemistry covers the ways in which metabolic pathways are modified to suit the environmental needs of the animal and the variations in the details of cofactor requirements and molecular structure. The invariant features of biochemistry emphasise the biochemical similarities between living organisms, and the variant aspects highlight the differences. A comparative approach to the biochemistry of animals or a group of animals, such as will be taken in this book, will tend to emphasise the differences between animals, rather than dwell on the similarities.

Much of the interest in parasite biochemistry comes from the ways in which the metabolic pathways have been modified to suit the highly specialised parasitic mode of life. In addition to this intrinsic interest, parasite biochemistry has great practical importance through chemotherapy and vaccine production. The development of successful vaccines against parasitic helminths necessitates routine *in vitro* culture, and for this an intimate knowledge of parasite biochemistry is required. In chemotherapy, parasite biochemistry can contribute to the development of new drugs and to the elucidation of the mode of action of compounds already discovered. The increased awareness of the possible dangerous side-effects of drugs has led to renewed interest in the mode of action of anthelmintics. For this, the basic biochemistry of parasites must be understood before the specific biochemical lesions caused by drugs can be identified. However, few if any anthelmintics have been reported to have one single mode of action, most of them appearing to disrupt several different cellular activities at once. Anthelmintics, by their very nature, are toxic to parasites, and perhaps it is not surprising that, in the dying parasite, many different metabolic processes become disrupted. So, identifying the primary effect of an anthelmintic (if indeed there is only one) is not a straightforward process. Commercially, the discovery of new anthelmintics involves the screening of large numbers of random compounds, in the hope that a new drug will be found. This empirical approach is, needless to say, very expensive and time-consuming (only 1 in 10 000 compounds screened shows any activity). It has often been felt that, with the increase in knowledge in parasite biochemistry over the last twenty years, a more rational approach to helminth chemotherapy should be possible, the idea being that any differences between the biochemistry of parasites and that of their mammalian hosts are potential sites for chemotherapy. Once such a difference has been identified, specific inhibitors for the parasite pathway could then be synthesised. Many biochemical differences between parasitic helminths and mammals are now known, but the rational approach to parasite chemotherapy has yet to produce a successful compound. Possibly, in comparison with the empirical method, the rational approach has not had a sufficiently long trial. More promising, perhaps, is the semi-rational approach in which knowledge, gained from the mode of action of empirically discovered drugs, is used as a basis for the synthesis of improved compounds.

1.1. THE PARASITE'S ENVIRONMENT

Animal environments can be divided into aquatic, terrestrial and parasitic. The environment of a parasite is, of course, the body of another animal, and this seems to be a relatively difficult environment to invade. However, those organisms which have done so have often been remarkably successful, both in terms of numbers of species and numbers of individuals.

An outstanding feature of many parasites is their complex life-cycles, which can involve up to four different hosts, interspersed with free-living phases. A parasite may be faced with a succession of different environments, ranging from the free-living, to the tissues of an invertebrate, to the tissues of an ectothermal vertebrate, to the tissues of an endothermal vertebrate. Even within the vertebrate host, helminths often undergo extensive migrations, passing, say, from the gut, to the bloodstream, to the lungs and back again to the gut. The change from one phase of the life-cycle to the next in parasites is often extremely rapid and there is little time for acclimatisation. The different environments occupied by a parasite during its life-cycle necessitate different biochemical (and structural) adaptations. So, the life-cycle of a parasitic helminth involves a regular sequence of metabolic switches; the extent of the biochemical changes occurring at each phase depends on the degree of difference between the two environments involved. The actual metabolic switches that take place during the life-cycle of parasitic helminths, and the control of these switches by environmental and genetic factors, will be dealt with in Section 5.2.

Parasites can invade almost every part of the vertebrate and invertebrate body, although some organs are more commonly parasitised than others. In vertebrates, the most favoured habitats are the alimentary system, the bloodstream and the respiratory system, in that order. The number of parasitic habitats in invertebrates is much fewer, and only the alimentary canal, its associated structures and the haemocoel are invaded to any great extent.

A detailed account of all of the different possible parasitic sites in vertebrates and invertebrates would involve a description of virtually every organ system and is obviously outside the scope of this book. Instead, we shall look briefly at the major physico-chemical factors that are especially important in influencing parasite metabolism and development in the different sites.

1.1.1. Oxygen Tension

The oxygen tension in the parasite's environment is important in relation to the possibility of aerobic or anaerobic metabolism. Oxygen tension in different parasite habitats can vary widely (*Table 1.1*). In general, reasonable amounts of oxygen are present in the tissues and body fluids of vertebrates, but in the alimentary canal and excretory system the oxygen tensions are low and rather variable. In the vertebrate gut, the partial pressure of oxygen is much higher at the mucosal surface than in the centre of the lumen, where it can fall to zero. In addition, intestinal pO_2 varies with the feeding cycle, being higher during fasting than after a meal. Gut micro-organisms may create localised anaerobic conditions, and obligate anaerobes like *Trichomonad*

Table 1.1 Oxygen tensions in vertebrate tissues

Habitat	Species	O_2 tension (mmHg)
Swim bladder	Fish	> 760
Skin	Mammals	50–100
Subcutaneous tissues	Mammals	20–43
Arterial blood	Mammals, birds and fish	70–100
Venous blood	Mammals and birds	40–66
	Fish	15–20
Peritoneal cavity	Mammals	28–40
Pleural cavity	Mammals	12–39
Urine	Mammals	14–60
Bile	Mammals	0–30
Stomach	Mammals (gases)	0–70*
Small intestine	Mammals (gases)	0–65*
	Mammals and birds (contents)	0.5–30†
Large intestine	Mammals (gases)	0–5

*High values due to swallowed air.   †Highest values near mucosa.

protozoa are able to survive in what would appear to be aerobic sites, such as the mouth, because of these local regions. Gut parasites, like hookworms, which feed on blood, may be able to get some oxygen from their blood meal.

The oxygen tension in invertebrates has not been measured and it is usually assumed that the tissues of small invertebrates are reasonably aerobic. Some insects only open their spiracles periodically and in these the pO_2 can drop to 20 mmHg when the spiracles are closed. The presence of obligate anaerobes in the intestines of several invertebrate species suggests that there are at least localised anaerobic regions in the gut. The oxygen tension in free-living habitats can also be very variable, anaerobic conditions frequently being found in stagnant water, mud and fermenting faeces.

During their life-cycles, parasites may have to face wide variations in oxygen availability. Many parasitic habitats have very low oxygen tensions and these are often described as being micro-aerobic. However, no parasitic site can really be described as totally anaerobic and all parasites probably have at least some oxygen available to them, although they may have to cope with extensive periods of anaerobiosis.

1.1.2. Carbon Dioxide Tension and Other Gases

Carbon dioxide levels play an important role in parasitic helminths. In many parasites, carbohydrate breakdown involves carbon dioxide fixation (Section 3.1.2), and pCO_2 plays a major part in the activation of trematode cysts, in the hatching and exsheathment of nematode eggs and larvae and in enhancing the hatching and activation of acanthocephalan eggs and cystacanths. Carbon dioxide is also one of the factors which attracts plant parasitic nematodes to developing roots.

In air, the pCO_2 is extremely low, 0.3 mmHg, but the levels in animal tissues, however, are very much higher (*Table 1.2*). In the blood and tissues of terrestrial vertebrates, the pCO_2 is around 40 mmHg, and in aquatic vertebrates, because of the high solubility of carbon dioxide in water, the pCO_2 is lower, 2-10 mmHg. Few measurements are available from invertebrates, but in insect tissues pCO_2 values of 23 to 48 mmHg have been recorded.

Table 1.2 Carbon dioxide tensions in vertebrate tissues

Habitat	Species	CO_2 tension (mmHg)
Blood	Mammals	34–42
	Birds	21–26
	Reptiles	27–38
	Fish	1.3–10
Small intestine	Non-ruminant mammals and birds	20–600
	Ruminant mammals	500–700

The intestines of mammals have extremely high pCO_2 levels, particularly ruminants where partial pressures of carbon dioxide as high as 700 mmHg have been reported. These excessively high levels of carbon dioxide must pose severe acid/base regulation problems for intestinal helminths (Section 3.2.10). It has also been suggested that the carbon dioxide fixing pathways found in helminths may have arisen in response to the high environmental carbon dioxide levels and are not necessarily adaptations to low oxygen levels (Section 3.7).

Animal tissues are characterised by relatively high carbon dioxide levels, and carbon dioxide may be an important factor in delineating the parasitic environment from the free-living one.

A number of other gases occur in the vertebrate intestine, particularly methane and hydrogen, but it is not known if they play any role in parasite development or metabolism.

1.1.3. Oxidation–Reduction Potential

Low oxidation–reduction (redox) potentials (reducing conditions) are required to initiate hatching or excystment in a number of nematode and trematode life-cycles.

The redox state will also have a bearing on the functioning of helminth cytochrome chains.

Oxidation–reduction potentials are difficult parameters to measure and there is little information available on different environments. For aerobic cells, the oxidation–reduction potential usually lies between −150 and +200 mV. The values for liver and brain are low, about −100 mV, those for muscle and nervous tissue somewhat higher, −50 to +100 mV. In the mammal, the stomach contents tend to be oxidised, around +150 mV, whilst the intestinal contents are reduced, −100 mV. The gut contents of insects are usually positive (up to +200 mV), but reducing conditions do occur, in *Blattela* (−100 mV) and in Mallophaga and clothes moths (−200 mV). In these last two groups, low redox conditions are necessary for the digestion of keratin.

Whether it is really possible to talk about a single redox potential for a particular tissue or environment is, however, questionable. Within tissues or cells there are many different redox couples which are not necessarily in equilibrium, so there is really no single redox value. Some redox couples will interact directly with metal electrodes, and can be measured by redox electrodes. Other systems will react with redox dyes and can be measured in that way. Still other systems do not react with either dyes or electrodes. One very important redox system, the thiol group system, is essentially irreversible and so, although extremely important, cannot be measured. Yet a possible mechanism for the action of reducing agents in the activation of helminth eggs and cysts is the need to keep thiol groups in the reduced form. A single redox value for a tissue or habitat, although it gives a convenient label, does not adequately express the oxidation–reduction states of the different possible redox couples.

1.1.4. Hydrogen Ion Concentration

The pH of parasitic habitats can vary widely. In body fluids and tissues, the pH is usually about neutral (pH 6.8–7.4), although minor fluctuations do occur; for example, in active muscle, lactic acid accumulation can cause a drop of 0.1 to 0.3 pH units. In the vertebrate gut, the stomach is extremely acidic (pH 1–3), whilst in the small intestine it is nearly neutral (pH 5–7.8). As the acidic stomach contents pass into the small intestine, there is a transitory drop in pH. In invertebrates, there is usually no acidic gastric phase in digestion. Instead, in insects the mid-gut is usually neutral to alkaline (pH 6–8) and may be as high as pH 10 in Lepidoptera. The hind-gut is usually more acidic due to excretions from the malpighian tubules and there may also be localised acidic regions. Values for intestinal pH in other invertebrates are, for crustacea pH 4.7–6.6, for annelids pH 6–7.8 and for molluscs pH 5.5–7.6.

External pH usually only slowly affects intracellular pH and, in general, the metabolism of invertebrates is relatively unaffected by external changes in pH over a limited range. Nevertheless, the extremely acidic vertebrate stomach is a major obstacle for parasites which must traverse it, and the low pH of the stomach is possibly the main reason why relatively few parasites are found there.

1.1.5. Osmotic Pressure

The osmotic pressure of the environment determines the amount of osmotic work that an organism has to do. Changes in osmotic pressure also trigger hatching in a number of helminth eggs. An example of this is *Schistosoma mansoni*; the eggs of this trematode pass out in the faeces and hatching is inhibited at osmotic pressures above about $\Delta = -0.5\,°C$. On dilution of the faeces by water, there is a massive hatching of eggs.

Table 1.3   Osmoconcentration in different parasite environments

Habitat	$\Delta\,(°C)$	Animal	Body fluid $\Delta\,(°C)$
Fresh water	−0.01	Molluscs	−0.08 to −0.22
		Crustacea	−0.8
		Fish	−0.5 to −0.55
		Amphibia	−0.45
Brackish water	−0.2 to −0.5	Euryhaline invertebrates	−0.5 to −1.8
Sea water	−1.85	Invertebrates	−1.8 to −1.85
		Elasmobranchs	−1.85 to −1.92
		Teleosts	−0.65 to −0.7
Terrestrial		Annelids	−0.3 to −0.4
		Molluscs	−0.5
		Insects	−0.5 to −1.0
		Reptiles	−0.6 to −0.7
		Mammals	−0.5 to −0.58

The range of osmotic pressures found in different free-living environments and in the tissues of different hosts is summarised in *Table 1.3*. During its life-cycle, a parasite may have to cope with a wide range of osmotic pressures, passing, say, from the tissues of a mammal ($\Delta = -0.58\,°C$), to fresh ($\Delta = -0.01\,°C$) or sea water ($\Delta = -1.85\,°C$), to the tissues of a marine or freshwater invertebrate ($\Delta = -0.08\,°C$ to $-1.85\,°C$). In general, tissue parasites are isosmotic with their environments, gut parasites slightly hypotonic. In the mammalian gut, the osmolarity of the contents tends towards that of the plasma ($\Delta = -0.58\,°C$). However, the volume of the free water in the gut varies with the feeding cycle, there being almost no fluid present in the fasting intestine.

1.1.6. Temperature

Temperature affects the rates of chemical reactions and the stability of biological macromolecules. Parasites of endotherms are subject to dramatic temperature changes during the course of their life-cycles. When an infective stage invades its mammalian or avian host, there is a sudden increase in environmental temperature to 35–43 °C. Conversely, when parasite eggs or larvae are shed from their endothermic host, there is an equally sudden drop in ambient temperature. These extensive temperature changes pose major problems for the functioning of metabolic pathways and for the stability of lipid membranes and cell proteins. The effects of temperature change on the properties of enzymes and on the composition of parasite lipids will be considered in detail in Section 5.2. For parasites of endotherms, a temperature above about 35 °C is usually required before infective stages can be activated.

1.1.7. Bile Salts

Bile salts are steroid derivatives and are involved in the hatching of helminth eggs, in the activation of trematode cysts and in the evagination of cestode scoleces. The role of bile salts in triggering these different events is probably related to their surfactant properties, and in many cases it can be mimicked by detergents.

The composition of bile varies substantially within different vertebrate groups and in some cases, at least, these differences may play a part in determining host specificity. In the vertebrate, there is a correlation between diet and the type of bile salts produced, herbivores having mainly dihydroxy and monohydroxymono-keto bile salts, and carnivores having trihydroxy bile salts.

Bile salts are not found in invertebrates. However, surfactant agents, such as sarcosyltaurine, occur in the intestines of crustaceans and possibly other higher invertebrates. Whether these compounds are involved in the activation of helminth stages in the invertebrate intestine is not known.

1.1.8. Other Factors

Environmental factors such as pCO_2, pO_2, temperature, pH and E_h act as developmental triggers in helminth life-cycles. These factors also influence metabolism directly; carbon dioxide and oxygen are substrates for carboxylating and oxidase reactions, respectively, temperature affects a variety of enzyme parameters (Section 5.2.3), as does pH, whilst E_h influences redox-linked reactions. Osmotic pressure and the presence or absence of bile salts also act as major environmental stimuli in different helminths. In addition, there are a number of other physico-chemical parameters which change from environment to environment and may act as developmental stimuli or necessitate specific metabolic adaptations.

Hosts, both vertebrate and invertebrate, mount, or attempt to mount, an immune response to invading parasites. The immune response can involve phagocytic and cytotoxic cells, specific antibodies and non-specific agglutinins and lysins. For the parasite, coping with the immune response involves tegumental modifications and in some cases the production of immunosuppressive or immunodisruptive compounds (Section 2.8.2). Hormones are another host product which affects parasites. Some helminths are able to respond to host hormone changes and in this way integrate their reproductive cycles with those of their hosts (Section 2.8). In other situations, parasites need to remain unaffected by host endocrine changes.

Intestinal helminths must protect themselves against digestion by host enzymes (Section 4.1.3), but partial digestion by host enzymes is necessary for hatching in a number of helminth eggs and cysts. For acanthocephalans and cestodes, which produce no digestive enzymes of their own, the activity of host enzymes is essential for providing nutrients of low molecular weight.

Within their hosts, parasites occupy high-nutrient habitats, although there are both quantitative and qualitative differences between sites. For example, intestinal amino acid ratios may be different in different hosts (Section 4.1.8) and, because of fermentation in the rumen, carbohydrate levels in the intestines of ruminants are much lower than those in non-ruminants. The nutritional requirements of helminths are poorly understood (Section 4.9) and the extent to which the availability of a particular nutrient or group of nutrients limits the distribution of helminths is not known. In general, it is probably the overall nutritional requirements that limit a parasite to a particular host or host group, rather than the requirement for a specific metabolite. Examples of specific requirements in parasitic helminths are rare; some shark tapeworms need urea for normal development, and several of the minor orders of tapeworms accumulate large amounts of vitamin B_{12} (Section 2.7.1). Egg hatching in the plant parasitic nematode *Globodera rostochiensis* is greatly stimulated by root exudates from host plants. The active factor in root exudate has been named ecleptic acid, and is an unstable lactone with an empirical formula of $C_{18}H_{24}O_8$.

Two other environmental factors that can affect parasites are the viscosity of the medium, which is important in locomotion and attachment, and light. A number of trematode and cestode eggs require light for hatching. Although action spectra have been constructed for the hatching of *Diphyllobothrium latum* eggs, the nature of the photosensitive pigment is not known.

The presence of a parasite in a particular site within a host may result in changes in the physico-chemical and biotic parameters of that site. A good example of this is the rat tapeworm *Hymenolepis diminuta*. The presence of this parasite causes a rise in intestinal redox potential, pCO_2 and pO_2 and a fall in intestinal pH and water; the number of micro-organisms in the intestine is reduced and the proportions of the different species altered. The physiology of the infected host is thus often different from the physiology of the uninfected host.

1.2. PARASITES AS INVERTEBRATES

Parasitic helminths belong to four different phyla, the Platyhelminthes, the Nematoda, the Nematomorpha and the Acanthocephala. Of these, two, the Nematomorpha and the Acanthocephala are totally parasitic groups. The platyhelminths and nematodes have both parasitic and free-living members and, in these two groups, parasitism has arisen independently on more than one occasion. So taxonomically, parasitic helminths represent a very miscellaneous collection of organisms and one would not necessarily expect their biochemistry to be very similar. On the contrary, it is perhaps remarkable that in many cases the metabolism of the different groups of parasitic helminths is often so alike.

The biochemistry of free-living invertebrates has not been extensively studied, so it is frequently not clear to what extent the metabolism, for example, of parasitic nematodes differs from that of their free-living relatives. Considerable emphasis in parasite biochemistry has been placed on the ways in which the biochemistry of helminths differs from that of their mammalian hosts. However, such differences are not necessarily adaptations to parasitism and may, instead, reflect basic differences between the biochemistry of invertebrates and the biochemistry of mammals. In steroid synthesis, for example (Section 4.3.3), parasitic helminths cannot synthesise steroids *de novo*, whilst mammals do. Free-living platyhelminths and nematodes (and many other invertebrates) are also unable to synthesise steroids. So the lack of steroid synthesis in parasitic helminths is not related to parasitism but is a peculiarity of the phyla (and invertebrates generally). From the point of view of chemotherapy, what is important is that there is a difference between the biochemistry of the host and the biochemistry of the parasite. Often the metabolism of free-living and parasitic helminths is very similar. So an investigation of the basic differences between invertebrate and mammalian systems could yield useful pointers to the ways in which the biochemistry of parasitic helminths might differ from that of their mammalian hosts. This presents the possibility that free-living helminths (such as the free-living nematodes *Caenorhabditis elegans* or *Turbatrix aceti*) could be used in preliminary screens for anthelmintics.

1.3. TECHNICAL PROBLEMS IN PARASITE BIOCHEMISTRY

Metabolic studies with parasitic helminths present a number of special problems due, first, to the fact that the habitat of a parasite is the tissues of another animal and, secondly, to the small size of the majority of helminths.

Parasites are in a state of dynamic equilibrium with their hosts, and this is particularly true of cestodes with their complex tegumental transport mechanisms (Section 4.1.6). Removal of a parasite from its host for *in vitro* experiments destroys this balance, although *in vitro* culture techniques do, to a certain extent, mimic the conditions inside the host. So, during *in vitro* work, there is always the criticism that the parasite, if not actually moribund, is not in its normal physiological state.

In vivo experiments with parasitic helminths, on the other hand, are very difficult to interpret. One often cannot be sure if a particular treatment is affecting the parasite directly or whether it is affecting the host and this in turn affects the parasite.

There is some evidence that parasites from different host species or different strains of host may show slight differences in their metabolism (Section 4.1.8). The sex and circadian rhythm of the host can also influence parasite metabolism. Parasitic helminths themselves often exist as a number of different strains, which again may differ, often quite considerably, in their biochemistry. So, apparent discrepancies between different groups of workers may have a variety of causes and for reproducible results the same strain and sex of parasite should be used. Moreover, it may have to be maintained in hosts of the same age, sex and strain and be isolated at the same time of day.

Most parasitic helminths are relatively small and often only limited numbers can be obtained from natural or even laboratory infections. The small size of most parasitic helminths means that only in a few cases is it possible to isolate specific tissues. For the majority of species, enzyme assays and biochemical analyses have to be performed on homogenates and extracts of whole animals. This means that differences between the various tissues of the parasite are obscured. A low enzyme activity in a whole homogenate could, for example, be due to a low activity throughout the animal or represent a high activity in some tissues and no activity in others. Another danger is that pathways can be proposed involving enzymes, which actually occur in different tissues.

1.4. SUMMARY AND CONCLUSIONS

Phylogenetically, parasitic helminths are a diverse group of organisms, all of which are adapted for a specialised mode of life.

The metabolism of parasitic helminths often shows considerable differences from that of its host, and these differences can be exploited by chemotherapy. The extent to which the metabolism of parasitic helminths differs from that of their free-living relatives is not so well known, there being comparatively little information on the biochemistry of free-living lower invertebrates. However, in many cases, the metabolism of free-living and parasitic helminths may be very similar.

The different parasitic sites within hosts offer unique combinations of physico-chemical and biotic factors, and parasites can be thought of as parasitising the homeostatic mechanisms of their hosts. The outstanding feature of parasite life-cycles is that they involve a series of rapid transitions from one habitat to the next. The different environments occupied by a parasite can include the tissues of an invertebrate, the tissues of a cold-blooded vertebrate and the tissues of a warm-blooded vertebrate, with free-living stages between. The different phases of the life-cycle occupy sites with widely differing physico-chemical characteristics and this can entail extensive metabolic adaptations. The metabolic switches which accompany the transition from one stage of the life-cycle to the next in parasites are under both genetic and environmental control and will be discussed in detail in Section 5.2.

1.5. GENERAL READING

Mettrick, D. F. and Podesta, R. B. (1974). 'Ecological and physiological aspects of helminth–host interactions in the mammalian gastrointestinal canal'. *Adv. Parasitol.,* **12**, 183–278

Crompton, D. W. T. (1973). 'The sites occupied by some parasitic helminths in the alimentary tract of vertebrates'. *Biol. Rev.,* **48**, 27–83

Crompton, D. W. T. and Nesheim, M. C. (1976). 'Host–parasite relationships in the alimentary tract of domestic birds'. *Adv. Parasitol.,* **14**, 95–194

Kurelec, B. (1975). 'Molecular biology of helminth parasites'. *Int. J. Biochem.*, **6**, 375–86

Lackie, A. M. (1975). 'The activation of infective stages of endoparasites of vertebrates'. *Biol. Rev.*, **50**, 285–323

Smyth, J. D. (1976). *Introduction to Animal Parasitology*, 2nd edn. London; Hodder and Stoughton

2 Biochemical Constituents

Living organisms are all made of the same kinds of molecules and, in general, have similar gross chemical compositions. However, animals or groups of animals often contain specialised or unique constituents. The possibility of unique or unusual compounds in parasitic helminths is particularly interesting, since the presence of unique compounds implies the presence of unique pathways, and the latter are potential sites for chemotherapy.

The biochemical constituents of an organism are in a state of dynamic equilibrium, constantly being synthesised and broken down; the half-lives of biochemical molecules range from a few minutes to several days. Gross biochemical analyses of tissues tend to give a static impression and do not emphasise this constant turnover of cellular components. The biochemical composition of an organism can, therefore, be regulated by the relative activities of the different synthetic and degradative pathways. So, in reality, the biochemical constituents of animals should not be considered in isolation, but as part of a dynamic system.

2.1. INORGANIC COMPOUNDS

In helminths, the dry weight is usually some 10–20% of the wet weight, depending on the tissue and its physiological state. Inorganic compounds normally constitute 5–10% of the dry weight, except in cestodes, where the presence of calcareous corpuscles may push this up to 40%. Some helminths, such as the muscle larvae of *Trichinella spiralis*, become enclosed in a calcareous capsule, but this is of host origin.

The inorganic composition of parasites does not seem in any way to be unusual and is normally similar to that of their host. In particular, the trace element composition of host and parasite often show marked similarities. There are a few exceptions: iron and copper are found in relatively high levels in blood-feeding parasites and cobalt levels are high in *D. latum* and *Haemonchus contortus* (probably due to vitamin B_{12} accumulation). The liver fluke *Fasciola hepatica* is said to have a higher zinc and cobalt content than host liver, but a lower manganese and uranium content. In the body fluids of *Ascaris lumbricoides*, the chloride levels are low, bicarbonate and amino acids providing the bulk of the anions.

The extent to which the inorganic composition of parasitic helminths depends on the host is not certain. Helminths can be readily shown to accumulate labelled ions which have been fed to or injected into their hosts. The uptake of ^{32}P has been demonstrated in nematodes, cestodes and acanthocephalans, ^{65}Zn has been shown to be both accumulated and released by *S. mansoni*, and the cuticular uptake of ^{131}I has been demonstrated in *Ascaridia galli, Heterakis gallinae* and *A. lumbricoides*. The latter species can also take up gold and silver ions. In addition, all helminths show a certain degree of permeability to Na^+, K^+ and Cl^- (Section 4.1.12). So, there may be a considerable flux of inorganic ions between host and parasite.

Calcareous Corpuscles

The parenchyma of many adult and larval cestodes contains large numbers of calcareous corpuscles. These corpuscles are produced intracellularly in corpuscle-forming cells and there are suggestions that they may be formed from mitochondria. The organic matrix of calcareous corpuscles consists of concentric rings with a double outer envelope. In vertebrates, calcification is normally associated with collagen, but the protein component of calcareous corpuscles is non-collagenous. The main inorganic components of calcareous corpuscles are calcium, magnesium, phosphorus and carbonate. The phosphorus and magnesium content is variable, and there is always a series of minor elements present that probably depend on the host's diet. The calcareous corpuscles are usually amorphous, but can be made crystalline by heating. The crystal forms produced vary with the species of parasite and the treatment.

In addition to the inorganic salts, calcareous corpuscles often contain small amounts of lipid (triacylglycerols, cholesterol, phospholipids, carotenoids) as well as RNA, DNA, glycogen and mucopolysaccharides. Alkaline phosphatase has also been demonstrated in the calcareous corpuscles of several species.

The mechanism of mineralisation of calcareous corpuscles is not known. The incorporation of calcium, phosphate and trace elements into calcareous corpuscles has been shown in various species. In *Mesocestoides corti*, the calcareous corpuscles concentrate a variety of ions from the incubation medium, including chromium, copper, calcium, indium, titanium, zinc and zirconium. It has been suggested that the phospholipids in calcareous corpuscles are involved in calcium mobilisation.

The physiological function of calcareous corpuscles is not really known, although there has been no lack of suggestions. They may function either as reserves of phosphate or of alkaline buffering capacity. The phosphate content of corpuscles varies with the nutritional state, and phosphate reserves do occur in protozoa in the form of polyphosphates, whilst phytin (inositol hexaphosphate) has been found in mesozoans. As an alkali reserve, calcareous corpuscles may help to neutralise the organic acids produced by carbohydrate catabolism (Section 3.1.4). There is some evidence in molluscs that, during anaerobic periods, calcium is used to neutralise the accumulating organic acids. In larval cestodes, the corpuscles could counteract the acid conditions during passage through the host's stomach and also provide a buffer reserve to cope with the high carbon dioxide levels in the gut lumen (Section 1.1.2).

A second possibility is that calcareous corpuscles are in fact excretory and store carbon dioxide or excess calcium from the diet. In marine invertebrates, bodies rather similar to calcareous corpuscles are involved in sequestering toxic elements, although there is no evidence of this in helminths.

Calcareous corpuscles may also have an immunological role. It has been shown that they can absorb antigens and in *Echinococcus granulosus* and *Echinococcus multilocularis* the calcareous corpuscles show anticomplement activity[1]. Other suggestions for the function of calcareous corpuscles include a role in lipid metabolism, tissue repair, osmotic balance and rudimentary skeletal structures.

Inclusions, very similar to cestode calcareous corpuscles, occur in the excretory system of trematodes. The trematode calcareous corpuscles have not been studied in much detail and seem to consist mainly of calcium carbonate with some phosphate. In trematodes, the corpuscles often accumulate in the metacercariae and disappear on infection.

Nematode Inclusions

A variety of granules and crystalline bodies have been described in the intestinal cells and intestinal lumen of nematodes. Originally, the granules were all thought to be the end-products of haemoglobin digestion. Later they were considered to be inorganic and were variously identified as calcium phosphate, calcium sulphate or even, in one case, as zinc sulphide! However, it is now thought that the majority of them are primarily protein or lipoprotein in composition[2,3], although many of them do contain iron, probably derived from haemoglobin. The granules in the intestinal cells of *Trichuris muris* and *Trichuris suis* are, however, mostly inorganic and are composed of calcium and phosphate with traces of magnesium, iron and potassium[4].

The biochemical role of intestinal inclusions in nematodes is again uncertain. Large numbers of inclusions are often found in the intestine of arrested fourth-stage larvae (Section 5.2.6). There is, however, no evidence that inclusions have any role in the control of delayed development, and it is now thought that the majority of these intestinal bodies may be the result of degenerative changes in the intestinal epithelium[88]. In *Nematodirus battus*, for example, the development of intestinal crystals closely parallels the development of the host's immune response.

Experimentally, calcium deposits superficially similar to calcareous corpuscles, and also iron deposits, can be produced in *A. lumbricoides* by the injection of calcium hydroxide or iron salts.

Micro-distribution of Elements

Not a great deal is known of the detailed distribution of elements in the tissues of helminths, but the development of x-ray microanalysis techniques is likely to lead to an increased interest in this field. There have been several studies following the uptake and fate of radioactive iron (either as ferric chloride or as haemoglobin) in trematodes. Iron appears to be accumulated in the intestinal epithelium, in the tegument, in the myoblasts and in the walls of the excretory tubules. In *F. hepatica*, the distribution of iron was closely matched by the distribution of ascorbic acid (vitamin C). This suggests that in these tissues the iron may be in the form of a soluble ferric hydroxide/ferrous ascorbate complex.

The distribution of calcium has been studied in the cercariae of schistosomes, where it occurs in high quantities in the preacetabular glands (Section 4.1.2). In adult schistosomes, the vitelline cells contain a large number of calcareous corpuscles. These corpuscles, which contain Ca^{2+}, Mg^{2+}, K^+, PO_4^{2-} and S, appear to be formed in the cysternae of the endoplasmic reticulum. The vitelline cells are passed into the egg, but most of the calcareous corpuscles are not incorporated into the miracidium and are left behind in the debris of the hatched egg[80].

2.2. CARBOHYDRATES

Carbohydrates perform three main functions in tissues. They are a major energy reserve, they form important structural components and, as phosphorylated inter-mediates, they are crucial to energy metabolism. The metabolic role of carbohy-drates will be dealt with in Chapter 3. In addition, carbohydrates are constituents of nucleotides, glycolipids and glycoproteins.

2.2.1. Reserve Carbohydrates

Carbohydrate is the major energy reserve in adult parasitic helminths, although lipid is often more important in the free-living phases. The levels of carbohydrate reserves in helminths depend, of course, on the nutritional state of the parasite and may change during the life-cycle. In addition, there may be differences between males and females and there can be both diurnal and annual cycles in carbohydrate content. In cestodes, for example, there are daily fluctuations in glycogen content.

The levels of free glucose in animal tissues are, in general, low and parasites are no exception, glucose usually forming less than 1% of the dry weight. Small amounts of galactose have been tentatively identified in *Macracanthorhynchus hirudinaceus* and what appears to be maltose has been isolated from the sporocysts of *Micro-phallus pygmaeus*. However, the principal reserve carbohydrates in parasitic hel-minths are trehalose and glycogen.

Trehalose

This is a non-reducing disaccharide formed from two glucose molecules joined through the 1 carbon (*Figure 2.1*). Trehalose is widely distributed in helminths, forming up to 5% of the dry weight of nematodes and acanthocephalans. Small amounts of trehalose have also been reported in cestodes and trematodes. In adult male *A. lumbricoides*, trehalose forms 70–80% of the total carbohydrate in the testis and seminal vesicle. The highest levels of trehalose (7.9% of the dry weight) are found in *A. lumbricoides* eggs. When the egg is fully developed, the trehalose is found almost exclusively in the perivitelline fluid. The eggs of the plant parasitic nematode *G. rostochiensis* contain 5.3% trehalose (0.34 M)[81].

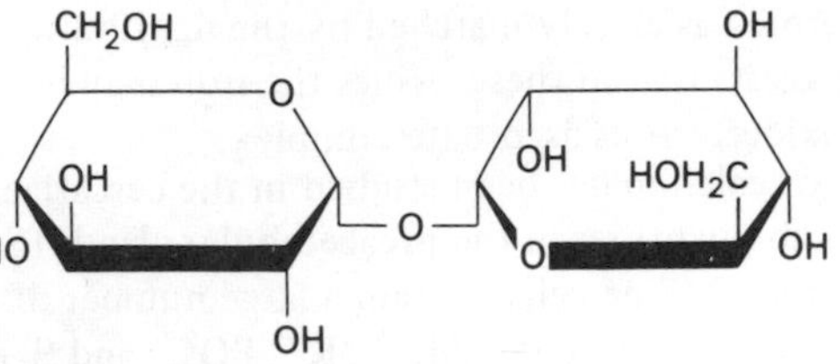

Figure 2.1 The structure of trehalose.

The biochemical significance of trehalose is not clear. The only other organisms which contain large amounts of trehalose are the arthropods (insects and crustacea). Trehalose is a method of transporting glucose as an inert low molecular weight compound and it may be a tissue-specific metabolite (Section 3.1.1). In infective *A. lumbricoides* eggs, the trehalose in the perivitelline fluid could have an osmotic role in hatching, or may act as an 'antifreeze'. Alternatively, the high osmotic pressure may dehydrate the infective larva and so keep it quiescent until hatching. Trehalose will, of course, also contribute to the osmotic pressure of helminth body fluids. An alternative role for trehalose is in glucose uptake (Section 4.1.7). By converting free glucose to trehalose in the pseudocoelom, nematodes and acanthocephalans can maintain a favourable inward gradient for glucose transport.

Glycogen

The main reserve polysaccharide in helminths (and mesozoans) is glycogen. Glycogen may constitute up to 40% of the dry weight of some cestode plerocercoids, but 10-20% of the dry weight is probably a more general figure for parasitic helminths. Glycogen levels are, however, low in filarial worms, in the ectoparasitic monogeneans and temnocephalans and in the free-living stages of nematodes where lipid is the main energy reserve. The larvae of the nematodes *Eustrongylides ignotus* and *Porrocaecum decipiens* live in the tissues of fish and up to 58% of the dry weight is glycogen. However, in general, there seems to be no obvious correlation between glycogen content and habitat in parasitic helminths.

In cestodes and trematodes, glycogen is stored primarily in the parenchyma, and in nematodes it is stored mainly in the lateral lines and muscles. Glycogen has been described in the pseudocoelomic fluid of *A. lumbricoides*, but this may well turn out to be a glycoprotein. There is also quite a lot of glycogen in the intestinal cells of nematodes, but apparently very little in the intestinal cells of trematodes.

Glycogen is a highly branched glucose polymer, with α 1-4 and α 1-6 bonds. The ratio of 1-4 links to 1-6 links varies from 12:1 to 15:1. Glycogen is also a very polydispersed molecule, with molecular weights ranging from several hundred thousand to over a hundred million. As a reserve polysaccharide, glycogen has a number of advantages. It is non-diffusable, it exerts a low osmotic pressure and the highly branched structure provides large numbers of chain ends for enzymes to work on. Lastly, glycogen can be catabolised both aerobically and anaerobically.

The physical properties of helminth glycogen and chemical properties such as the lengths of the external and internal branches are similar to those of mammalian glycogen[5]. The molecular weight distribution of glycogen has been investigated in several helminths. In *A. lumbricoides*, the glycogen can be separated more or less equally into two varieties, one with an average molecular weight of 50 million, the other 450 million. On the other hand, in *F. hepatica* most of the glycogen forms a low molecular weight peak, with the rest (30%) forming a continuum from the low molecular weight fraction to the very high molecular weight fraction. There is also a continuum of molecular weights in *H. diminuta* glycogen from high (average molecular weight 900 million) to low (average molecular weight 60 million). In this parasite, 30% of the glycogen falls into the very high fractions, 60% into the low fractions, with very little in the intermediate weights. The spectrum of molecular weights of *H. diminuta* glycogen varies to a certain extent during development. Whether the different molecular weight forms of glycogen can be correlated with the different types of glycogen particle seen under the electron microscope (α, β and γ) is questionable.

It has been suggested, by several workers, that the high and low molecular weight forms of glycogen in helminths may have different metabolic roles and different turnover rates. Both high and low molecular weight fractions decrease during starvation in *F. hepatica* and *H. diminuta*, and both fractions increase rapidly again on feeding. Isotope experiments with *H. diminuta*[6] showed that glucose incorporation was higher in the high molecular weight limit dextrin than in the low molecular weight limit dextrin. The highest incorporation, however, was into the intermediate weight limit dextrins, although this is the smallest glycogen fraction. Incorporation into the limit dextrin, that is internal to the α 1-6 branch points, shows that it is not just chain lengthening involved, but also activity of the branching enzyme (Section 4.2.3).

Glycogen granules normally contain a small amount of amino nitrogen. This may be due to a binding protein which confers stability on the granule and also to enzymes involved in glycogen synthesis and degradation. Apparently homogeneous glycogen/protein complexes containing a high proportion of protein have been isolated from a number of cestodes (*H. diminuta, Moniezia expansa, Taenia saginata, Raillietina cesticillus*). Two complexes have been prepared from *M. expansa* and have been called baerine (contains 60% glycogen) and moniezine (contains 11% glycogen). Four or five such complexes have been isolated from other tapeworms. What these glycogen/protein complexes are, whether or not they are artefacts and whether or not they have any physiological function has not been investigated.

There have been several studies on the distribution of lyoglycogen ('free' glycogen) and desmoglycogen ('bound' glycogen) in parasitic helminths. However, it is now thought that lyo- and desmoglycogen are artefacts, and the same may prove true of the glycogen/protein complexes of cestodes.

2.2.2. Structural Carbohydrates

Structural carbohydrates can be divided into the homopolymers (such as chitin and cellulose) and the heteropolymers or mucopolysaccharides. The latter will be dealt with in the next section.

Chitin

The egg shells of nematodes and acanthocephalans both contain chitin layers. In nematodes, the chitin layer (probably α-chitin) is laid down by the fertilised egg, not by the uterus of the female. In *T. suis* eggs, the chitin layer has a lamellate appearance, consisting of a helicoidal chitin/protein complex[7]; in other nematode eggs, the chitin fibres may be randomly arranged. Helminth chitin shows minor differences (in optical properties and higher flexibility) from typical arthropod chitin[82]. These differences probably reflect differences in the associated protein components of the different types of chitin.

2.2.3. Mucopolysaccharides

Mucopolysaccharides are heteropolysaccharides that contain amino sugars (glucosamine, galactosamine, *N*-acetylglucosamine, *N*-acetylgalactosamine) and uronic acids (glucuronic, galacturonic). In addition, the sugars may be sulphonated. Many mucopolysaccharides occur in complexes with proteins and are usually referred to as mucoproteins or glycoproteins. In mammals, mucoproteins frequently contain 6-deoxy-L-galactose (fucose) and sialic acids. The latter are derivatives of neuraminic acid, *N*-acetylneuraminic acid being a common sialic acid.

Histochemically, mucopolysaccharides have been found to be widely distributed in the tissues of parasitic helminths. Mucopolysaccharides frequently occur in association with the egg membranes of trematodes, cestodes and nematodes, and they form an important part of the cyst wall of trematode metacercariae. The egg coat protein of *A. lumbricoides* is also a glycoprotein (Section 2.5.1). The teguments of trematodes, cestodes and acanthocephalans all contain mucopolysaccharides, and mucopolysaccharides have been described in cercarial gland cells, in the excretory system and general body tissues of nematodes, in the uterus of cestodes and in Mehlis' gland in trematodes.

However, very little is known either of the biochemistry of helminth mucopolysaccharides or of their function. Mucopolysaccharides are major components of connective tissue matrix and cell coats. The mucopolysaccharide molecules are extremely long, fairly random coils, which makes them good lubricants; the molecules can also contain up to 500 times their own weight of water. Use is made of this latter property of mucopolysaccharides in trematode egg hatching. In the eggs of *F. hepatica*, there is a viscous cushion composed of mucopolysaccharide lying beneath the operculum. The hydration and accompanying swelling of this viscous cushion causes the pressure inside the egg to rise during hatching and so burst open the operculum. The viscous cushion is surrounded by a membrane, and a change in permeability of this membrane allows water to enter the viscous cushion. It is not clear whether the permeability change in the membrane is induced by enzymes or by mechanical damage from the active miracidium (Section 4.1.2). In gut parasites, mucopolysaccharides may protect the parasite from host digestive enzymes (Section 4.1.3).

At the biochemical level, polysaccharide–protein complexes containing *N*-acetylglucosamine, N-acetylgalactosamine, glucosamine, galactosamine, glucose and galactose have been isolated from the cysticerci of *E. granulosus* and *Taenia taeniaeformis*. Acid mucopolysaccharides containing uronic acids and sulphonated sugars have also been purified from trematodes, cestodes and nematodes[8] and a glycoprotein containing hexosamines and N-acetylhexosamines has been found in the pseudocoelomic fluid of *A. lumbricoides*[9].

Sialic acids and fucose (6-deoxy-L-galactose), characteristic components of mammalian mucoproteins, have rarely been positively identified in helminths. Fucose has been reported associated with *A. lumbricoides* collagen (Section 2.5.1), and rhamnose (6-deoxy-L-mannose) has been identified in extracts of *F. hepatica*, whilst unidentified deoxypentoses have been found in *E. granulosus* cysts. There is, however, histochemical evidence for sialic acids in the egg shell of the nematode *Capillaria hepatica*.

2.2.4. Immunologically Active Polysaccharides

Antigenic polysaccharides or polysaccharide/protein complexes have been isolated from trematodes, nematodes and cestodes. In *S. mansoni*, for example, an antigenic polysaccharide, molecular weight 30–50×10^3, is released by the gut cells, whilst three major antigenic glycoproteins have been isolated from the eggs. The chemical nature of helminth polysaccharide complexes is uncertain and many, if not all, of the antigenic fractions described from helminths are probably not discrete chemical entities. In several cases, they are heteroproteins complexed with glycogen (Section 2.2.1). Some antigenic fractions have been shown to contain deoxymannose and unidentified pentoses, deoxypentoses and aldohexoses as well as amino sugars. The presence of pentoses may indicate contamination of some of these fractions with nucleic acids.

Attempts have been made to use some of these antigenic polysaccharides in skin tests and they have also been used, so far unsuccessfully, to try to develop effective vaccines.

2.3. LIPIDS

Lipids are a heterogeneous group of compounds with similar physical properties, being relatively insoluble in water but soluble in organic solvents. The total lipid content of helminths is very variable, but is usually between 10 and 30% of the dry weight.

Lipids have a variety of functions in tissues. They are major structural components of cell membranes and, in many organisms, triacylglycerols are an important energy reserve. Other lipids are associated with enzyme reactions as activators or glycosyl carriers and lipid components form part of the cytochrome chain and membrane transport mechanisms. Prostaglandins and steroid and prenoid hormones also play a crucial role in metabolic regulation. Finally, lipids occur in association with proteins and carbohydrates in lipoproteins and glycolipids.

Table 2.1   Classification of lipids

Fatty acids	Saturated acids, unsaturated acids, branched and cyclopropane acids, prostaglandins
Acylglycerols	Mono-, di- and triacylglycerol, diacylglycerol alkyl ether, diacylglycerol alk-1-enyl ether, glycosylacylglycerol, glyceryl ether
Phosphoglycerides	Phosphatidic acid, phosphatidylcholine, phosphatidylethanolamine, phosphatidylserine, phosphatidylinositol, phosphatidylglycerol, aminoacylphosphatidylglycerol, cardiolipin (diphosphatidylglycerol), plasmalogens, phosphatidyl alkyl ethers, lysophosphoglycerides
Sphingolipids	Ceramides, sphingomyelin, cerebrosides, sulphatides, gangliosides
Ascarosides	Free and esterified ascarosides
Waxes	Free and esterified long chain alcohols, long chain aldehydes, hydrocarbons
Terpenes	Farnesol, squalene, carotenoids, polyprenols, ubiquinones
Steroids	Free and esterified steroids

The varied chemical structure of lipids means that there is no generally agreed method of classification; the scheme used in this section is outlined in *Table 2.1*.

2.3.1. Fatty Acids

A great variety of saturated and unsaturated fatty acids ranging from C_{10} to C_{24} has been found in helminth lipids. Fatty acids can be written in a short-hand form; palmitoleic acid, for example, is $C_{16:1(7)}$, the 16 being the number of carbon atoms, the 1 after the colon being the number of double bonds and the 7 in parentheses being the position of the double bond counting from the carboxyl carbon. The double bonds are in the *cis*-configuration unless otherwise indicated. Fatty acids occur in helminth tissues both as free fatty acids and esterified as a component of complex lipids.

Free Fatty Acids

The levels of free fatty acids in animal tissues are normally low (less than 1% of the total lipids). However, abnormally high levels of free fatty acids have been reported in some helminths. Amongst the nematodes, free fatty acid levels of 40% and 67% of the total lipids have been found in the parasitic females and infective larvae, respectively, of *Strongyloides ratti*, and values of 60% and 20% have been recorded for the infective larvae and adults of *Nippostrongylus brasiliensis*. The egg lipids of *S. mansoni* have 45% free fatty acids (18% in *Schistosoma japonicum*). Free fatty acids are also the major lipid component in the cercariae of *Glypthelmins pennsylvaniensis* and the metacercariae of *Echinostoma revolutum*. Levels of between 2 and 15% of the total lipids have been reported for free fatty acids in a variety of trematodes[10] including *S. mansoni*, the adults of *Polymorphus minutus*, the cysticerci of *Taenia hydatigena* and the larvae of *Spirometra mansonoides*.

The significance of the high levels of free fatty acids in these helminths is not clear, nor is it known if the fatty acids are indeed free or if they are bound to carrier proteins. Free fatty acids are important metabolic intermediates, but they do not usually occur in such high levels, even in tissues with an active lipid metabolism. In larval helminths, the high levels of free fatty acids might be related to the lipid changes which take place during infection (Section 5.2.3). It is also quite probable that the high levels of fatty acids reported in helminths may, in part, be an artefact due to the hydrolysis of complex lipids during extraction and analysis.

Esterified Fatty Acids

The various lipid fractions of an organism usually have different and often characteristic fatty acid compositions. The same lipid class, isolated from different tissues in the same organism, can also show variations in fatty acid composition. In helminths, there is a large literature on the fatty acid composition of whole lipid extracts and isolated lipid fractions from a wide range of parasites. As in other organisms, the different lipid classes have different and often characteristic fatty acid compositions, and the same lipid class from different tissues of the same parasite may show variations. In *A. lumbricoides*, for example, the ovarian triacylglycerols have a different fatty acid composition to the body-wall triacylglycerols. Whilst in *H. diminuta*, the fatty acid composition of polar lipids from isolated tegumental components (brush borders and vesicles) differs considerably from that of polar lipids prepared from whole worms[11].

In general, a similar range of fatty acids is found in free-living organisms and parasitic helminths, and the major fatty acids in both are usually C_{16} and C_{18}. Compared with mammals, parasitic helminths tend to have a lower proportion of C_{16} acids in their lipids and rather more C_{18}. Of the C_{18} acids, the principal one in most mammals and in insects, planarians and free-living nematodes is oleic ($C_{18:1}$). Oleic acid is also the main C_{18} acid in most parasitic helminths. There are exceptions, and in *H. diminuta* linoleic ($C_{18:2}$) is the major C_{18} acid, whilst stearic ($C_{18:0}$) is the predominant C_{18} acid in *F. hepatica* and larval *T. spiralis*. Helminths also tend to have a higher percentage of unsaturated C_{18} acids ($C_{18:1}$, $C_{18:2}$, $C_{18:3}$) than do mammals. In mammals, unsaturated C_{18} acids are usually 30–40% of the total acids, whilst in helminths they form 40–70%.

The high degree of unsaturation of helminth fatty acids has attracted a certain amount of attention. The degree of unsaturation can be expressed either as the percentage of acids with double bonds or as the average number of double bonds per molecule. In mammals, approximately 50–60% of the fatty acids are unsaturated (0.7–0.8 double bonds/molecule). Most parasitic helminths also fall within this range, although some helminths have markedly higher levels of unsaturated fatty acids: 80% in *H. diminuta*, *Moniliformis dubius* and *M. hirudinaceus* (1.2–1.5 double bonds/molecule), 75% in *A. lumbricoides* (1.1 double bonds/molecule). The presence of high levels of unsaturated fatty acids in these helminths is

enigmatic since, at the raised body temperature of the host, one might expect
a drop in the proportion of unsaturated fatty acids (see below and Sections 4.3.1
and 5.2.3). The fatty acids of insects and of free-living and plant parasitic nematodes also show a high degree of unsaturation (up to 90%). So, a high proportion
of unsaturated fatty acids may be a common feature of invertebrates and not just
a peculiarity of parasites.

Helminth lipids, like the lipids from other animals, usually contain a small
proportion (less than 1%) of odd-numbered (C_{15}, C_{17}) and branched chain acids.
Exceptions are the adult filarial worms, *Dirofilaria immitis, Dipetalonema viteae*
and *Litomosoides carinii* where branched chain acids form 7.4–8.6% of the total
(mostly C_{17} branched). Odd-numbered fatty acids tend to be rather more abundant
in marine invertebrates.

Volatile fatty acids (C_2–C_6), derived from carbohydrate breakdown (Section 3.1)
are found in the neutral lipids (but not the phospholipids) of *A. lumbricoides,
Ascaris columnaris* and *Parascaris equorum*. No hydroxy or cyclopropane acids have
been reported from helminth lipids.

In free-living organisms, the overall fatty acid composition is strongly influenced
by two factors, the fatty acids present in the diet and the ambient temperature.

Influence of Diet

Changes in dietary fatty acids usually result in changes in fatty acid composition,
and there is often quite a close correspondence between the fatty acid composition
of an organism and the fatty acid content of its diet. The incorporation of dietary
fatty acids into the different lipid fractions is nevertheless a regulated process, and
animals are able to maintain the physical properties of their different lipid components despite variations in fatty acid composition.

In parasitic helminths, the relationship between diet and fatty acid composition
is particularly marked in cestodes. Fatty acid analyses are usually expressed as moles
per cent and this is not very suitable for most statistical comparisons, since the
values are not independently variable. One way of comparing these kinds of data is
to use the mean square distance[12] or a non-parametric method such as the Spear-
man rank correlation coefficient. These enable a quantitative comparison to be
made between different fatty acid compositions. When this is done, it is found that
there is a highly significant rank correlation between the total fatty acid compositions of *H. diminuta* and rat intestinal contents, *R. cesticillus* and chicken intestinal
contents, and between shark tapeworms and their hosts (*Calliobothrium verticillatum, Dasyrhynchus giganteus, Grillotia simmonsi, Lacistorhynchus tenuis,
Orgymatobothrium musteli, Poecilancistrium caryophyllum, Thysanocephalum
cephalum*). The similarity between host and parasite fatty acids is especially noticeable in the shark tapeworms, since sharks characteristically contain large amounts
of C_{20} and C_{22} polyunsaturated acids. These acids are also found in high concentrations in shark tapeworms, and occur in all the lipid classes. In *H. diminuta*,
modifying the rat host's dietary fatty acids results in a corresponding change in the
tapeworm lipids[13]. However, although there is a significant correlation between the

total fatty acid composition of a variety of tapeworms and their hosts' gut lipids, the same is not necessarily true for all of the individual lipid classes. In *H. diminuta*, there is a high correlation between the fatty acid composition of the host's diet and the fatty acid composition of the triacylglycerol and sterol ester fractions. The fatty acid content of the phosphatidylcholine and phosphatidylethanolamine fractions show a lower, but still statistically significant, correlation with the diet. There is, however, no significant rank correlation between dietary fatty acids and the free fatty acid fraction of *H. diminuta* or with the phosphatidylinositol, phosphatidylserine or cerebroside fractions. So, as in other animals, it is the 'depot fats', the triacylglycerol fraction, that most closely mirrors the dietary fatty acids, whilst the structural phospholipids have a more conservative fatty acid composition. A similar relationship can be shown in *C. verticillatum*, where again there is a high correlation between triacylglycerol composition and dietary lipids, rather less correlation for phosphatidylcholine and phosphatidylethanolamine and very little correlation for the other phospholipids[14].

This similarity between host and parasite fatty acids is not so prominent in other groups of helminths. The fatty acid composition of the lung fluke *Haematoloechus medioplexus* is similar to that of host lung tissue[12], but there is no correlation between liver lipid fatty acids and *F. hepatica*, nor between host blood and *S. mansoni* lipids. In the nematodes there is, similarly, no correlation between the fatty acid composition of *T. spiralis* larvae and host muscle, nor between host serum fatty acids and the filarial worms *D. immitis*, *D. viteae* or *L. carinii*.

Influence of Temperature

The second factor that affects fatty acid composition is the ambient temperature. Free-living organisms respond to a drop in environmental temperature by increasing the proportion of unsaturated fatty acids in their lipids, and to a rise in ambient temperature by increasing the proportion of saturated fatty acids. Unsaturated fatty acids have a lower melting point than the corresponding saturated acids. Branched chain acids also have a lower melting point than their straight chain analogues, and in bacteria the proportion of branched chain acids in the lipids decreases as the ambient temperature increases. The melting point of a fatty acid also depends on its chain length: the longer the chain, the higher the melting point. Straightforward changes in the average chain length of the fatty acids does not, however, appear to be a significant factor in temperature adaptation in animals. The effect, on melting point, of altering the fatty acid chain length is relatively minor compared to the effects of introducing double bonds. Going from C_{16} to C_{18} raises the melting point of the fatty acid by 33 °C, but putting a double bond into C_{18}, to give $C_{18:1}$, lowers the melting point by 55 °C, and introducing two double bonds to give $C_{18:2}$ lowers it by 80 °C. In many species of fish, a decrease in environmental temperature is accompanied by an increase in the proportions of polyunsaturated C_{22} acids (particularly $C_{22:6}$), the effects of increased chain length being more than outweighed by the effect of the double bonds.

During their life-cycles, parasitic helminths, and particularly parasites of endotherms (birds and mammals), are subjected to wide temperature fluctuations

(Sections 1.1.6 and 5.2.3). However, nothing is really known of the sorts of modifications which take place in the lipid composition of parasites in response to the change from a free-living stage (at ambient temperatures) to the adult parasite in the tissues of a mammal or bird (at 35-43 °C). At the moment, fatty acid analyses are available for the adult and larval stages of only two parasitic helminths, the trematode *S. mansoni* and the cestode *S. mansonoides*. In both cases, it is the adult that has the highest levels of unsaturated fatty acids and not the larval stages as might have been expected. The average chain length of the fatty acids in larval and adult *S. mansoni* and larval and adult *S. mansonoides* are not significantly different. So, in neither of these two parasitic helminths can infection of the final host be correlated with changes in fatty acid composition. It has been suggested that the presence of large amounts of free fatty acids in some trematode cercariae and infective nematode larvae could be related to possible changes in lipid composition during infection. A similar role could be proposed for the branched chain fatty acids, frequently found in helminth lipids. There is, however, no experimental evidence for either of these two suggestions. The temperature changes accompanying infection (and also the release of eggs or infective larvae from an infected host) are virtually instantaneous. It is quite possible that the lipids of these intermediate stages are adapted to function over a wide temperature range. So, the processes of infection or egression need not necessarily be accompanied by changes in lipid composition.

Utilisation of Fatty Acids

The effect of starvation on fatty acid composition has been studied in a number of parasitic helminths. No significant changes in fatty acid composition were found when adult *A. lumbricoides*, adult *H. diminuta* or larval *T. spiralis* were incubated *in vitro* in non-nutrient media. This is not unexpected, as these helminths all appear to lack a functional β-oxidation sequence (Section 3.3.1). In contrast, the free-living stages of helminths can catabolise fatty acids, and this has been followed in the infective larvae (L_3) of *S. ratti* and in the developing eggs of *A. lumbricoides*. In *S. ratti* L_3, all of the fatty acid fractions except C_{12} decrease during starvation, but $C_{18:1}$ decreases the most. In *A. lumbricoides* eggs, all of the fatty acid fractions are again catabolised, the volatile fatty acids (Section 2.3.2) showing the highest rate of utilisation.

Prostaglandins

These are formed by the cyclisation of C_{20} unsaturated fatty acids. In vertebrates, prostaglandins have profound physiological effects; however, they have yet to be demonstrated in helminths (or any other invertebrate apart from insects).

2.3.2. Acylglycerols

These are all lipids which have glycerol as the backbone. The structure of the main acylglycerols is summarised in *Figure 2.2*.

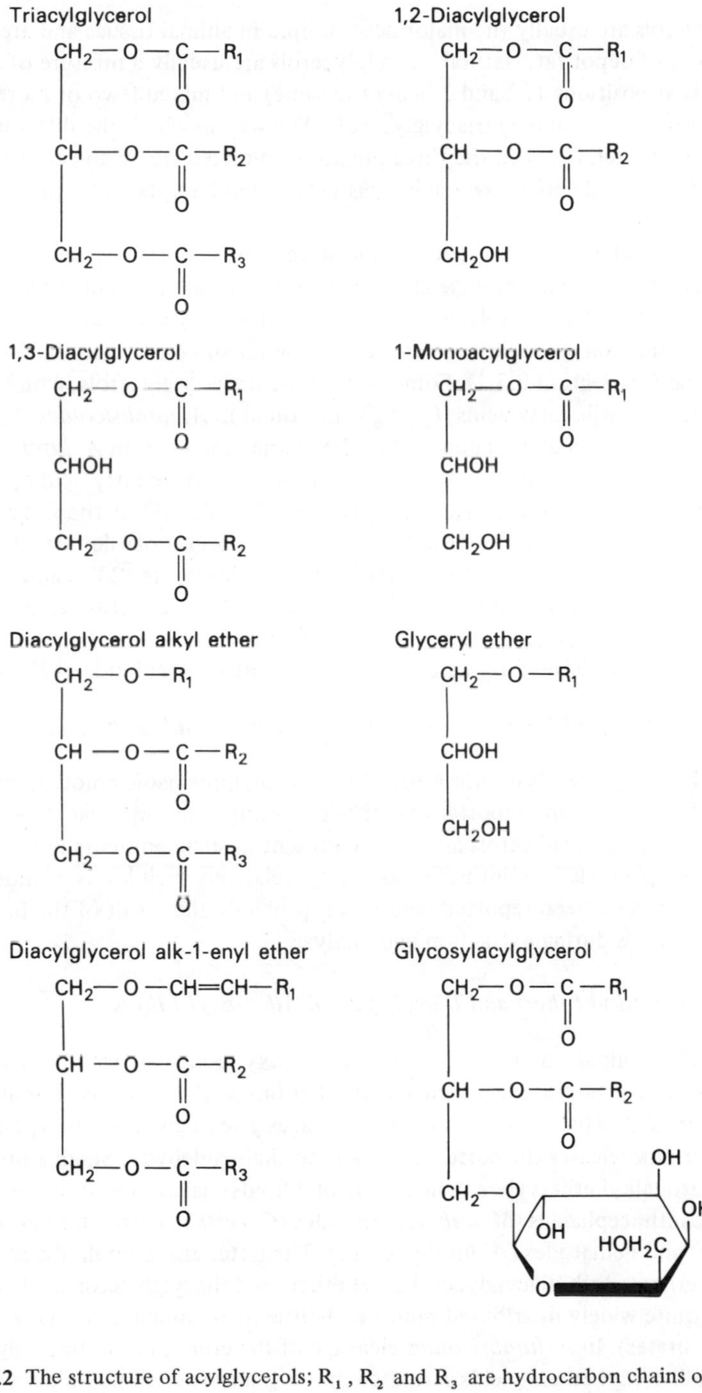

Triacylglycerol

$$CH_2-O-C-R_1$$
$$\quad\quad\quad \| $$
$$\quad\quad\quad O$$

$$CH-O-C-R_2$$
$$\quad\quad\quad \|$$
$$\quad\quad\quad O$$

$$CH_2-O-C-R_3$$
$$\quad\quad\quad \|$$
$$\quad\quad\quad O$$

1,2-Diacylglycerol

$$CH_2-O-C-R_1$$
$$\quad\quad\quad \|$$
$$\quad\quad\quad O$$

$$CH-O-C-R_2$$
$$\quad\quad\quad \|$$
$$\quad\quad\quad O$$

$$CH_2OH$$

1,3-Diacylglycerol

$$CH_2-O-C-R_1$$
$$\quad\quad\quad \|$$
$$\quad\quad\quad O$$

$$CHOH$$

$$CH_2-O-C-R_2$$
$$\quad\quad\quad \|$$
$$\quad\quad\quad O$$

1-Monoacylglycerol

$$CH_2-O-C-R_1$$
$$\quad\quad\quad \|$$
$$\quad\quad\quad O$$

$$CHOH$$

$$CH_2OH$$

Diacylglycerol alkyl ether

$$CH_2-O-R_1$$

$$CH-O-C-R_2$$
$$\quad\quad\quad \|$$
$$\quad\quad\quad O$$

$$CH_2-O-C-R_3$$
$$\quad\quad\quad \|$$
$$\quad\quad\quad O$$

Glyceryl ether

$$CH_2-O-R_1$$

$$CHOH$$

$$CH_2OH$$

Diacylglycerol alk-1-enyl ether

$$CH_2-O-CH=CH-R_1$$

$$CH-O-C-R_2$$
$$\quad\quad\quad \|$$
$$\quad\quad\quad O$$

$$CH_2-O-C-R_3$$
$$\quad\quad\quad \|$$
$$\quad\quad\quad O$$

Glycosylacylglycerol

$$CH_2-O-C-R_1$$
$$\quad\quad\quad \|$$
$$\quad\quad\quad O$$

$$CH-O-C-R_2$$
$$\quad\quad\quad \|$$
$$\quad\quad\quad O$$

$$CH_2-O$$

Figure 2.2 The structure of acylglycerols; R_1, R_2 and R_3 are hydrocarbon chains of fatty acids.

Triacylglycerols (Triglycerides)

Triacylglycerols are usually the major neutral lipid in animal tissues and are the normal form of depot fat. Natural triacylglycerols are usually a mixture of simple (fatty acids at positions 1, 2 and 3 being the same) and mixed (two or more fatty acids at positions 1, 2 and 3) triacylglycerols. The way in which the different fatty acids are distributed between the three positions in mixed triacylglycerols has been the subject of considerable research but, as yet, no hard-and-fast generalisations can be made.

    Triacylglycerol is the major neutral lipid in the vast majority of helminths. Exceptions include the larval stage and occasionally the adult of some trematodes (*E. revolutum*[15]), where sterols, or in some cases free fatty acids, are the major neutral lipid fraction. Free fatty acids are also the major constituent in certain nematode larvae (Section 2.3.1). Some very unusual triacylglycerols, which contain esterified volatile fatty acids (C_2–C_6), are found in *A. lumbricoides*[16]. These acylglycerols are particularly abundant in the ovaries and eggs. In *A. lumbricoides* ovaries, 80% of the triacylglycerols contain 1 mole of volatile fatty acid esterified at one of the three positions; triacylglycerols with 2 moles of volatile fatty acid are present in only very small amounts. The main glyceride volatile fatty acids in *A. lumbricoides* are 2-methylvalerate (70%), 2-methylbutyrate (23%) and *n*-valerate (7%), traces of acetate, propionate, isobutyrate and *n*-butyrate also being found. Triacylglycerols containing 2-methylbutyrate have been found in the related *A. columnaris*[17] and volatile fatty acids also occur in the neutral lipids of *P. equorum*.

Monoacylglycerols and Diacylglycerols (Monoglycerides and Diglycerides)

Mono- and diacylglycerols do not normally occur in appreciable amounts in animal tissues, although they are important synthetic intermediates. Monoacylglycerols and 1,2- and 1,3-diacylglycerols are usually present in small amounts in most lipid extracts from parasitic helminths. Occasionally, relatively high levels of mono- and diacylglycerols have been reported, and this is probably the result of the breakdown of triacylglycerols during extraction and analysis.

Diacylglycerol Alkyl Ethers and Diacylglycerol Alk-1-enyl Ethers

These are glycerolipids, in which two of the hydroxy groups are esterified with fatty acids, whilst the third is joined via an ether link with a long alkyl or alkenyl chain (*Figure 2.2*). Hydrolysis of the ester linkages gives a glyceryl ether, cleavage of the ether link releases the corresponding long chain aldehyde. Small amounts of diacylglycerol alkyl ethers (less than 1% of total lipids) have been found in the lipids of acanthocephalans (*M. dubius*), cestodes (*C. verticillatum*), trematodes (*E. revolutum*) and nematodes (*A. lumbricoides*). The latter also contain diacylglycerol alk-1-enyl ethers. Both diacylglycerol alkyl ethers and diacylglycerol alk-1-enyl ethers are quite widely distributed minor constituents of animal lipids (vertebrates and invertebrates). In *A. lumbricoides* cleavage of the ether link of diacylglycerol alkyl and alk-1-enyl ethers yields saturated and α–β unsaturated C_{18} aldehydes.

Glycosylacylglycerols

These occur in nervous tissue, but have not been reported in parasitic helminths.

2.3.3. Phosphoglycerides

The parent compound of phosphoglycerides is phosphatidic acid (*Figure 2.3*). This is a glycerol molecule where one of the primary hydroxyl groups is esterified with phosphoric acid, whilst the other two are esterified with fatty acids. In addition, there is a polar head group which is an alcohol (X-OH in *Figure 2.3*), the hydroxyl group of which is esterified to the phosphoric acid. Each of the different classes of phosphoglyceride exists as many different chemical species, depending on the fatty acid composition. Most phosphoglycerides have one saturated fatty acid and one unsaturated acid, the latter being in the 2 position.

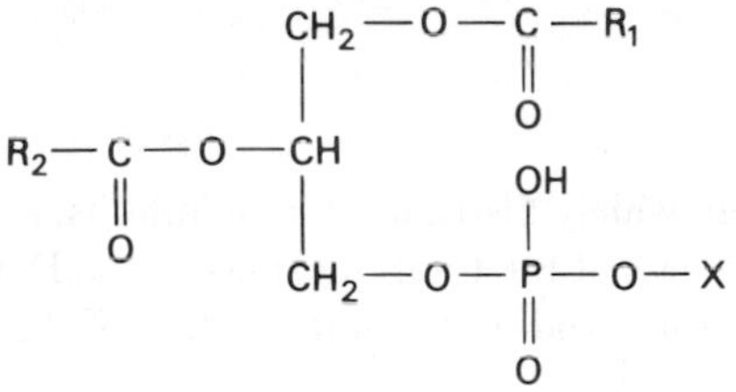

$$
\begin{array}{l}
CH_2-O-\overset{\overset{\displaystyle O}{\|}}{C}-R_1 \\[2mm]
R_2-\overset{\overset{\displaystyle \|}{O}}{C}-O-CH \qquad OH \\[2mm]
CH_2-O-\overset{\overset{\displaystyle \|}{O}}{P}-O-X
\end{array}
$$

Figure 2.3 The structure of phosphoglycerides; R_1 and R_2 are hydrocarbon chains of fatty acids, X is a polar head group. Phosphatidic acid, X=H; phosphatidylcholine, X=choline; phosphatidyl-ethanolamine, X=ethanolamine; phosphatidylserine, X=serine; phosphatidylinositol, X=inositol; phosphatidylglycerol, X=glycerol; aminoacylphosphatidylglycerol, X=lysylglycerol; cardiolipin, X=phosphatidylglycerol.

Phosphatidic Acid

Although it is an important intermediate and also the parent compound of phospho-glycerides, phosphatidic acid is usually only present in very small amounts in animal lipids. In helminths, it has been identified in *H. diminuta* and in the nematodes *A. lumbricoides, D. immitis* and *Setaria cervi*.

Phosphatidylcholine

This is usually the major phospholipid present in animal tissues and the same holds for parasitic helminths. Exceptions are the infective larvae of *S. ratti* and adult *Ancylostoma caninum*, where phosphatidylethanolamine predominates. In the cysticerci of *T. hydatigena*, there is also more phosphatidylethanolamine than phosphatidylcholine, but the major phospholipid component is claimed to be phosphatidylinositol. Not surprisingly, phosphatidylcholine has been found in all helminths so far investigated (trematodes, cestodes, acanthocephalans and nema-todes). In *H. diminuta*, fatty acid analyses of the phosphatidylcholine fraction suggests that, as is usual in mammalian tissues, there is one saturated fatty acid and one unsaturated fatty acid per mole. In marked contrast, the phosphatidylcholine fraction from *T. taeniaeformis* larvae seems to consist largely of the dipalmitate compound.

Phosphatidylethanolamine

Again, phosphatidylethanolamine appears to be universally distributed in animal tissues and has been found in trematodes, cestodes, acanthocephalans and nematodes. Together, phosphatidylethanolamine and phosphatidylcholine usually make up about 70% of the total phospholipids.

Phosphatidylserine

Phosphatidylserine is normally present in helminth lipids (trematodes, cestodes, acanthocephalans and nematodes) and usually constitutes about 10% of the total phospholipids.

Phosphatidylinositol

This phospholipid is again widely distributed in helminths, although it is only a minor component (5% or less of the total phospholipids). However, in *T. hydatigena* larvae, phosphatidylinositol is said to account for 40% of the phospholipids.

Phosphatidylglycerol and Aminoacylphosphatidylglycerol

These are, primarily, lipids of bacterial cell membranes and have not been found in helminths.

Cardiolipin (Diphosphatidylglycerol)

Cardiolipin is again found in bacterial cell membranes, but is also a major constituent of the inner mitochondrial membrane. Small amounts of cardiolipin have been identified in lipid extracts from a variety of trematodes, cestodes and nematodes. Curiously, no cardiolipin could be found in the eggs of *F. hepatica*, although it is present in the adult.

Plasmalogens

These are phosphoglycerides in which the 1-hydroxyl group is joined via an ether link to a long alk-1-enyl chain, instead of esterified to a fatty acid. Plasmalogens are the phosphoglyceride equivalent of the diacylglycerol alk-1-enyl ethers (Section 2.3.2). Plasmalogens occur widely in the tissues of vertebrates and invertebrates, and in mammals they can constitute up to 10% of the total phospholipids. In most organisms, the major plasmalogen is ethanolamine plasmalogen, with lesser amounts of choline plasmalogen. Plasmalogens have been demonstrated in several helminths: *F. hepatica, H. diminuta, M. dubius, M. hirudinaceus, A. lumbricoides, D. immitis* and *L. carinii*. Unusually high levels of plasmalogens occur in some parasitic nematodes. In *A. lumbricoides* and *L. carinii*, plasmalogens constitute about 20% of the total phospholipids and in isolated muscle tissue from *A. lumbricoides* 30-38% of the phospholipids are plasmalogens. In both *A. lumbricoides* and *L. carinii* ethanolamine plasmalogens predominate, as they also do in *D. immitis* and *H. diminuta*, with lesser amounts of choline plasmalogens. In *F. hepatica*, ethanolamine and choline plasmalogens occur in more or less equal amounts.

Hydrolysis of the α-β unsaturated ether link in *A. lumbricoides* plasmalogens yields a variety of saturated and unsaturated aldehydes, ranging from C_{12} to C_{18}, including some branched chain isomers. The major aldehydes from *A. lumbricoides* are, however, unsaturated C_{18} compounds. In contrast, in mammals, the predominant plasmalogen aldehyde is usually palmitate (C_{16} saturated).

Phosphatidyl Alkyl Ethers

These have a saturated, rather than an α-β unsaturated, ether link at the 1-hydroxyl group and are the phosphoglyceride equivalent of diacylglycerol alkyl ethers (Section 2.3.2). Like plasmalogens, phosphatidyl alkyl ethers are found as minor components in both vertebrate and invertebrate lipids. In *A. lumbricoides* and *L. carinii*, they occur in relatively large amounts, constituting about 10% of the total phospholipids. As in the plasmalogens, ethanolamine-containing phosphatidyl alkyl ethers predominate, with lesser amounts of choline ethers, and C_{18} is the major aldehyde.

Lysophosphoglycerides

These are formed from the corresponding phosphoglyceride by the removal of one of the fatty acids. Lysophosphoglycerides are important intermediates in phosphoglyceride metabolism (Section 4.3.5) and, like phosphatidic acid, they usually occur in tissues in relatively low amounts (less than 1% of total lipids). Lysophosphatidylcholine is usually the major lysophosphoglyceride and small amounts of lysophosphatidylcholine are usually present in lipid extracts from helminths. However, a number of parasites have been found to contain relatively large amounts (5 to 10% of the phospholipids) of lysophosphatidylcholine (*F. hepatica, T. hydatigena* larvae, *S. cervi, A. caninum*) or lysophosphatidylethanolamine (*T. spiralis* larvae, *Dipylidium caninum, S. mansoni* eggs). In *A. lumbricoides* lipids, lysophosphatidylcholine, lysophosphatidylethanolamine and lysophosphatidylserine each comprise about 3% of the total phospholipids. The possible biochemical significance of these high levels of lysophosphoglycerides in parasitic helminths is discussed in Section 4.3.5. However, it must also be remembered that lysophosphoglycerides can arise by hydrolysis of the corresponding phosphoglycerides during extraction and analyses.

2.3.4. Sphingolipids

Sphingolipids are important components of cell membranes and are particularly abundant in nervous tissue. As a backbone, sphingolipids have sphingosine (*Figure*

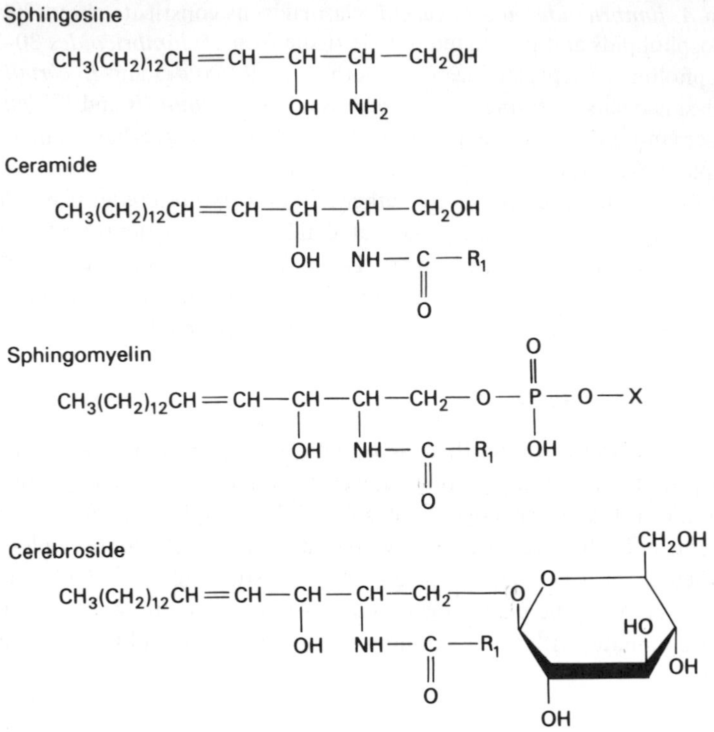

Sphingosine

$$CH_3(CH_2)_{12}CH\!=\!CH\!-\!\underset{\underset{OH}{|}}{CH}\!-\!\underset{\underset{NH_2}{|}}{CH}\!-\!CH_2OH$$

Ceramide

$$CH_3(CH_2)_{12}CH\!=\!CH\!-\!\underset{\underset{OH}{|}}{CH}\!-\!\underset{\underset{NH-\underset{\underset{O}{\|}}{C}-R_1}{|}}{CH}\!-\!CH_2OH$$

Sphingomyelin

$$CH_3(CH_2)_{12}CH\!=\!CH\!-\!\underset{OH}{CH}\!-\!\underset{NH-\underset{O}{\overset{}{C}}-R_1}{CH}\!-\!CH_2\!-\!O\!-\!\overset{O}{\underset{OH}{\overset{\|}{P}}}\!-\!O\!-\!X$$

Cerebroside

Figure 2.4 The structure of sphingolipids; R_1 is a hydrocarbon chain of a fatty acid, X is a polar head group.

2.4) or a closely related base. Some 30 or so different amino alcohols have been found in the sphingolipids of organisms; in mammals, the major bases are sphingosine and sphinganine, whilst many marine invertebrates have 4,8-sphingadiene. There has been no work on the nature of the base in helminth sphingolipids. Sphingosine has been identified in *M. expansa* and sphinganine has been found in the larvae of *T. taeniaeformis*. In the latter case, it is not known if sphinganine is actually part of the sphingolipids, as it is also an intermediate in sphingosine synthesis (Section 4.3.5).

In addition to the complex organic base, sphingolipids all contain a fatty acid molecule, attached via an amide link and a polar head group.

Ceramides (N-acylsphingosine)

Ceramides are composed of the base plus a fatty acid (*Figure 2.4*). Ceramides are intermediates in sphingolipid synthesis and are normally only present in trace amounts. Ceramides have been detected in the tissues of two trematodes, *F. hepatica* and *Paramphistomum microbothrium*[18].

Sphingomyelins

These are usually the most abundant of the sphingolipids and consist of a ceramide with phosphorylethanolamine or phosphorylcholine attached to the terminal hydroxyl group (*Figure 2.4*). Helminth lipids normally contain measurable amounts of sphingomyelins, usually 2 to 5% of the total. There have, however, been conflicting reports on the presence of sphingomyelin in *F. hepatica.*

Cerebrosides

Cerebrosides have a monosaccharide (glucose or galactose) as a head group, attached by a β-glycoside link to the terminal hydroxyl group of a ceramide (*Figure 2.4*). Amongst parasitic helminths, cerebrosides have only been identified with any regularity in cestodes. The cerebrosides from *M. expansa* and larval *T. taeniaeformis* contain galactose, whilst the cerebroside from *H. diminuta* contains glucose. In mammals, galactose cerebrosides are characteristic of nervous tissue, glucose cerebrosides of non-nervous tissue. Cerebrosides have also been identified in the lipids of *F. hepatica, P. microbothrium, A. caninum* and in the eggs, but not the adults, of *S. mansoni*. Cerebrosides were also not detected in larval *T. spiralis*. Characteristically, cerebrosides contain long chain, saturated and mono-unsaturated fatty acids, and in mammals hydroxy acids are common. The cerebrosides of *H. diminuta* contain the characteristic $C_{24:0}$ and $C_{24:1}$ fatty acids, but hydroxy acids have not been found.

Ceramides can also have sulphated sugars as head groups and these glycosphingolipids are known as sulphatides. Sulphatides have been tentatively identified in the lipids of *A. caninum, F. hepatica, P. microbothrium* and *D. caninum*[19,20]. Other neutral glycosphingolipids have di-, tri- and tetrasaccharide chains as head groups and are called dihexosides, trihexosides and tetrahexosides, respectively. These sphingolipids have not been reported from helminths.

Gangliosides

The gangliosides are glycosphingolipids which have oligosaccharide head groups containing one or more sialic acid residue. Again, gangliosides have not been reported from helminths.

2.3.5. Ascarosides

The ascarosides are a series of unique α-glycosides, which have been isolated from the eggs and female reproductive tract of ascarid and oxyurid nematodes (*P. equorum, A. lumbricoides, A. columnaris, A. galli, Toxocara cati, Passarulus* sp.[17]). The ascarosides can be grouped into three related classes: the monol ascarosides, the diol ascarosides and the diol diascarosides (*Figure 2.5*). In all cases, the glycone (sugar moiety) appears to be the same, and is 3,6-dideoxy-L-arabinohexose (ascarylose), a sugar not found in any other eukaryote. Ascarylose has only been unambiguously identified in the ascarosides of *P. equorum* and *A. lumbricoides*,

Monol ascaroside

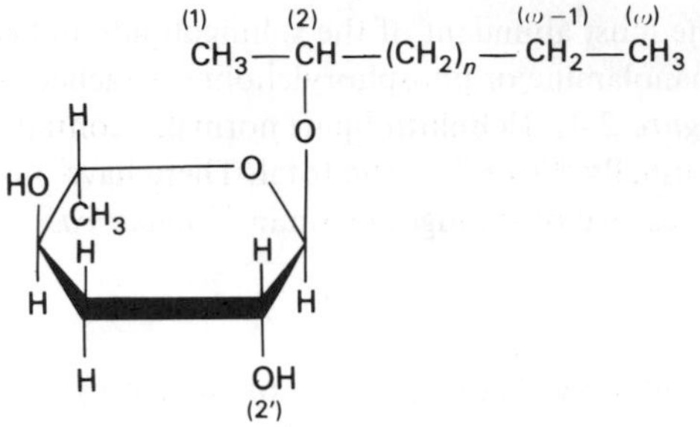

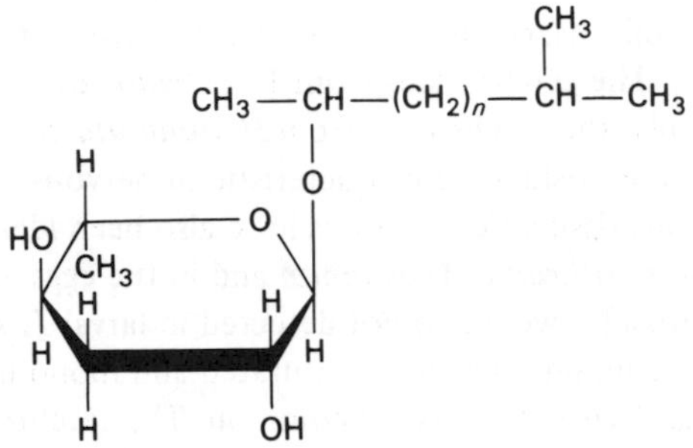

$$CH_3 - CH - (CH_2)_n - CH_2 - CH_3$$

with positions (1), (2), $(\omega-1)$, (ω) labeled and (2') below.

$$CH_3 - CH - (CH_2)_n - CH - CH_3$$
with a CH_3 branch.

Diol ascaroside

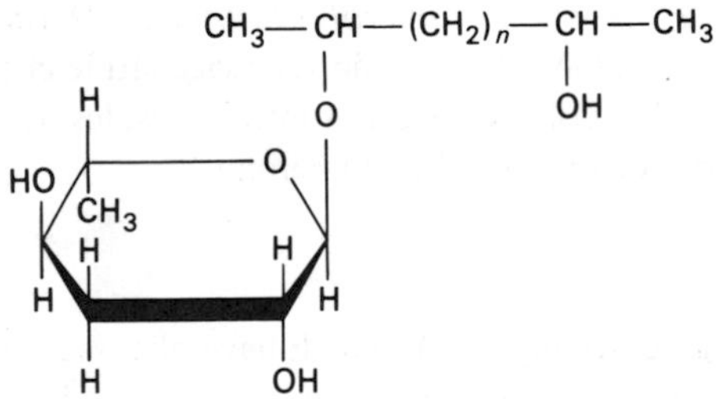

$$CH_3 - CH - (CH_2)_n - CH - CH_3$$
with OH.

Diol diascaroside

$$CH_3 - CH - (CH_2)_n - CH - CH_3$$

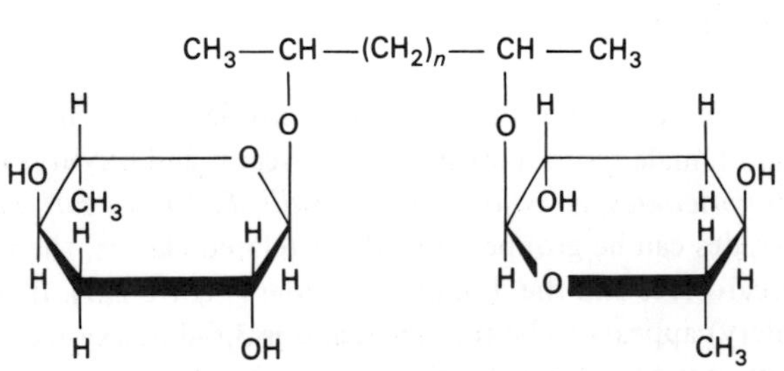

Figure 2.5 The structure of ascarosides.

but there is fairly good evidence that it is the glycone in the other species as well.

The aglycones of the monol ascarosides are a mixture of long chain secondary alcohols, with the hydroxyl group on carbon 2 (L-2-alkanols). In *A. lumbricoides*, the monol aglycones contain 25–32 carbon atoms, C_{29} being the most abundant[21]. About a quarter of the *A. lumbricoides* monol aglycones have an even number of carbon atoms (largely C_{30}) and are branched, the branch consisting of a methyl group on the second carbon of the opposite end to the hydroxyl group ($\omega - 1$ position). The distribution of aglycone chain lengths and the percentage of branched monol aglycones varies in the different species. In *P. equorum*, the monol aglycones range from C_{26} to C_{30}, the latter predominating, whilst in *A. galli*, they range from C_{25} to C_{34}, with C_{31} as the major component.

The aglycones from the diol ascaroside and the diol diascaroside are a mixture of unbranched, long chain diols. Originally, it was thought that the hydroxyl groups were on carbons 2 and 6 of the long chain diols. However, recent work[22] has shown that the diols are, in fact, symmetrical molecules with the hydroxyl groups at the 2 and ($\omega - 1$) positions (*Figure 2.5*). The diol ascarosides have one glycoside link and one free hydroxyl group per mole, whilst the diol diascarosides have two glycoside links per mole. Again, the distribution of the carbon chain lengths varies slightly between species. In *A. lumbricoides*, the diol aglycones range from C_{29} to C_{33}; in the diol ascarosides C_{31} and C_{33} are equally abundant, whilst in the diol diascarosides C_{33} is the most common chain length.

Ascaroside Esters

In ovarian tissue, the ascarosides occur almost entirely as esters, the two hydroxyl groups of ascarylose and the free hydroxyl group of the diol ascaroside aglycone being esterified. In *A. lumbricoides*, the esters contain 95 moles per cent acetate and only 5 moles per cent propionate. When present, propionate always occurs in the 2′ position of the sugar. Of the ovarian ascarosides in *A. lumbricoides*, 90% are completely esterified, the remainder having a free hydroxyl group on the sugar or on the diol[21]. The 2′ position of the sugar is, however, always esterified and ascaroside esters with more than one free hydroxyl group are extremely rare.

The ascaroside esters of other species have not been characterised in detail. Acetate and propionate residues occur in the ascaroside esters of *P. equorum* and *A. columnaris*; all of the other species investigated contain only acetate esters (*A. galli*, *T. cati*, *Passarulus* sp.). It is interesting that in *A. lumbricoides*, *A. columnaris* and *P. equorum*, although volatile fatty acids (C_5 and C_6) occur in the ovarian neutral lipids, they are not present in the ascaroside esters. The absence of 2-methylbutyrate and 2-methylvalerate residues from the ascaroside esters of ascarids, despite their abundance in ovarian triacylglycerols and waxes, suggests considerable biochemical specificity.

Free Ascarosides

The only known function of ascaroside esters is the formation of the ascaroside membrane of the egg shell (Section 4.3.4). Some 75% of the ascaroside layer of

A. lumbricoides eggs consists of free ascarosides, the remainder being protein with traces of sterol. Hydrolysis of the protein in the ascaroside membrane of *A. lumbricoides* yields lysine, arginine, glutamic acid, serine, glycine, cystine, aspartic acid, threonine, alanine, valine, tyrosine, leucine, isoleucine, tryptophan, phenylalanine and proline. The protein from *A. lumbricoides* ascaroside membranes is, however, not particularly rich in proline[23]. This is in contrast to *P. equorum*, where proline-rich refringent granules, which are thought to contribute to the ascaroside layer, are found in the oocyte. The ascaroside layer is responsible for the extreme chemical resistance of *A. lumbricoides* eggs. It is normal, for example, to store the eggs in 0.1 N sulphuric acid and they will even embryonate successfully in 12% formalin. In *A. lumbricoides*, the ascarosides of the egg membrane consist of 12% monol ascaroside, 10% diol ascaroside, 8% diol diascaroside and 70% diol ascaroside in which the free hydroxyl group of the aglycone is acetylated.

2.3.6. Waxes

Most natural waxes consist of a mixture of long chain hydrocarbons, long chain aldehydes and free and esterified long chain alcohols. The waxes from parasitic helminths, however, are all esterified long chain alcohols.

Esterified Alcohols

The most remarkable example of wax esters in parasitic helminths occurs in the cystacanths of the acanthocephalan *P. minutus*. The cystacanth, which develops in the haemocoel of Gammarids, is an infective resting stage and, like the infective stages of many other parasites, it contains large amounts of lipid. However, 80% of its lipids are wax esters (long chain alcohols esterified with long chain acids). In contrast, wax esters are not found in any significant amounts in the adult parasite. The wax esters of *P. minutus* cystacanths contain predominantly saturated long chain alcohols (C_{12} to C_{20}), mostly C_{16} and C_{18}, esterified with long chain fatty acids (C_{12}–C_{22}), with C_{16} and $C_{18:1}$ predominating. The significance of the enormous amounts of wax esters in the cystacanths of *P. minutus* is obscure. Wax esters function as storage lipids in some protozoa and in a number of marine invertebrates, particularly copepods. In marine organisms, wax esters may have a buoyancy function, since they have a lower density than the corresponding triacylglycerols. In the cystacanths of *P. minutus*, the buoyancy of the wax esters might affect the balance of the intermediate host. Wax esters also have a lower melting point than the corresponding triacylglycerols and this might be important in *P. minutus* in relation to the temperature changes that accompany infection (Section 5.2.3).

   Wax esters have also been found in the cestode *C. verticillatum* and in the nematodes *A. lumbricoides, A. columnaris* and *A. galli*. In *A. lumbricoides*, the wax esters are extremely unusual in that they consist of a long chain alcohol esterified, not with a long chain acid, but with a short chain volatile fatty acid[16]. The alcohol fraction of *A. lumbricoides* wax esters is mostly C_{18}, with small amounts of C_{16}, C_{17} and C_{19}. The acid component is largely 2-methylbutyrate with small amounts of acetate, propionate and *n*-valerate and traces of *n*-butyrate and 2-methylvalerate. The wax esters of *A. columnaris* similarly consist largely of C_{16} and C_{18} alcohols, esterified with 2-methylbutyrate, acetate and propionate. In contrast, the wax esters of *A. galli* contain long chain alcohols and long chain acids[17].

Nothing is known of the biosynthesis of wax esters in helminths. The distribution of chain lengths in the alcohol moiety of helminth waxes (mostly C_{16} and C_{18}) strongly suggests that, as in other organisms, the alcohols are formed by the direct reduction of the corresponding fatty acids. However, there is always the possibility, particularly in the cystacanths of *P. minutus*, that the wax esters may not be synthesised *de novo* by the parasite, but are obtained from the host.

2.3.7. Terpenes

Terpenes contain multiple isoprene units (2-methyl-1,3-butadiene) and can either be linear or cyclic molecules, or both.

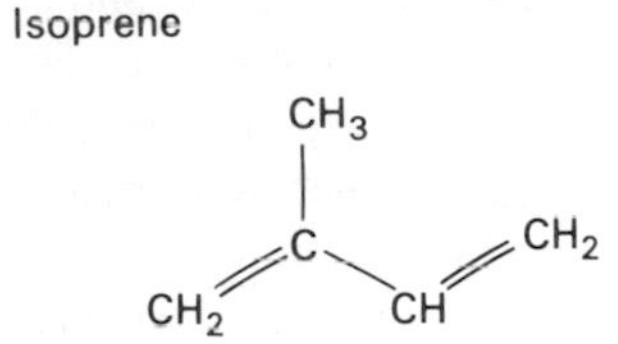

Isoprene

Terpenes are often classified according to the number of isoprene units in the molecule. The monoterpenes have two isoprene units, the sesquiterpenes have three, and the di-, tri- and tetraterpenes have four, six and eight isoprene units, respectively. Farnesol is a sesquiterpene, squalene a triterpene, whilst higher terpenes include carotenoids, polyprenols and the ubiquinones.

Farnesol

The tapeworm *H. diminuta* contains measurable amounts of 2-*trans*,6-*trans*-farnesol (*Figure 2.6*)[24]. Farnesol is a precursor of higher prenoids (Section 4.3.3), and it is also a juvenile hormone mimic. A compound similar to, and possibly identical with,

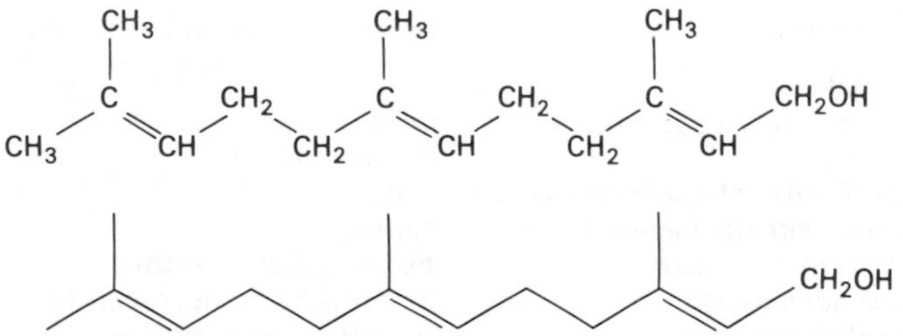

Figure 2.6 The structure of 2-*trans*,6-*trans*-farnesol.

2-*trans*,6-*trans*-farnesol has also been identified in the protoscoleces of *E. granulosus* and the cysticerci of *T. hydatigena*. Farnesol has not so far been reported from nematodes, trematodes or acanthocephalans. The possibility of farnesol having a hormonal function in cestodes is discussed in Section 4.3.3.

Squalene

The triterpene, squalene, is a precursor of cholesterol (Section 4.3.3). Normally, squalene is fairly widely distributed in tissues, but it has not been found in helminths. The absence of squalene in parasitic helminths correlates with their inability to synthesise sterols *de novo* (Section 4.3.3).

Carotenoids

The carotenoids are red or yellow pigments, most of which are alicyclic molecules, formed from eight isoprene units. Carotenoids occur widely in invertebrates and have been found in nematodes, trematodes, cestodes and acanthocephalans (*Table 2.2*). The acanthocephalans, in particular, often contain large amounts of carotenoid, and the pigment gives the worms their characteristic red or yellow colours. In addition to the species in *Table 2.2*, β-carotene and lutein occur in the larval stages of several trematodes (sporocysts, rediae and cercariae) and some seven different carotenoid fractions have been found in the filarial worm *Foleyella funcata*. Differ-

Table 2.2   The carotenoids found in parasitic helminths

Species	Carotenoid
Cestodes	
Ligula intestinalis (plerocercoid)	Astaxanthin, astaxanthin ester, cryptoxanthin, taraxanthin, 4-keto-α-carotene
Schistocephalus solidus (plerocercoid)	γ-Carotene derivatives, canthaxanthin, ketocarotenoid?
Taenia saginata	Esterified astaxanthin, isozeaxanthin, α-cryptoxanthin, ξ-carotene oxide?, γ-carotene oxide, 4-hydroxy-4-keto-carotene
Trematodes	
Fasciola hepatica	β-Carotene, lutein, echinenone, zeaxanthin
Acanthocephalans	
Arhythmorhynchus comptus	β-Carotene?
Filicollis anatis	β-Carotene
Macracanthorhynchus hirudinaceus	Lutein
Neoechinorhynchus pseudemydis	Lutein
Nipporhynchus ornatus	Esterified astaxanthin
Pallisentis nagpurensis	β-Carotene oxide, α-carotene oxide
Polymorphus minutus	Esterified astaxanthin
Pomphorhynchus laevis	β-Carotene
Pseudoacanthocephaloides galaxis	Lutein

ent species of helminth have different carotenoids and it is not clear whether this has any phylogenetic significance or whether it is related to the host's diet.

Animals cannot synthesise carotenoids *de novo* and must obtain them from their diet. Parasitic helminths must obtain their carotenoids from their hosts. The range of carotenoids present in helminths does not necessarily appear to reflect the range of carotenoids available in the host's diet. So, some form of selective uptake of carotenoids is probably involved. This is particularly noticeable in the Acanthocephala where most species contain only one major carotenoid. Selective uptake of carotenoids has also been found in free-living invertebrates; for example, some polychaetes take up only β-carotene, and certain molluscs preferentially absorb hydroxycarotenoids. The uptake of carotenoids by helminths may also be associated with the uptake of other compounds, such as lipids or proteins, in the form of lipocarotenoid complexes or carotenoproteins.

The ability of helminths to interconvert carotenoids has not been investigated and it is not known, for example, if they are able to insert hydroxyl or keto groups into the carotenoid molecule or if they can convert β-carotene to astaxanthin. It has, however, been suggested that *F. hepatica* may be able to hydroxylate carotenes and *A. lumbricoides* can cleave β-carotene to vitamin A (Section 4.7).

The role of carotenoids in parasitic helminths is not clear. Endoparasites, living in the dark, would appear to have no need for coloration, although this may not be true of the free-living and intermediate stages. In the acanthocephalan *P. minutus*, both the adults and the intermediate acanthor and cystacanth stages are bright red, due to the presence of esterified astaxanthin. The intermediate host of *P. minutus*, *Gammarus pulex* is relatively transparent and the cystacanth is clearly visible, through the body wall, as a bright red spot. It is possible that this makes infected gammarids more readily visible to water fowl, which are the final host. Another brightly coloured infective stage is the metacercarial-containing sporocyst of the trematode *Leucochloridium* which are found in the tentacles of their snail hosts (*Succinea* sp.). Mature sporocysts have alternating red, green or brown bands and are clearly visible through the wall of the tentacle, and again this may attract the final bird host. The pigments in this case have not been characterised.

Possible biochemical functions for carotenoids in parasitic helminths include acting as antioxidants, or as a source of vitamin A, or they may be involved in oxidative metabolism. It has been suggested in molluscs, for example, that carotenoids can act as alternative electron acceptors under anaerobic conditions, thus allowing the cytochrome chain to function anaerobically. There is, however, no evidence in parasitic helminths that carotenoids act as a terminal electron acceptor (Section 3.2). In many organisms, carotenoids appear to be associated with reproduction, occurring in high concentrations in the ovaries and eggs. Whether the carotenoids of helminths are also involved in reproduction is not known.

Despite all of these different possibilities, it is not at all certain what function carotenoids have in helminths, or if they have any at all. Carotenoids have never been shown to be essential in parasitic helminths, the concentration of carotenoids can vary widely from individual to individual, and they are completely absent from many species.

Polyprenols

These are long chain, linear polyisoprenoid compounds, with a terminal, primary alcohol group. One of the functions of polyprenols is as a cofactor in glycosyl transferase reactions (Section 4.2.3). The most common polyprenol in animal tissues is dolichol (contains 19 isoprenoid units). Although phosphorylated iso-prenols occur in the tegument of S. mansoni (Section 4.2.3), the only polyprenol which has been fully characterised from helminths is solanesol, a nine isoprenoid unit compound found in A. lumbricoides.

Solanesol

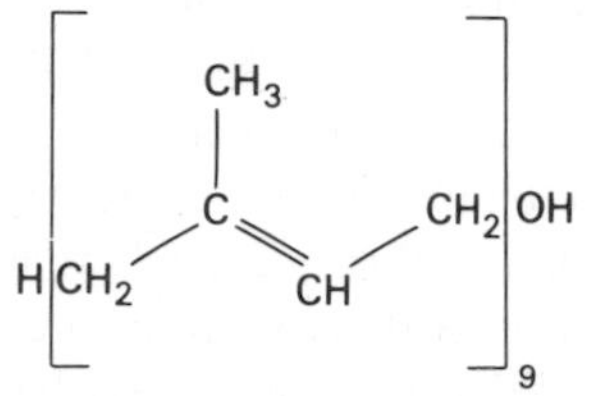

Ubiquinones (Coenzyme Q)

The ubiquinones (UQ) are a group of compounds (*Figure 2.7*) that act as hydrogen carriers in biological systems and are intimately involved in the cytochrome chain. They consist of a substituted quinone ring with a long isoprenoid chain. The most common ubiquinone in animals is ubiquinone-10 (UQ_{10}) (10 isoprenoid units in the side chain), although ubiquinones with 9, 11 and 12 isoprenoid units are quite common. Not a great deal of information is available on the ubiquinones of hel-minths and it is restricted to nematodes and cestodes. Ubiquinone has been

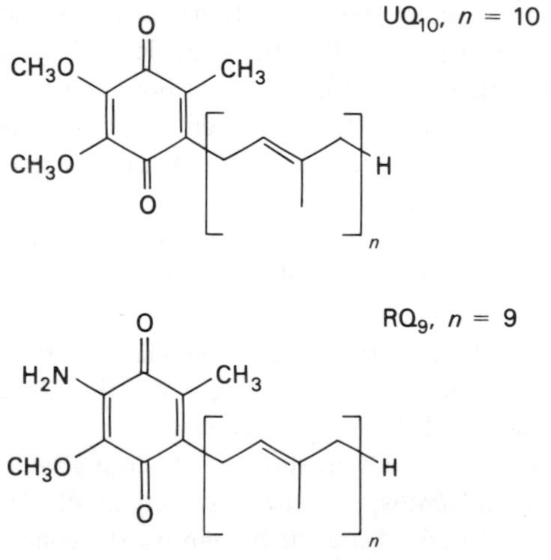

Figure 2.7 The structure of ubiquinone (UQ) and rhodoquinone (RQ).

identified in a variety of nematodes (Section 3.2.1). In *Metastrongylus elongatus*, the ubiquinone is UQ_9, whether the ubiquinone in the other species of nematode is also UQ_9, or the more usual UQ_{10}, is not known. A number of nematodes and cestodes contain rhodoquinone-9 (RQ_9), either instead of, or as well as, UQ (Section 3.2.1). Since rhodoquinone does not occur in mammals, its presence in helminths is of interest from the point of view of chemotherapy. Micro-organisms can convert ubiquinone to rhodoquinone, but whether ubiquinone is the precursor of rhodoquinone in helminths is unknown. Indeed, it is not even known if helminths can synthesise ubiquinones *de novo*. The immediate precursor of ubiquinones (and steroids) is farnesol. However, parasitic helminths cannot convert farnesol to squalene (the next step in steroid synthesis) and a similar block could be present on the ubiquinone pathway. Insects are in a comparable situation, as they are unable to synthesise squalene *de novo* (Section 4.3.3), but in this case ubiquinone synthesis has been demonstrated.

2.3.8. Steroids

Steroids are all derivatives of the complex heterocyclic hydrocarbon perhydrocyclopentanophenanthrene. In tissues, steroids occur free and in the form of steroid esters. Steroids and their derivatives are major components of cell membranes and, in many organisms, steroids play an important role in metabolic regulation.

Free Steroids

The major steroid found in helminths is cholesterol. Indeed, in the majority of helminths, it seems to be the only steroid present. Cholesterol usually constitutes around 10% of the parasite's lipids, but the figure varies from 2 to 26% in different species. In the trematode *E. revolutum*, for example, cholesterol is the major neutral lipid fraction. Two derivatives of cholesterol, cholestanol and cholestane (*Figure 2.8*), occur in helminths. Cholestane has been found in the trematodes *E. revolutum* and *S. mansoni*, whilst cholestanol occurs in *A. lumbricoides*, *M. hirudinaceus* and *M. dubius*.

In addition to cholesterol, two plant steroids, campesterol and β-sitosterol, together with their reduction products, campestanol and stigmastanol, have been found in *A. lumbricoides*, *M. dubius* and *M. hirudinaceus*. Campesterol and β-sitosterol differ from cholesterol in having an extra methyl or ethyl group, respectively, at C_{24} on the side chain. These three helminths probably obtain the phytosterols from the host's intestinal contents.

Steroid Esters

A variable proportion of the tissue cholesterol is esterified with long chain fatty acids. In helminths, free steroids usually predominate, with about a third of the steroid fraction being esterified.

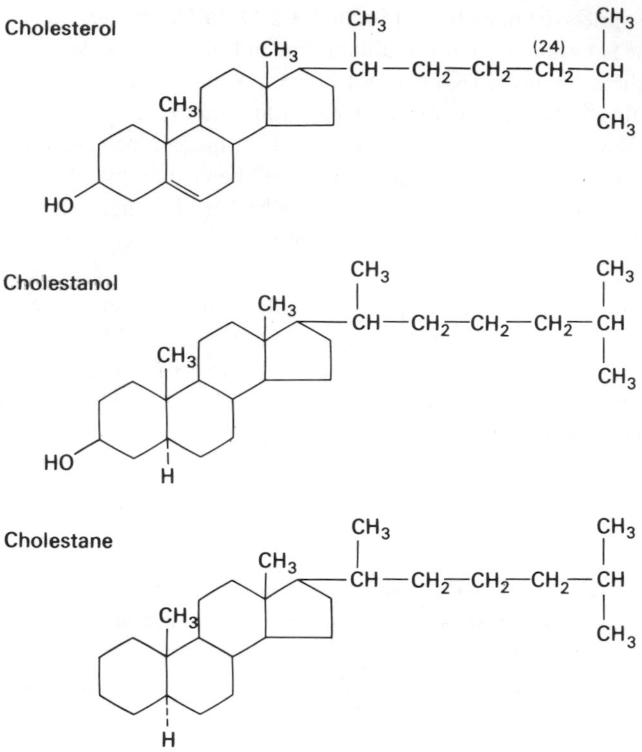

Figure 2.8 The structure of cholesterol and some of its derivatives.

Steroid Hormones

In many animals, steroid derivatives have important hormonal functions. The only steroid hormone so far identified in helminths is β-ecdysone, minute quantities of which have been isolated from *A. lumbricoides*. Many plants contain steroids with ecdysone-like activity (phytoecdysones) and the traces of ecdysone found in *A. lumbricoides* may well be derived from plant material present in the host gut (Section 4.3.3).

There is, at the moment, no evidence for steroid hormones occurring in parasitic helminths, although the sex attractant of the parasitic nematode *N. brasiliensis* and in the trematode *Leucochloridiomorpha constantiae* may well be steroidal, possibly cholesterol.

2.3.9. Distribution of Lipids

With the exception of ascarosides, which are unique to certain nematodes, the different lipid classes found in parasitic helminths are the same as those found in free-living organisms. The relative amounts of the various lipid fractions are also fairly similar. In parasitic helminths, the proportion of phospholipids is usually between

20 and 50% of the total lipids and this is perhaps rather higher than in most free-living invertebrates. An extreme value for phospholipids of 72% of the total lipid has been claimed in larval *T. spiralis*. As in free-living organisms, phosphatidyl-choline and phosphatidylethanolamine are the major phospholipids in parasitic helminths, with lesser amounts of phosphatidylserine. Significant quantities of sphingolipids are found in helminths, even though there are only relatively small amounts of nervous tissue in parasites. The rather sporadic reports of cerebrosides and sulphatides in parasitic helminths probably reflects the fact that these sphingo-lipids are usually only present in small amounts in tissues.

Some rather unusual features of parasitic lipids are the high levels of lysophospho-glycerides and the high levels of plasmalogens in certain species. Free fatty acids are also found in unusually large amounts in some helminths, particularly in the larval stages. High levels of free fatty acids would have a disruptive effect on cell membranes, so possibly in helminths the free fatty acids are bound to a carrier protein. Although high levels of free fatty acids do not usually occur in vertebrate tissues, even those with an active lipid metabolism, there are reports from free-living invertebrates (molluscs and annelids) of similar high free fatty acid levels.

The distribution of lipids in the different tissues of parasitic helminths has been extensively studied histochemically. In tapeworms, lipid occurs primarily in the parenchyma, although lipid droplets are found in or around the excretory canals. When ripe proglottides are shed, the lipid in the parenchyma is essentially being excreted, as it is not used by the adult, nor by the eggs. In some cases, it is conceivable that the lipid in the proglottides might attract the intermediate host to eat it. There have been reports of a gradient in lipid content along the length of cestodes and the lipid content also varies with age. Trematodes, in general, contain relatively little lipid. Lipid droplets occur in and around the excretory vessels and lipid excretion by trematodes has been well documented (Section 3.3.3). In nematodes, lipid occurs in the lateral cords, muscles, intestine and reproductive organs. The intestine is a particularly prominent site of lipid storage in infective larvae. Finally, in the acanthocephalans, most of the lipid occurs in the body wall, and the fluid in the lacunar canal system may well be lipoidal. An interesting feature of lipid distribution in helminths (nematodes, cestodes and trematodes) is that much of the lipid in the eggs is extra-embryonic, occurring in the space between the embryo and the egg shell. When the eggs hatch, the lipid is discarded.

2.4. AMINO ACIDS AND THEIR DERIVATIVES

There are twenty common or standard amino acids found in proteins (alanine, arginine, asparagine, aspartate, cysteine, glutamine, glutamate, glycine, histidine, isoleucine, leucine, lysine, methionine, phenylalanine, proline, serine, threonine, tryptophan, tyrosine, valine), and there are also a number of rare amino acids, such as 4-hydroxyproline, 5-hydroxylysine and ϵ-N-methyl-lysine which only occur in specialised proteins. In addition, there are some 150 known non-protein α-amino acids, compounds such as ornithine, citrulline, taurine and 4-aminobutyric acid.

These amino acids do not occur naturally in proteins, and are often metabolic intermediates or, in some cases, neurotransmitters.

2.4.1. Free Amino Acid Pools

The free amino acid fraction in tissues is small compared with the protein amino acids. In vertebrate tissues, the free and protein amino acids often resemble one another fairly closely. The free amino acid pools of invertebrates, however, are often dominated by one or two amino acids. The levels of free amino acids are also usually much higher in invertebrates than in vertebrates. In birds and mammals, free amino acid levels range from 10 to 50 mg/100 g fresh weight, figures for invertebrates are from 300 to 2000 mg/100 g fresh weight, to as high as 3000 mg/100 g fresh weight for marine invertebrates. Parasitic helminths come in the lower part of the invertebrate range, with free amino acid pools of 50–400 mg/100 g fresh weight. In free-living invertebrates, free amino acids are important regulators of intracellular osmotic pressure. It is not clear if amino acids fulfill the same function in parasitic helminths, although there are claims that proline is an osmotic effector in the larval stages of the trematode *Himasthla quissetensis*[25] and that amino acid transport may be involved in osmoregulation in *H. diminuta*[89].

The amino acid pool is not necessarily a single entity, and there may be several independent amino acid pools in tissues. In cestodes, for example, there is some evidence of separate pools for amino acids which have just been absorbed and for synthetic intermediates.

Cestodes

In cestodes, the free amino acid pool sizes range from about 100 to 400 mg/100 g fresh weight, the highest values being for the shark tapeworm *Lacistorhynchus* sp. Tapeworms do not appear to be able to regulate, to any great extent, the amino acid flux across their teguments and are at the mercy of environmental fluctuations (Section 4.1.8). In the rat tapeworm *H. diminuta*, there is even a positive rank correlation between intestinal amino acids and the parasite's free amino acid pool. Diurnal variations in the size of the free amino acid pool have been reported for *H. diminuta*.

The major free amino acid in *H. diminuta* is alanine, in the procercoids of *Triaenophorus nodulosus* it is proline, and in *Lacistorhynchus* sp. the main free amino acids are glycine and taurine. Taurine often occurs in high levels in the tissues of marine animals. In addition to taurine, a variety of non-protein amino acids, β-alanine, citrulline, ornithine, 3-aminoisobutyrate and 4-aminoisobutyrate have been found in the free amino acid pools of cestodes.

Trematodes

In the trematodes, free amino acid pools range from 112 mg/100 g fresh weight for *S. mansoni* to 300 mg/100 g fresh weight for *F. hepatica* and 522 mg/100 g fresh weight for *Paragonimus westermani*.

Alanine and glutamate are the major free amino acids in *S. mansoni*, whilst the main free amino acids in *F. hepatica* are proline and alanine, and in *P. westermani*, proline and arginine. Five non-protein amino acids, taurine, ornithine, citrulline, 2-aminobutyrate and 4-aminobutyrate have been found in the free amino acid pools of trematodes[26]. Proline and alanine are also the major free amino acids in the parasitic turbellarian *Syndesmis franciscana*[27].

High levels of proline have again been found in the free amino acid pools of monogeneans[28]. The free amino acid pools of monogeneans range from 400 mg/100 g fresh weight for freshwater forms to 2600 mg/100 g fresh weight for marine species, and proline may constitute up to 70% of the total free amino acids. The biochemical role of these high proline levels is not clear. Proline is not particularly abundant in the monogenean diet, there is no evidence that it is acting as an osmotic effector in these species, and nor does it appear to be catabolised as an energy source. In the digenean *F. hepatica*, it seems likely that proline is an end-product of amino acid catabolism (Section 3.4.2).

Nematodes

Compared with trematodes and cestodes, there is very little information on the free amino acid pools of parasitic nematodes. The free amino acid pool in *A. lumbricoides* is relatively small, about 20 mg/100 g fresh weight. In the perienteric fluid, serine and alanine are the main free amino acids[29], although some workers have reported large amounts of glutamate and proline to be present. The major free amino acids in the ovaries of *A. lumbricoides* are alanine and glutamate, whilst lysine predominates in seminal fluid[29]. The basic amino acid, lysine, may be having a histone-like function in the sperm.

The non-protein amino acid, 4-aminobutyrate, causes muscle strips of *A. lumbricoides* to relax, and this can be used for the bioassay of 4-aminobutyrate[30]. However, there is no evidence to show that 4-aminobutyrate is an inhibitory neurotransmitter *in vivo*. A number of non-protein amino acids, 3-aminoisobutyrate, citrulline, ornithine, 2-aminoisobutyrate and β-alanine, have been isolated from larval *Anisakis*[31].

2.4.2 Amino Acid Derivatives

The role of amino acids in biosynthesis is summarised in *Table 4.10* and is discussed in detail in Section 4.4.2.

2.5. PROTEINS

Proteins have many different biological functions, they are ubiquitous in their distribution and there is really no satisfactory scheme of classifying them. The largest group of proteins are the enzymes, of which nearly 2000 different ones have been described. Proteins are also involved in contractile systems, in transport, as protective agents, toxins, hormones, amino acid reserves and as important structural components. Organisms usually show a complex pattern of soluble proteins and protein polymorphism is used in taxonomy.

In parasitic helminths, protein usually constitutes between 20 and 40% of the dry weight, but values as high as 70% of the dry weight have been reported for *M. hirudinaceus* and the infective larvae of *N. brasiliensis*. It has also been suggested that an amino acid storage protein may be present in the intestine of larval Mermithids. A variety of specific proteins have been isolated from parasitic helminths and some of them have been studied in detail.

2.5.1. Structural Proteins

Several structural proteins have been found in helminths, including collagen, cuticlin, keratin and sclerotin. Histochemically, a protein resembling resilin, the arthropod rubber-like protein, has been found in the pharynx of nematodes. The structural protein elastin has only recently been reported from parasitic helminths.

Collagen

Collagen is usually the most abundant structural protein in animals, forming in some cases as much as one-third of the total body protein. In parasitic helminths, collagen has been found in the cuticle, gut-basement membrane and possibly the egg shells of nematodes and in the teguments of trematodes and acanthocephalans. Characteristically, collagen contains about 30% glycine and appreciable amounts of proline (12%), 4-hydroxyproline (10%) and 5-hydroxylysine (5%). Invertebrate collagens, however, often show quite a range of amino acid compositions. In vertebrates, the collagen sub-unit (tropocollagen) is composed of three polypeptide chains (α-chains), twisted round one another to form a superhelix. Most collagens have, associated with them, variable amounts of carbohydrate bound to the hydroxylysine residues. However, there is no correlation between the number of hydroxylysine residues and the carbohydrate content. Collagens from vertebrates tend to contain relatively little carbohydrate (0.3 to 0.5%), whilst invertebrate collagens usually have between 5 and 15% carbohydrate. Vertebrate collagens also contain a variable number of inter- and intramolecular covalent links, formed by the aldol condensation of a lysine side chain with another lysine or histidine residue.

The most extensively studied collagens from parasitic helminths are the body-wall and gut-basement membrane collagens of *A. lumbricoides*. Two different collagens can be isolated from the body wall, one from the cuticle and the other from the muscles. The x-ray diffraction pattern of *A. lumbricoides* cuticle collagen shows the typical 2.86 Å meridional spacing characteristic of collagen. The cuticle collagen is attacked by bacterial collagenase, and an unusual feature of the action of collagenase on *A. lumbricoides* collagen is that digestion is greatly accelerated by calcium ions[32]. Under the electron microscope, *A. lumbricoides* cuticle collagen does not show the 640 Å banding characteristic of native vertebrate collagen.

Compared with vertebrate collagens, *A. lumbricoides* cuticle collagen has a low glycine content (26%), a high proline content (29%) and relatively low hydroxyproline and hydroxylysine levels (2% combined). There are, however, significant levels of half-cystine (2%) in *A. lumbricoides* cuticle collagen. Unlike most invertebrate collagens, the carbohydrate content of *A. lumbricoides* cuticle collagen is very low, 0.04%. The sub-unit of *A. lumbricoides* cuticle collagen has a molecular weight of 900 000, considerably higher than vertebrate tropocollagen (300 000). The polypeptide chains from *A. lumbricoides* cuticle collagen are, however, smaller than vertebrate α-chains, 52 000 molecular weight as opposed to 95 000. Each of the *A. lumbricoides* polypeptide chains is thought to be folded back on itself to form a hydrogen-bonded, three-stranded superhelix. The *A. lumbricoides* cuticle collagen sub-unit consists of a series of individual polypeptide chains, held together by sulphydryl bridges (*Figure 2.9*). The structure of *A. lumbricoides* cuticle collagen

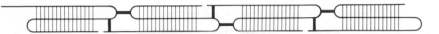

Figure 2.9 Proposed structure of *Ascaris lumbricoides* cuticle collagen. Each polypeptide chain is back-folded to form a three-stranded hydrogen-bonded superhelix. Thick bars represent sulphydryl bridges, and thin lines represent triple helical region.

is unique, in that no other collagen has been found to be stabilised by sulphydryl bridges, nor has the back-folded polypeptide structure been found in any other natural collagen. The cuticle collagen of *A. lumbricoides* has been found to be a useful model for studying the effects of cross-linking on the thermal stability of collagens[33].

Recently[34], the polypeptide chains from *A. lumbricoides* cuticle collagen have been resolved into three types, A, B and C. There is no stoichiometric relationship between the three chains, and they probably represent three different types of collagen and not the three chains of the superhelix. Also present in the cuticle are two fragments, C_1 and C_2, which represent two-thirds and one-third of the C chain, respectively. The C_1 and C_2 fragments are presumably formed by proteolytic cleavage of the C chain. Native cuticle collagen from *A. lumbricoides* and its sub-units are both strongly immunogenic and this may be related to the unique polypeptide configuration.

In marked contrast to the cuticle collagen, the muscle layer collagen from *A. lumbricoides* is a typical invertebrate collagen. Amino acid analysis gives 32% glycine, 10% proline, 12% hydroxyproline and 4% hydroxylysine. There is no evidence of stabilisation by sulphydryl links, although there is 0.3% half-cystine present. As in most invertebrate collagens, the carbohydrate content is high, 12.6%. The *A. lumbricoides* muscle collagen resembles vertebrate collagen in that the carbohydrate is linked to hydroxylysine residues and not to serine or threonine as in some other invertebrates. The muscle collagen of *A. lumbricoides* can be isolated as a complex with a non-collagen component[35]. The collagen and non-collagen components occur in the approximate ratio of 1:1 and they may possibly be linked by sulphydryl bonds.

Basement membranes are composed of a specialised form of collagen, with a complex carbohydrate composition. The basement membrane of the intestine of

A. lumbricoides has been studied in some detail[36,37,38,83]; it is essentially collagenous, but has a higher proportion of polar amino acids than vertebrate basement membrane collagen and a lower hydroxyproline and glycine content. The basement membrane collagen from *A. lumbricoides* contains 4.9% carbohydrate but, unlike vertebrate basement membranes, there is no sialic acid. Under the electron microscope, neither vertebrate nor *A. lumbricoides* basement membranes show the characteristic 640 Å collagen periodicity.

The basement membrane collagen of *A. lumbricoides* has been separated into a series of polypeptides, 17 in all (molecular weights 22 500 to 400 000), the amino acid compositions of which show varying degrees of relatedness to collagen. Several of these polypeptides have carbohydrate side chains attached to hydroxylysine residues. In the glycopeptides from *A. lumbricoides* basement membrane, there appear to be two sorts of side chain, one a disaccharide composed of glucose and galactose, and the other an oligosaccharide containing fucose, galactose, mannose, galactosamine and glucosamine.

Collagen has been prepared from two other species of helminth, the acanthocephalan *M. hirudinaceus* and the trematode *F. hepatica*. The collagen of *M. hirudinaceus* has a sub-unit molecular weight of 329 000 and a fairly typical amino acid composition: 31% glycine, 7.7% proline, 6% hydroxyproline, 4% hydroxylysine and 5.5% carbohydrate.

The collagen from *F. hepatica* has an intermediate sub-unit molecular weight of 500 000 and, again, a fairly typical amino acid composition: 30% glycine, 11% proline, 9.5% hydroxyproline, 2.6% hydroxylysine and 12.8% carbohydrate. Glucose–galactose side chains have been shown to be attached to the hydroxylysine residues[84]. The sub-units of *F. hepatica* collagen are extremely labile and have not been further characterised. There is no evidence for cystine cross-links in either *M. hirudinaceus* or *F. hepatica* collagens.

Collagens usually show a relationship between thermostability and body temperature, this relationship also holding for parasitic helminths (*Table 2.3*). The melting temperature (T_m) of collagen is the temperature at which half of the helical structure has been lost, and this is usually a few degrees above body tem-

Table 2.3 The relationship between thermostability and environmental temperature for different collagens

Source	T_s	T_m	Environmental temperature ($^{\circ}$C)
Ascaris lumbricoides			
cuticle	—	52	37
muscle layer	—	45	37
Macracanthorhynchus hirudinaceus	68	46	37
Fasciola hepatica	—	36.6	37
Earthworm	—	22	5–20
Cow skin	65	39	37
Cod skin	40	16	10–14
Antarctic fish	27	6	0–5

perature. The shrinkage temperature (T_s) is the comparable figure for the native collagen fibre, and $T_s - T_m$ is usually about 25 °C. Many collagens show a linear relationship between thermostability and imino acid content (proline + hydroxyproline). However, the collagens of *M. hirudinaceus* and *A. lumbricoides* cuticle do not fall onto this straight line (*Figure 2.10*), presumably because of covalent links in the molecule.

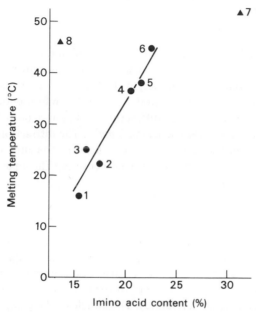

Figure 2.10 Correlation between melting temperature (T_m) of collagen and imino acid content (proline + hydroxyproline): 1, cod skin; 2, earthworm; 3, sea anemone; 4, *F. hepatica*; 5, cow skin; 6, *A. lumbricoides* muscle; 7, *A. lumbricoides* cuticle; 8, *M. hirudinaceus*.

Cuticlin

In addition to collagen, a second structural protein, cuticlin, has been extracted from *A. lumbricoides* cuticles[39]. Cuticlin has a high proline content (30%), but only a low glycine content (15%), it does not give the characteristic collagen x-ray diffraction pattern and it is not attacked by collagenase.

Cuticlin contains dityrosine linkages[40].

Dityrosine

Dityrosine occurs in a number of other structural proteins such as resilin, elastin, fibroin and keratin. Histochemically, dityrosine has been detected in the tegument of cestodes, in the spines of *F. hepatica* and in the egg shells of some monogeneans. *In vitro*, tyrosine dimers can be produced by the action of hydrogen peroxide and peroxidase on tyrosine. The mechanism for the biosynthesis of dityrosine is not known, but may be similar.

Keratin

Sulphur-rich, keratin-like proteins have been reported in the tegument and egg shells of acanthocephalans, in the cuticle and egg shells of some nematodes, in the cysts, tegument and spines of digenetic trematodes, in the hook sclerites of monogenetic trematodes, in the scolex hooks of cestodes and in the embryophore blocks of Taenioid tapeworms. The only x-ray diffraction studies have been on the hook sclerites of the monogenean *Entobdella diadema*[85]. The diffraction pattern from the hook sclerites showed some resemblance to keratin. The amino acid composition of keratins can be quite variable, but whether or not these parasite proteins are 'true keratins' is debatable.

Sclerotin

Quinone-tanned proteins are the principal component in the egg shells of pseudophyllidean cestodes, most monogenetic trematodes and many digenetic trematodes. One of the layers of the trematode metacercarial cyst is quinone-tanned, as may also be some nematode egg shells (the eggs of oxyurids, strongyloids and the tertiary egg envelope of *A. lumbricoides*). The cuticle of the plant parasitic nematode *G. rostochiensis* contains sclerotin, but quinone-tanning in the cuticles of other species of parasitic nematode is questionable.

In quinone-tanning, *O*-diphenols are oxidised by phenolase to *O*-quinones (Section 3.2.7). The *O*-quinones then react with terminal amino groups, the ϵ-amino groups of lysine and sulphydryl groups, to produce a cross-linked stable protein. The brown colour of sclerotin is due, in part, to the polymerisation of excess quinones, giving melanins. An alternative form of cross-linking involves activation of the β-position on the phenol side chain (the carbon atom closest to the ring), which is then linked to the proteins[41].

Phenolase and phenolic substances occur widely in the vitellaria of trematodes (monogeneans and digeneans) and in the vitellaria of pseudophyllideans. In monogeneans and digeneans, the phenolase may be present as an inactive prophenolase (Section 3.2.7). There is some evidence that quinone-tanning in trematode eggs does not necessarily involve free phenols and, instead, a process of autotanning may take place—tyrosine, bound to the protein, being oxidised to quinones, which can then react directly with free amino and sulphydryl groups. The vitelline globules of *F. hepatica* are rich in tyrosine. However, autotanning has never been chemically proven and there would be considerable problems of steric hindrance. The nature of the possible binding of tyrosine to the vitelline protein is also uncertain. Tyrosine might be incorporated into the backbone, with the aromatic side chain available for oxidation. Alternatively, it could be linked covalently to a backbone amino acid through a dityrosine link or via a free amide link in the form of a substituted diphenol. In some insects, the phenols involved in tanning the cuticle are transported bound to protein and the phenol–protein complex may be the tanning substrate.

Quinone-tanning makes egg shells resistant to enzymatic digestion, and it has been suggested that there might be a correlation between egg tanning and having to pass through the host gut. Several nematode eggs, including *A. lumbricoides*, appear to tan in the host gut and there are some indications that host digestive enzymes may be required to initiate the tanning process.

Ascaris Egg Coat Protein

The outer layer (tertiary envelope) of *A. lumbricoides* eggs is secreted by the uterus of the female. The tertiary envelope is composed of a sticky glycoprotein, molecular weight 10 000, which in solution rapidly forms aggregates[54]. During passage through the gut, it is this outer layer that may become tanned.

2.5.2. Haemoglobin

Haemoglobins are iron metalloporphyrin proteins that can combine reversibly with oxygen, the iron remaining in the ferrous state. Haemoglobins vary in molecular weight and amino acid composition, but probably all consist of a number of monohaem units of molecular weight approximately 17 000. Vertebrate haemoglobin has a molecular weight of about 70 000 and consists of four polypeptide chains. Several different polypeptide chains are known (α, β, γ), and they combine together in pairs to give the various types of vertebrate haemoglobin ($\alpha_2 \beta_2$, $\alpha_2 \gamma_2$, and so on). It is not known if a similar variety of chain types occur in invertebrates or if they combine together in simple ratios.

Distribution and Properties

Haemoglobin appears to occur randomly throughout the animal kingdom. Amongst the parasitic helminths, it has been found in representatives of the Trematoda (monogenea and digenea) and Nematoda, but has not been found in cestodes or acanthocephalans. Interestingly, apart from haemoglobin, no other respiratory pigments (such as haemocyanin, haemerythrin or chlorocruorin) have been found in parasitic helminths.

Where they have been examined in detail, the parasite haemoglobins are always distinct from those of their hosts (see, for example, References 42 and 43). The haemoglobin in parasitic helminths occurs in the tissues, and in nematodes it is also found in solution in the perienteric fluid (but not in corpuscles). Occasionally, haemoglobin is located preferentially in certain regions of the parasite; for example, in *F. hepatica*, it is found primarily around the vitellaria and uterine coils, and in the nematode, *Mermis subnigrescens*, it is the pigment in the anterior chromotrope (light-sensitive organ). The association of haemoglobin with the vitellaria in *F. hepatica* may be related to the oxygen requirement of egg tanning (Section 2.5.1).

Parasites frequently contain multiple haemoglobins. In the Trematoda, the haemoglobins of *Fasciola gigantica, Dicrocoelium dendriticum, Philophthalmus megalurus* and *E. revolutum* can be separated into two components, but *Fasciolopsis buski* has only one haemoglobin. In the nematodes, different haemoglobins occur in the perienteric fluid and body wall of *A. lumbricoides*. There is also some evidence that the body-wall haemoglobin of *A. lumbricoides* may be further separable into two components. The gape worm, *Syngamus trachea*, has only one haemoglobin[44], but there are three haemoglobins in *Tetrameres confusa*, five in *Ostertagia* sp. and six in *Obeliscoides cuniculi*. The body wall of *O. cuniculi* contains three haemoglobins, the perienteric fluid two and there is one in the gut. Developing fourth- and fifth-stage larvae of *O. cuniculi* have been reported to contain yet another different haemoglobin. In *T. confusa*, only the females have haemoglobin and in *Spirocamallanus cricotus*, the haemoglobins from males and females have different isoelectric points[43].

The free-living stages of parasitic nematodes, however, do not appear to contain haemoglobin and, in the development of *O. cuniculi*, haemoglobin first becomes detectable in the parasitic fourth-stage larva. Haemoglobin is found in larval *T. spiralis* and larval *E. ignotus*, but both of these larvae are tissue parasites.

Table 2.4 Physical and kinetic properties of *Ascaris lumbricoides* body-wall and perienteric fluid haemoglobins

	A. lumbricoides		
	Perienteric fluid	Body wall	Sheep
Molecular weight	328 000	40 600	70 000
Haem groups/mol	8	1	4
Sub-units	8	1	4
Oxygen			
K'(on) $(M^{-1} s^{-1})$ (at 20 °C)	1.53×10^6	1.19×10^6	1.5×10^6
K(off) (s^{-1}) (at 20 °C)	0.004	0.23	12
$p_{50}O_2$ (mmHg) (at 20 °C)	0.0015	0.108	20
Carbon monoxide			
K'(on) $(M^{-1} s^{-1})$ (at 20 °C)	1.7×10^5	2.17×10^5	4×10^5
K(off) (s^{-1}) (at 20 °C)	0.017 (at 27.5 °C)	0.038	0.07
$p_{50}CO$ (mmHg) (at 20 °C)	0.063 (at 27.5 °C)	0.132	0.1
KCO/O_2	0.075	0.82	200

With the exception of *A. lumbricoides* (*Table 2.4*), the physical properties of parasite haemoglobins have not been extensively studied. The only values so far available for the molecular weight of helminth haemoglobins are: *F. hepatica*, 17 500; *F. buski*, 15 000; *D. dendriticum*[45], 15 500; *S. trachea*[44], 38 400; and *A. lumbricoides*, perienteric fluid haemoglobin 328 000, body-wall haemoglobin

40 600. Generally, in invertebrates, intracellular haemoglobins have a relatively low molecular weight, extracellular haemoglobins having a high molecular weight.

An important parameter of haemoglobins is the oxygen affinity. The oxygen tension at half saturation, the p_{50}, is generally used as a convenient index of oxygen affinity and the p_{50} for several parasite haemoglobins is summarised in *Table 2.5*. For comparison, the p_{50} of horse haemoglobin and myoglobin are also

Table 2.5 Oxygen affinities of haemoglobin from parasitic helminths

Species	$p_{50}O_2$ (mmHg)	n
Horse haemoglobin	26	2.9
Horse myoglobin	3.2	1
Ascaris lumbricoides		
body wall	0.49	
perienteric fluid	0.01	1
Camallanus trispinosus	7	
Dicrocoelium dendriticum	0.1	1
Haemonchus contortus	0.05	1
Nematodirus sp.	0.05	1
Nippostrongylus brasiliensis	0.1	1
Syngamus trachea	8.8	
Strongylus sp.	< 0.1	
Trichinella spiralis		
(adult)	7.6	

included. All of the parasitic haemoglobins show a high oxygen affinity and there may be an inverse relationship between p_{50} and environmental oxygen tension, the mammalian gut parasites all having a low p_{50}, whilst *S. trachea* (from the trachea of birds) and *Camallanus trispinosus* (from reptiles) have higher p_{50} values. In *A. lumbricoides*, the perienteric fluid haemoglobin has a higher oxygen affinity than the body-wall haemoglobin. Usually, where two haemoglobins are present in an animal, the reverse situation exists, with the tissue haemoglobin having the highest affinity, thus enabling oxygen to be transferred from the circulating fluid to the tissues. The affinity of *A. lumbricoides* perienteric fluid haemoglobin for oxygen (p_{50} = 0.01 mmHg at 37 °C) is the highest oxygen affinity reported for any haemoglobin, and is a reflection of the extremely small dissociation constant (*Table 2.4*). Use has been made of the extreme stability of the perienteric fluid oxyhaemoglobin to study the reactions of haem compounds with hydrogen peroxide[46]. Data on the rates of oxygenation and deoxygenation are also available for the haemoglobin of *Anisakis*[47].

Although p_{50} gives a measure of the oxygen affinity, it does not describe the shape of the oxygen dissociation curve for the haemoglobin. In mono-haem pigments, such as myoglobin, the oxygen dissociation curve is hyperbolic. In multi-haem pigments, the haem groups can interact with one another and the oxygen dissociation curve becomes sigmoidal (*Figure 2.11*). A numerical value for the extent of the haem–haem interaction is given by the Hill constant n. The Hill

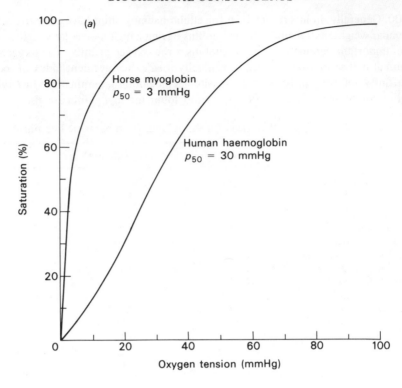

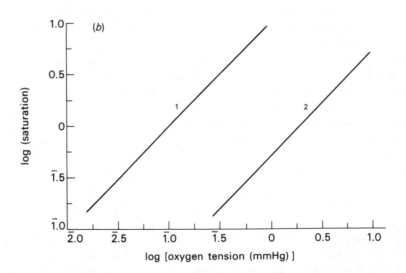

Figure 2.11 (*a*) Oxygen equilibrium curves for vertebrate myoglobin (1 haem) and haemoglobin (4 haem). (*b*) Oxygen equilibrium curves: 1, *Nippostrongylus brasiliensis* haemoglobin; 2, horse myoglobin.

constant, which is characteristic for each haemoglobin, is derived from the Hill equation:

$$\log\left(\frac{\overline{Y}_S}{1 - \overline{Y}_S}\right) = \log K + n \log[S]$$

where $\overline{Y}_S$ is the fractional saturation of the protein with substrate S. When $n = 1$, there is no haem–haem interaction and the curve is hyperbolic, but as n increases, so the curve becomes more sigmoidal. All of the parasite haemoglobins so far studied have an n value of 1, indicating that there is no haem–haem interaction. Some parasite haemoglobins, such as the *A. lumbricoides* body-wall one, are mono-haem pigments, but others, like perienteric fluid haemoglobin, are multi-haem pigments. No explanation has been put forward to account for the absence of haem–haem interactions in parasite multi-haem pigments.

In vertebrate haemoglobins, there is usually a marked reduction in oxygen affinity as the pH decreases, that is, acidification increases oxygen dissociation (positive Bohr effect). In contrast, many invertebrates show no, or only a small, Bohr effect and in some cases there is a reverse Bohr effect, acidification increasing oxygen affinity. In parasitic helminths, the haemoglobin of *S. trachea* shows a small positive Bohr effect, whilst the body-wall and perienteric fluid haemoglobins of *A. lumbricoides* show a small reverse Bohr effect. A reverse Bohr effect may be of adaptive value for an animal living in an environment low in oxygen and high in carbon dioxide (such as the vertebrate gut).

Another modulator of oxygen affinity in vertebrate haemoglobins is organic phosphates (2,3-diphosphoglycerate in mammals, inositolhexose phosphate or inositolpentose phosphate in birds and turtles and adenosine-5'-triphosphate (ATP) in reptiles and amphibians). The role, if any, of organic phosphates in modulating invertebrate haemoglobins has not been studied.

Physiological Role of Haemoglobins

Oxygen-binding pigments, such as haemoglobin, have two distinct functions. They either help to maintain a continuous supply of oxygen to the tissues, or they can act as an oxygen reserve. In addition, intracellular haemoglobins can facilitate the passage of oxygen through tissues at low oxygen tensions. The haemoglobin-modulated facilitated diffusion of oxygen through a static solution is called the Scholander effect and it may be an important function of invertebrate tissue haemoglobins.

All of the helminth haemoglobins that have been studied in detail have high oxygen affinities and probably remain fully oxygenated *in vivo*. This makes it un-likely that these haemoglobins are functioning in oxygen transport, and poisoning the haemoglobins of *H. contortus* or *N. brasiliensis* with carbon monoxide, for example, does not reduce oxygen uptake. However, under anaerobic conditions, the haemoglobins of *C. trispinosus, E. ignotus, H. contortus, N. brasiliensis* and *Nematodirus* sp. all become deoxygenated. In these nematodes, the haemoglobins would seem to be acting as oxygen reserves, or they may only act as oxygen transporters, at very low tensions. The body-wall haemoglobin of *A. lumbri-coides* is also slowly deoxygenated by the parasite under anaerobic conditions. The nematode is, however, unable to deoxygenate the perienteric fluid haemoglobin and this can only be deoxygenated by chemical means (dithionite). The perienteric fluid haemoglobin of *Strongylus* sp. similarly can only be deoxygenated by chemical treatment.

The extremely high oxygen affinities of *A. lumbricoides* and *Strongylus* peri-enteric fluid haemoglobin, and the inability of the parasite to deoxygenate these haemoglobins, makes it unlikely that the perienteric fluid haemoglobins function in oxygen transport or as oxygen reserves. It has also been shown that the perienteric fluid haemoglobin of *A. lumbricoides* does not give a Scholander effect. If the peri-enteric fluid haemoglobin is not involved in oxygen transport, oxygen storage or the facilitated diffusion of oxygen, then what is its function? It could, of course, be a functionless by-product, but this seems unlikely. The perienteric haemoglobin could be a store, either of haem or iron, or even possibly amino acids. The female *A. lumbricoides* produces large numbers of eggs, about 0.5 g/day and the eggs con-tain haem compounds. The haematin content of one day's output of eggs is more or less equal to the total haematin content of the female's perienteric fluid. In female *A. lumbricoides*, the perienteric fluid may be a source of haematin for the eggs. This does not, however, explain what the haemoglobin does in males!

Haemoglobin, like all haem compounds, catalyses the decomposition of hydrogen peroxide. In *A. lumbricoides*, hydrogen peroxide is formed during respiration (Section 3.2.1) but this parasite, like most parasitic helminths, appears to be deficient in catalase (Section 3.2.8). The pseudoperoxidase activity of the haemo-globins may prevent toxic levels of hydrogen peroxide from accumulating. It has been suggested, in *A. lumbricoides*, that hydrogen peroxide might be produced in the hypodermis and then diffuse into the deeper tissues, where it could be decom-posed by pseudoperoxidases to release oxygen. In this way, oxygen could get to the deeper tissues of the parasite. However, the toxic nature of hydrogen peroxide makes this scheme extremely unlikely.

A final property of haemoglobins which may be relevant is their buffering capacity. Intestinal helminths, such as *A. lumbricoides*, have to cope with high environmental carbon dioxide levels, and consequent tissue acidification. These parasites also excrete large amounts of organic acids. The high buffering capacity of haemoglobin would help to minimise pH changes. However, the overall contribu-tion of proteins to the buffering capacity of *A. lumbricoides* perienteric fluid is relatively low (Section 3.2.10).

Bile Pigments

Bilirubin and an unidentified metalloporphyrin have been found in *A. lumbricoides* (Section 4.4.2). The intramolluscan larvae of trematodes contain a variety of pig-ments which have not been characterised, but may include bile pigments and also chlorophyll derivatives, the latter, of course, derived from the host's diet.

2.5.3. Contractile Proteins

The contractile proteins of *A. lumbricoides* muscle have been studied in some detail.
The muscles of *A. lumbricoides* are obliquely striated, and at the ultrastructural
level, 10 to 12 thin filaments surround each thick myosin filament, rather than the
more familiar hexagonal arrangement of vertebrates. Actomyosin only represents
about 10% of the *A. lumbricoides* muscle protein (in mammals it represents about
55%).

Actin

The actin extracted from *A. lumbricoides* muscle is very similar to rabbit actin,
both in molecular weight (42 000) and amino acid composition (93% sequence
homology)[48,86]. The actin and tropomyosin extracted from the free-living nematode *C. elegans* are also very similar to rabbit actin and tropomyosin. Actin, and
contractile proteins in general, seem to have a highly conserved structure throughout the animal kingdom.

Myosin

The myosin from *A. lumbricoides* is again identical in molecular weight and shape
to rabbit myosin. However, the ATPase activity of *A. lumbricoides* myosin is three
to four times lower than that of rabbit myosin. The properties of *A. lumbricoides*
myosin ATPase resemble those of mammalian striated or cardiac muscle, rather
than smooth muscle[49]. In actomyosin preparations, *A. lumbricoides* myosin con-
tracts at lower ATP levels than mammalian myosin[50]. It has been suggested that
this is an adaptation to the relatively low ATP production in helminths
(Section 3.1).

The myosin from *A. lumbricoides* can be separated into one heavy and two light
chains (molecular weights 220 000, 16 000 and 18 000, respectively), which seem
similar to the heavy and light chains of vertebrate skeletal myosin[51]. Mutations
which affect the structure of myosin have been found in the free-living nematode
C. elegans.

Troponin

Troponin has been demonstrated in the muscle of *A. lumbricoides* and a component functionally equivalent to vertebrate troponin occurs in *C. elegans*. In *A. lumbricoides*, as in most invertebrates, two systems are involved in the regulation of
muscle contraction, one myosin-linked, the other actin-linked[87]. In contrast, in
vertebrate muscles, control is solely actin-linked.

Paramyosin

Paramyosin was first discovered in molluscan 'catch' muscles (bivalve slow adductor
muscles) but is, in fact, widely distributed in invertebrates. Paramyosins, with

characteristic amino acid compositions, tactoid banding and molecular weights, have been isolated from *A. lumbricoides, H. diminuta*, the nematomorphans *Gordius robustus* and *Paragordius various* as well as the free-living nematode *C. elegans*[52,53]. In *A. lumbricoides* the paramyosin/myosin ratio is 0.25, and for the non-striated muscles of *H. diminuta* the ratio is 1.6. Generally, paramyosin/myosin ratios are higher in invertebrate smooth muscle than in striated muscles, the highest ratios, around 2.2, occurring in molluscan catch muscles. The high paramyosin content in *H. diminuta* raises the possibility that paramyosin-rich 'catch' muscles may be present in the adhesive organs of parasites. Like molluscan adductor muscles, the suckers of parasites have to remain contracted for long periods of time.

2.5.4. Ascaridine

Ascaridine is an unusual protein, isolated from the refringent bodies of ascarid sperm cells. It contains neither sulphur nor phosphorus, is insoluble in cold water, but dissolves suddenly at 50–51 °C. The exact nature and function of ascaridine is unknown, it may be formed as a nuclear inclusion, and there are indications that it is involved in the post-fertilisation synthesis of ribonucleoproteins.

2.5.5. Soluble Proteins

Fractionation of soluble proteins from helminths gives a variety of lipoprotein and glycoprotein conjugates. In cestodes, bile salt/protein complexes have also been found. Many of these complexes are antigenic, and much effort has gone into trying to isolate pure antigenic fractions (Section 2.2.4). One well characterised soluble protein is a lipoprotein from *F. hepatica*, which has a molecular weight of 193 000 and contains 47% lipid. This lipoprotein is probably the same as the lipoprotein produced by Mehlis' gland, and which forms part of the liver fluke egg shell. In addition to the lipoprotein, Mehlis' gland may also produce a surface active agent, which aids coalescence of the sclerotin precursor granules, and it may also be responsible for the activation of prophenolase.

Sperm-activating Substance (SAS)

In male *A. lumbricoides*, secretions from the glandular vas deferens cause the sperm to undergo morphological changes (coalescence of cytoplasmic droplets to give a single refringent body and fusion of membrane organelles with the plasma membrane). These changes, which are related to the acquisition of motility, can also be brought about by extracts of the glandular vas deferens[29]. The sperm-activating substance appears to be a heterogeneous group of proteins.

2.6. NUCLEIC ACIDS AND THEIR COMPONENTS

Nucleic acids are polymers of nucleotides, the latter consisting of a pentose sugar joined to a nitrogen base (purine or pyrimidine) and a phosphate group. In nucleic acids, the nucleotides are linked by phosphodiester bridges between the 3'-hydroxyl group of one unit and the 5'-hydroxyl group of the next. There are two types of nucleic acids, the ribonucleic acids (RNA) and the deoxyribonucleic acids (DNA). In RNA the pentose sugar is D-ribose and the bases are adenine, guanine, uracil and cytosine. DNA contains D-deoxyribose and the bases are adenine, guanine, thymine and cytosine. In addition, there are some 30 unusual bases which occur with low frequencies in both DNA and RNA.

Nucleic acids normally constitute about 5–15% of the dry weight of tissues and they are involved in the storage, transmission and translation of genetic information.

2.6.1. Deoxyribonucleic Acid

Most of the cell's DNA is found in the nucleus, associated with chromatin. However, DNA also occurs in certain cell organelles such as mitochondria (and chloroplasts in plants), and there is also evidence for DNA in centrioles and in the basal bodies of cilia. A small number of unusual methylated bases occur in some DNA molecules. Unlike other cell constituents, there is no turnover of DNA, but enzyme systems are present which carry out DNA repair and DNA replication (Section 4.6.4).

Nuclear DNA

In eukaryotes, the nuclear DNA is tightly bound to histones, these being highly basic proteins of which there are five major classes (H1, H2a, H2b, H3, H4). The occurrence and distribution of histones has not been studied in parasitic helminths, although basic proteins, associated with nuclear DNA, have been demonstrated histochemically in *A. lumbricoides*[55]. The cleavage of *A. lumbricoides* eggs is accompanied by a decrease in the basic nuclear proteins.

The base composition of nuclear DNA is very characteristic of an organism (or strain of organism) and is usually expressed as the percentage of guanine + cytosine (G + C) bases. The actual base composition varies quite widely. Mammals usually have about 40% G + C (38–43%), invertebrates tend to have rather lower values (30–40%), whilst the biggest range is found in protozoa (15–65%) and bacteria (25–75%). The G + C composition has been determined in a range of helminth DNA (*Table 2.6*) and it varies from 34 to 47%[56], with one cestode having a G + C content of 61%. With this last exception, the G + C content of helminth DNA is fairly similar to that of invertebrates generally. The significance, if any, of the different G + C contents is not known. One suggestion has been that organisms exposed to sunlight have evolved a high G + C content (and thus a low adenine + thymine content) as a means of reducing genetic damage from solar-radiation-induced thymine dimers. So, it might be expected that parasites, which have free-living stages and thus are exposed to sunlight, would have a higher G + C content than parasites with reduced free-living stages. The G + C content will also depend very much on the base composition of the repetitive DNA.

When vertebrate DNA is fractionated in a density gradient, there is usually a single large peak and then one or more small satellite peaks. The satellite DNA constitutes about 10% of the total DNA in mammalian cells and contains short

Table 2.6 The guanine + cytosine (G + C) content of helminth DNA

Species	G + C content (%)
Cestodes	
Orygmatobothrium sp.	61
Schistocephalus sp.	47
Lacistorhynchus tenuis	45
Phyllobothrium sp.	44
Echinococcus multilocularis	44
Hymenolepis microstoma	39
H. citelli	39
H. diminuta	38
Gyrocotylideans	
Gyrocotyle rugosa	45
G. maxima	43
G. parvispinosa	38
G. fimbriata	36
Trematodes	
Fasciola hepatica	47
Schistosoma mansoni	34
S. japonicum	34
Nematodes	
Ascaris lumbricoides	41
Acanthocephalans	
Moniliformis dubius	39

sequences (100–300 nucleotides) which are highly repetitive (10^7 copies). Satellite DNA appears to be concentrated in the centromere region of the chromosome. In whole-cell DNA preparations, mitochondrial DNA also appears as a satellite band.

In *A. lumbricoides*, four satellite bands have been detected[56], one of which is mitochondrial DNA. Hymenolepid cestodes (*Hymenolepis diminuta, Hymenolepis microstoma, Hymenolepis citelli*) also show four satellite DNA bands and, again, one of them represents mitochondrial DNA. Two satellite bands have been observed in Gyrocotylideans, but no satellite DNA was found in *S. mansoni* or *S. japonicum*. There is no evidence that the DNA from helminths contains any appreciable amounts of unusual bases.

In mammals, some 10% of the DNA is highly repetitive, and another 20% of the sequences are reiterated some 10^3 to 10^4 fold. So, about 70% of the DNA sequences are, therefore, unique or nearly unique. Estimates of the amounts of repetitive DNA in parasitic helminths reveals a range of values from 14 to 42% (*Table 2.7*). The amount of repetitive DNA in free-living helminths shows a similar range. In vertebrate DNA, the moderately repetitive and non-repetitive sequences are interspersed. However, in the free-living nematode *C. elegans*, the moderately repetitive sequences of DNA do not show this interspersion[57].

The total amount of DNA per nucleus can be very variable, depending on the amount of polyploidy. The gametic nuclei of *A. lumbricoides* contain about 0.8 pg of DNA, the germ cell nuclei of *P. equorum* similarly contain about 1 pg of DNA.

Table 2.7   The percentage of repetitive DNA in helminths

Species	Repetitive DNA (%)
Nematodes	
Ascaris lumbricoides	
(oocytes)	14
Trichinella spiralis	
(larvae)	42
Panagrellus redivivus*	46
Caenorhabditis briggsae*	9
Platyhelminths	
Hymenolepis diminuta	16
Dugesia tigrina*	50

*Free-living species.

Typical mammalian cells contain 5–6 pg of DNA, but values for invertebrate nuclei range from 0.1 to 3 pg.

Cytochemical studies indicate that in *A. lumbricoides* many of the somatic nuclei are polyploid. The intestinal cells usually show a low ploidy, whilst the cells of the uteri, pharynx and excretory system are highly polyploid (up to 150n). The nuclei of the somatic musculature do not, however, appear polyploid and DNA cannot be detected in these nuclei by standard Feulgen staining techniques. Polyploidy also occurs in acanthocephalans. During development, the cortical nuclei of acantho-cephalans increase dramatically in size from 5 or 10 μm in diameter, up to 100 μm. In some species, these giant nuclei persist in the adult, in other species the nuclei become dendritic and fragment. The formation of these giant nuclei may be related to massive RNA production associated with the formation of the complex tegument. Morphologically, these nuclei are very similar to the dendritic nuclei of spider silk glands. The formation of the latter is again thought to be related to massive RNA production, only this time for silk production. In *M. dubius*, an acanthocephalan in which the giant nuclei do not fragment, the DNA content of the giant nuclei cor-responds to a polyploidy of about 350n. For comparison, the polytene nuclei of Drosophila are 2000n.

Genome Size

The complexity or information content of an organism's genome is a measure of the number of DNA base pairs present in non-repeating sequences. This is usually expressed in terms of molecular weight (daltons), one base pair weighing approxi-mately 6×10^2 daltons. A reduction in the size of the parasite's genome could make the parasite dependent on the genome of its host. An even more intimate form of parasitism would arise if part of the parasite's genome were to become incorporated into that of the host. When compared with free-living animals, adult parasitic helminths show a reduction in biochemical abilities and a simplified mor-phology. These reductions, however, do not necessarily apply to the free-living and intermediate stages of parasites (Section 5.2). Estimates of the genome size of

Table 2.8   Genome size of helminths

Species	Genome (daltons)
E. coli	2.8×10^9
Calf thymus	9.9×10^{11}
Nematodes	
Ascaris lumbricoides	$1.5–2.8 \times 10^{11}$
Trichinella spiralis	1.6×10^{11}
Panagrellus redivivus*	0.46×10^{11}
Caenorhabditis briggsae*	0.81×10^{11}
Platyhelminths	
Hymenolepis diminuta	9.2×10^{10}
Dugesia tigrina*	4.6×10^{10}

*Free-living species.

parasitic and free-living helminths are given in *Table 2.8*. From these[58], it would appear that the genome of parasitic helminths is about twice as large as the genome of related free-living helminths. This is presumably correlated with the complex life-cycles of parasitic helminths. So, the biochemical and morphological reductions found in the adult parasitic helminth are the result of the repression, rather than the deletion, of genetic information. Interestingly, in parasitic plants (*Cuscuta*), which do not have complex life-cycles, the genome is only about one-half that of non-parasitic relatives. It is possible that the evolution of parasitism in helminths was first accompanied by a reduction in genome size, but that this was followed by an increase, as the life-cycles became more complex.

The degree of homology of nucleotide sequences in DNA from different sources can be estimated from the extent to which they form hybrid double-stranded DNA (heteroduplex formation). This technique is useful in taxonomy for determining the relatedness of species (particularly congeneric species) and it has been used to investigate the taxonomy of species of *Gyrocotyle*[59]. It would also be very interesting to see if there were any homologies between the DNA of parasites and the DNA of their hosts.

Chromosome Diminution

This is a remarkable process, which occurs during the early cleavage stages of ascarid embryos. It involves the loss of heterochromatic regions of the chromosome into the cytoplasm during mitosis, and it takes place in those cells which are destined to form the somatic tissue of the nematode, but not in the germ line. Chromosome diminution has been described in *A. lumbricoides, P. equorum* and *Toxocara canis*, but it is not known if it occurs in any other nematodes apart from ascarids. In *P. equorum*, chromosome diminution starts at the second division ($2 \rightarrow 3$ cell stage) and in *A. lumbricoides* at the third division ($4 \rightarrow 5$ cell stage). The cells from a diminution division do not undergo further diminution at subsequent divisions. In *P. equorum*, whether or not a division will be a diminution division depends on the distribution of cytoplasmic factors within the egg. The distribution of these factors can be altered by centrifuging the egg and this results in an abnormal pattern of diminution divisions[60].

Estimates vary as to the amount of DNA which is lost during chromosome diminution. In *A. lumbricoides* about 30–33% of the DNA is lost, and in *P. equorum* up to 80%. This amounts to about 0.2 pg of DNA/nucleus in *A. lumbricoides* or approximately 2×10^8 base pairs (enough to code for 1×10^5 proteins).

Chromosome diminution has been described in a variety of free-living organisms as well. It occurs, for example, in copepods, dipterans, heteropterans and in some marsupials (bandicoots), where there is selective elimination of one of the sex chromosomes. In the copepod *Cyclops furcifer*, 70% of the DNA is eliminated. Unfortunately, nothing is known of the molecular events which underlie chromosome diminution in these animals.

There have been several attempts to try to determine the nature and function of germ line limited DNA in *A. lumbricoides* and *P. equorum*. Germ line limited DNA is the DNA component found only in the germ line and is the fraction lost from the somatic line during diminution. There are three main possibilities. First, the chromosomes of these ascarids may be highly polyploid and chromosome diminution could represent the loss of extra copies. Secondly, chromosome diminution might involve the elimination of highly repetitive DNA from the genome. The genes coding for *r*RNA are often selectively amplified in oocytes and they could be being eliminated from the somatic line. Finally, chromosome diminution could involve the loss of unique DNA sequences. This would mean that the somatic and germ line cells of adult ascarids could differ in their information content. So in this system, differentiation would be accompanied by the actual loss of genetic information rather than by the repression of genetic information.

In ascarids, chromosome diminution is associated with the loss of one of the DNA satellites[56,61]. This satellite comprises about 23% of the total DNA in *A. lumbricoides* and 85% of the total in *P. equorum*. So, the relative amounts of this repetitive DNA correlates quite well with the estimated DNA loss during chromosome diminution. The G + C ratios in somatic and germ line DNA appear to be similar, although there have been reports to the contrary. Reassociation studies with *A. lumbricoides* DNA suggest that the somatic and germ line cells have similar genome sizes. However, some workers[62,63] have claimed that both unique and repetitive sequences are lost during diminution, in the ratio 1:1. So, the nature of the germ line limited DNA is still not clear, much of it is highly repetitive DNA, but some unique (or nearly unique?) sequences may be lost as well. It is very difficult to prepare ascarid nuclei free from contamination, and different subspecies of *A. lumbricoides* may have different karyotypes. In *A. lumbricoides* from the USA $n = 12$, in European strains $n = 24$, and in *P. equorum* races have been described where $n = 2$ and $n = 4$.

The function of the germ line limited DNA is not known. The evidence, so far, would suggest that much of the DNA which is being lost is highly repetitive. However, it has been shown that it is not amplified *r*DNA cistrons that are being lost[64]. The germ line limited DNA is obviously necessary to delineate the germ line, despite the fact that heterochromatic DNA is usually held to be inactive. There is, though, conflicting evidence for germ line limited DNA being transcribed *in vivo*. The germ line limited DNA in ascarids may have a regulatory function or could play a structural role in the chromosomes. The enzymatic mechanisms involved in diminution are unknown, but presumably the process will involve restriction endonucleases and possibly DNA modification enzymes (M–R systems).

Another interesting nuclear process found in nematodes and acanthocephalans is eutely or cell constancy. With the exception of the gonads, and possibly the intestine, the cells of the adult never divide and the number of nuclei in the different organs of the body is constant. This means that these animals have very limited powers of repair and regeneration.

Mitochondrial DNA

This normally constitutes 0.1 to 0.2% of the total cell DNA (up to 25% in *Trypanosomes*). In structure, mitochondrial DNA resembles prokaryote DNA and has a different G + C ratio to the nuclear DNA. The mitochondrial DNA molecule is circular (although, in some protozoa, it is said to be linear), about 5 μm long, it is not associated with histones and there are no highly repetitive sequences. Mammalian mitochondria usually contain four to six copies of the circular DNA molecule, presumably in readiness for mitochondrial division.

Mitochondrial DNA has been shown to code for some of the cytochrome and cytochrome oxidase sub-units and for some of the other inner membrane polypeptides. In addition, it probably also codes for the mitochondrial ribosomal RNA. During the life-cycle of a parasitic helminth, there are frequently major changes in mitochondrial function. The role of the cytochromes may be very different in the free-living and parasitic phases, and there are changes in the tricarboxylic acid cycle and β-oxidation sequence enzymes (Section 5.2). These aerobic/anaerobic transformations make the role of mitochondrial DNA in parasites particularly interesting.

Table 2.9 Mitochondrial DNA from parasitic helminths

Species	G + C (%)	Contour length	DNA/ mitochondrion (μg × 10^9)	DNA/ mitochondrion (mole)
Rat liver	44	5.15	13	8
Ascaris lumbricoides				
eggs	—	4.85	14.8	9
body muscle	31	4.95	1.8	1
Hymenolepis diminuta	31	4.76	—	—

The properties of helminth mitochondrial DNA are summarised in *Table 2.9*[65,66]. As in all other eukaryotes, the mitochondrial DNA from helminths consists of circular molecules with a contour length of about 5 μm. The G + C composition of helminth mitochondrial DNA is lower than that of mammalian mitochondrial DNA, but is within the range reported for other invertebrates (25–65%).

The mitochondria of *A. lumbricoides* muscle cells appear to contain only a single

DNA copy. This may be related to the fact that the somatic cells of nematodes do not divide.

It has been reported that, in the four-cell *A. lumbricoides* egg, mitochondrial DNA constitutes as much as 40% of the total, and branched DNA molecules, which are probably replicative intermediates, have also been found[67]. The value of 40% of the total is almost certainly much too high and is probably the result of contamination with other DNA fractions.

2.6.2. Ribonucleic Acid

There is usually two to eight times as much RNA in cells as DNA. There are three different types of RNA in cells, ribosomal RNA (*r*RNA), transfer RNA (*t*RNA) and messenger RNA (*m*RNA).

Ribosomal RNA

This constitutes about 70–80% of the total RNA. Ribosomes are the site of protein synthesis in the cell and they are composed of riboproteins, containing about 60% RNA. The actual role of *r*RNA in ribosomes is not known. A few *r*RNA bases are methylated.

In eukaryotes, the ribosomes vary in size from 73 to 83s, the ribosomes of prokaryotes are somewhat smaller (70s). Mitochondrial ribosomes are different from the cytoplasmic ones and tend to resemble those of prokaryotes.

Parasitic helminths have typical eukaryotic 80s ribosomes composed of 60s and 40s sub-units (Section 4.6.4). The G + C ratio of helminth *r*RNA is around 50% (*Table 2.10*), which is somewhat lower than mammalian *r*RNA, where the ratio is usually about 60%, but is similar to other invertebrate *r*RNA values.

Table 2.10   The guanine + cytosine content of helminth RNA

Species	G + C (%)
Ribosomal RNA	
Ascaris lumbricoides	
1-cell egg	52
gastrula	52
Panagrellus redivivus*	51
Caenorhabditis elegans*	51
Echinococcus granulosus	
protoscoleces	50 and 54
Transfer RNA	
Ascaris lumbricoides	
1-cell egg	64
Echinococcus granulosus	
protoscoleces	59

*Free-living species.

It has been claimed that there is a fundamental difference between the 28s
rRNA of protostomes and that of deuterostomes, in terms of thermostability. If
the 28s rRNA of molluscs or most insects is briefly heated, it undergoes an orderly
dissociation into two equal 18s units[68,69]. The 28s rRNA from mammals, on the
other hand, shows only a slight decrease in molecular weight on heating. The
orderly breakdown of protostome 28s rRNA is said to be due to the presence of a
primary 'nick' near the centre of the molecule. The 28s rRNA from *A. lumbricoides*
does not degrade on heating, whilst the 28s rRNA fractions from the free-living
nematode *Panagrellus redivivus* and the trematode *F. hepatica* also fail to dissociate
in an orderly way on heating. So there is no indication of a primary 'nick' in the
structure of helminth 28s rRNA. Some insects (aphids) also lack a primary break in
their 28s rRNA, and it has been suggested that the lack of a primary nick may be
correlated with high reproductive rates.

Transfer RNA

There are about 60 different species of tRNA and their function is to transport
activated amino acids in protein synthesis (Section 4.5.1). Transfer RNAs are small
molecules (4s), constituting about 10 to 15% of the total RNA, and up to 10% of
the tRNA nucleotides contain unusual bases.

Typical transfer RNA has been identified in the protoscoleces of *E. granulosus*,
larval *Taenia crassiceps*, *H. diminuta* and *A. lumbricoides* eggs (Section 4.6.4). The
G + C ratio of helminth tRNA is about 60% (*Table 2.10*), and the tRNA of mammals is also characterised by a relatively high G + C ratio (58%).

Messenger RNA

Messenger RNA carries information for protein synthesis from the nucleus to the
cytoplasm (Section 4.5.1). There are many thousands of species of mRNA, and
molecular weights range from 5×10^4 to 5×10^6 daltons (6-25s). The mRNA in
the cell is constantly turning over and it is usually the smallest of the RNA fractions,
comprising 5–10% of the total. Normally, there are very few methylated bases in
mRNA.

Typically, eukaryote mRNA has a chain of 200 polyadenylate bases at the 3'
end. A polyadenylate containing mRNA, which codes for the egg shell protein, has
been isolated from the uterine epithelium of *A. lumbricoides*[54]. Typical mRNA
fractions have also been demonstrated in *E. granulosus*, *T. crassiceps* and *H. diminuta* (Section 4.5.1).

2.6.3. Nucleotides and Nucleosides

Nucleotides are the basic building blocks of nucleic acids; nucleosides are nucleotides without the phosphate group:

nucleoside = base + sugar
nucleotide = base + sugar + phosphate

Nucleosides are not found free in the cell to any appreciable extent. Deoxyribo-nucleotides, the precursors of DNA, also do not occur in significant levels in tissues. Ribonucleotides, however, are important cellular components and occur not only as $5'$-monophosphates, but also as di-, tri- and cyclic-$3',5'$-phosphates. The nucleoside phosphates function as energy carriers, as coenzyme-like energised carriers of synthetic intermediates and as energy-rich precursors for nucleic acid synthesis. The cyclic nucleotides (cyclic-$3',5'$-AMP and cyclic-$3',5'$-GMP) are important 'second messengers' in metabolic regulation. These cyclic nucleotides are present in only minute amounts in tissues, in *A. lumbricoides* muscle there are about 0.4 nmoles of $3',5'$-cyclic-AMP per gram wet weight (Section 5.1.7), and in the free-living nematode *P. redivivus*, $3',5'$-cyclic-AMP is again about 0.4 nmoles/g wet weight, and $3',5'$-cyclic-GMP about 5 nmoles/g wet weight[70]. This last figure is some 30 times higher than values for the levels of $3',5'$-cyclic-GMP in mammalian tissue.

The content of ATP, ADP and AMP has been measured in a variety of parasitic helminths (Section 5.1.8) and, in general, the adenine nucleotide content of helminths is similar to that of mammalian tissue. The non-adenine nucleotides (GTP, ITP, UTP, CTP) are usually present in tissues at much lower concentrations than the adenine nucleotides. Small amounts of GTP and traces of GDP, ITP and IDP have been found in *A. lumbricoides* muscle[71] and traces of GTP and GDP have been demonstrated in *S. mansoni*[72]. However, in the fertilised eggs of *A. lumbricoides*, guanine nucleotides comprise 84% of the total[73,74]. The function of this extremely high level of guanine nucleotides is not clear. One possibility is that at least a part of the guanine nucleotides are utilised for DNA synthesis in the developing embryo. High levels of non-adenine nucleotides have been found in the eggs of a number of free-living invertebrates (*Artemia, Oncopeltus*) and it has been suggested that a high guanine, low adenine nucleotide ratio may be characteristic of dormant stages. An interesting guanine nucleotide found in *Artemia* eggs is diguanosine tetraphosphate. Diguanosine polyphosphates have not, however, been reported from helminths.

2.7. VITAMINS AND COFACTORS

The vitamin and cofactor content of parasites has not been studied in much detail. With the exception of vitamin B_{12}, which is accumulated by certain cestodes, the vitamin and cofactor composition of parasitic helminths is similar to that of other organisms.

2.7.1. Vitamins

Of the fat-soluble vitamins, vitamin A has been found in parasites, whilst vitamins D, E and K have not been looked for. Most of the B group vitamins (thiamine, riboflavin, biotin, nicotinic acid, folic acid, pantothenic acid, pyridoxine and cobalamin) have been found in parasitic helminths, as has vitamin C (ascorbic acid). Parasitic nematodes often accumulate B_{12} in their pseudocoelomocytes (*N. brasiliensis, A.*

caninum), and in the Cestoda, members of the Tetraphyllidea, Trypanorhyncha, Caryophyllidea, Diphyllidea, most of the Proteocephalidea and most of the Pseudophyllidea contain high concentrations of B_{12} (0.5 to 200 $\mu g/g$ dry weight)[75]. The Cyclophyllidean cestodes, on the other hand, do not store B_{12}. Accumulation of B_{12} may be a characteristic of the more primitive cestode groups. Vitamin B_{12} is a cofactor for methylmalonyl-CoA mutase, one of the enzymes involved in propionate synthesis (Section 3.1.4). Many of the helminths that accumulate B_{12} are propionate producers, and it has been suggested that the methylmalonyl-CoA mutase of these helminths only binds B_{12} very weakly, so high tissue levels of the cofactor are necessary.

2.7.2. Cofactors

Only a limited number of cofactors and prosthetic groups exists and there are only occasional variations in detail. In the few analyses that have been done on helminths, the tissue levels of NAD, NADP and CoA are similar to those reported for mammalian tissues.

2.8. HORMONES AND HORMONE ANALOGUES

Some helminths, for example the monogenean *Polystoma interregium*, are thought to respond to host hormones, and in this way are able to integrate their breeding cycle with that of their host. In order to respond to vertebrate hormones, the parasite must have the appropriate hormone binding protein. It would be extremely remarkable if an invertebrate possessed a specific binding protein for a vertebrate hormone. An alternative explanation is that the parasites do not respond directly to the host's hormones, but to the hormone-induced physiological changes in the host (Section 1.4).

Another interesting possibility is that parasites may produce hormones or hormone analogues which affect the host's metabolism, hopefully in a way adaptive for the parasite.

2.8.1. Invertebrate Hormones

Farnesol, and possibly other juvenile hormone mimics, have been found in parasitic helminths, as has β-ecdysone and ecdysone mimics (Sections 2.3.8 and 4.3.3). Juvenile hormone would prevent an insect host from moulting and preserve the larval environment, which might be particularly favourable for parasites. However, there is no evidence that juvenile hormone or ecdysone mimics are released by helminths, and the amounts present in parasite tissues are extremely small. It has also been suggested, but again never shown, that plant parasitic nematodes may produce the plant growth regulator indoleacetic acid (IAA), which could be responsible for giant cell and gall formation. Cytokinins have, however, been detected in the plant parasitic nematode *Meloidogyne incognita*. As there is no evidence that the nematode synthesises cytokinins, they must be of host origin instead, but since nematodes do not have breakdown enzymes for cytokinins, the hormones accumulate.

Infection of insects with mermithid nematodes often leads to sterility or feminisation of the host, or in social insects to caste changes. There are also reports of gigantism in molluscs infected with larval trematodes. These phenomena could have a hormonal basis, the parasite producing host hormone analogues or antagonists. Alternatively, they could result from nutritional effects or from the physical destruction of secondary endocrine organs. Destruction of the gonads might also be the cause of gigantism, since energy, which would normally have gone into gamete production, might be diverted into somatic growth. Many infected intermediate hosts show behavioural changes, which may help to increase the chances of the infective stage coming into contact with the final host. These behavioural changes could also have a hormonal basis.

2.8.2. Vertebrate Hormones

There are several reports of helminth parasites stimulating the growth of their vertebrate hosts. Mice infected with *T. spiralis* have an enhanced growth rate over controls, when they are maintained on an inadequate diet, and there are several claims that animals infected with *F. hepatica* gain weight faster than uninfected animals. However, the best known example of parasite-induced growth is the effect of plerocercoids (spargana) of the cestode *Spirometra mansonoides* on rodents[76]. Rats and mice, infected with *S. mansonoides* spargana, show a smooth and gradual increase in weight and skeletal growth over uninfected controls, and this effect can last throughout life. The spargana have been shown to produce a factor, sparganum growth factor (SGF), which is responsible for the stimulated growth and in a number of ways resembles mammalian growth hormone (GH). In the diabetic hypophysectomised rat, both SGF and GH promote growth and have a stimulatory effect on lymphoid tissue, but they have different effects on lipid metabolism[77,78]. The release of SGF by the parasite suppresses host growth hormone production. SGF is a protein, molecular weight approximately 50 000, and it is chemically distinct from growth hormone. Like growth hormone, SGF promotes somatomedin (sulphation factor) production by host tissues.

The biological role of SGF is not clear, nor is it produced by all strains of *S. mansonoides*. The natural intermediate host for *S. mansonoides* spargana are reptiles, not rodents, and there are no reports of enhanced growth in infected reptiles.

Another larval cestode which may affect the endocrine balance of its host are the plerocercoids of *Ligula intestinalis*. Fish infected with *L. intestinalis* become sterile and their pituitary glands show a reduction in the number and size of gonadotrophs. Whether this involves the production of hormone analogues by the parasite, or whether it is a stress response by the host is not clear. The plerocercoids of *Schistocephalus solidus* prevent spawning of their fish host, but in this case no changes in the pituitary have been reported and the effect may be nutritional.

Immunologically Active Factors

Lymphokinins, humoral factors which affect host white blood cell migration, have been isolated from *A. lumbricoides, T. taeniaeformis* and from the plerocercoids of *L. intestinalis* and *S. solidus*, and an eosinophilic chemotactic factor has also been demonstrated in larval *N. brasiliensis*[79] . The cysticerci of *T. taeniaeformis* contain an anticomplement factor and there is evidence that helminths may produce non-specific mitogens. These various immunologically active factors have not, however, been chemically characterised.

2.9. SUMMARY AND CONCLUSIONS

The chemical composition of an organism is dynamic, rather than static, and there is a constant turnover of cellular components. Many important constituents are present in tissues at only very low levels, although the total amount formed and destroyed in a 24 h period may be considerable.

In parasitic helminths, the levels of different chemical constituents may vary with the age, sex and strain of the individual and with the nutritional status of the host and the host species. Some components, such as glycogen, may show a diurnal rhythm.

The gross chemical composition of parasites is similar to that of free-living organisms, although several unusual compounds have been found. Amongst the nematodes, for example, the ascarosides are a unique group of compounds, as are the volatile fatty acid containing acylglycerols. The structure of *A. lumbricoides* cuticle collagen is again unique. The occurrence of rhodoquinone rather than ubiquinone in a number of helminths and the presence of calcareous corpuscles in larval trematodes and cestodes is also rather peculiar.

The composition of individual tissues is probably more informative than the overall chemical composition. However, it is only from the few very large helminths, such as *A. lumbricoides* or *F. hepatica*, that data on the tissue distribution of compounds are available.

An intriguing possibility is the production, by parasitic helminths, of analogues or antagonists of host hormones. Molecular mimicry, the idea that the proteins of parasites may have evolved such that they are identical, or at least immunologically identical, with those of their host, has often been proposed, particularly for parasitic nematodes. This would help to explain why so many hosts fail to mount an effective immune response against invading helminths—the parasites would not be recognised as foreign. It has also been suggested that the protein polymorphism, which is found in animals, is a response to molecular mimicry by pathogens; the host, as it were, trying to confuse the parasite. Unfortunately, however, there is no biochemical evidence whatsoever to support the idea of molecular mimicry in parasitic helminths.

2.10. GENERAL READING

von Brand, T. (1973). *Biochemistry of Parasites*, 2nd edn. New York; Academic Press

Fairbairn, D. (1957). 'The biochemistry of *Ascaris*'. *Exptl Parasitol.*, **6**, 491–554

Lee, D. L. and Smith, M. H. (1965). 'Haemoglobins of parasitic animals'. *Exptl Parasitol.*, **16**, 392–424

2.11. REFERENCES

1. Kassis, A. I. and Tanner, C. E. (1976). *Int. J. Parasitol.*, **6**, 25–35
2. Bird, A. F., Waller, P. J., Dash, K. M. and Major, G. (1978). *Int. J. Parasitol.*, **8**, 69–74
3. Martin, J. and Lee, D. L. (1976). *Parasitology*, **72**, 75–80
4. Jenkins, T., Erasmus, D. A. and Davies, T. W. (1977). *Exptl Parasitol.*, **41**, 464–71
5. Orpin, C. G., Huskisson, N. S. and Ward, P. F. V. (1976). *Parasitology*, **73**, 83–95
6. Roberts, L. S., Bueding, E. and Orrell, S. A. (1972). *Compar. Biochem. Physiol.*, **43B**, 825–36
7. Wharton, D. A. and Jenkins, T. (1978). *Tissue and Cell*, **10**, 427–40
8. Rahemtulla, F. and Løvtrup, S. (1974). *Compar. Biochem. Physiol.*, **49B**, 639–46
9. Fukushima, T. (1966). *Exptl Parasitol.*, **19**, 227–36
10. Yusufi, A. N. K. and Siddiqi, A. H. (1976). *Int. J. Parasitol.*, **6**, 5–8
11. Cain, G. D., Johnson, W. J. and Oaks, J. A. (1977). *J. Parasitol.*, **63**, 486–91
12. Cain, G. D. and French, J. A. (1975). *Int. J. Parasitol.*, **5**, 159–64
13. Overturf, M. and Dryer, R. L. (1968). *Compar. Biochem. Physiol.*, **27**, 145–75
14. Beach, D. H., Sherman, I. W. and Holz, G. G. (1973). *J. Parasitol.*, **59**, 655–66
15. Fried, B. and Boddorf, J. M. (1978). *J. Parasitol.*, **64**, 174–5
16. Tarr, G. E. and Fairbairn, D. (1973). *Lipids*, **8**, 303–10
17. Tarr, G. E. (1973). *Compar. Biochem. Physiol.*, **46B**, 167–76
18. Hazenjak, T. and Ehrlich, I. (1975). *Veterinarski Arhiv*, **45**, 299–309
19. Chopra, A. K., Jain, S. K., Vinayak, V. K. and Khuller, G. K. (1978). *Experientia*, **34**, 1457–8
20. Khuller, G. K., Jain, S. K. and Vinayak, V. K. (1977). *Experientia*, **33**, 1585
21. Tarr, G. E. and Fairbairn, D. (1973). *Lipids*, **8**, 7–16
22. Tarr, G. E. and Schnoes, H. K. (1973). *Arch. Biochem. Biophys.*, **158**, 288–96
23. Foor, W. E. (1967). *J. Parásitol.*, **53**, 1245–61
24. Fioravanti, C. F. and MacInnis, A. J. (1977). *Compar. Biochem. Physiol.*, **57B**, 227–33
25. Kasschau, M. R. (1975). *Compar. Biochem. Physiol.*, **51B**, 273–80
26. Bailey, R. S. and Fried, B. (1977). *Int. J. Parasitol.*, **7**, 497–9

27. Mettrick, D. F. and Boddington, M. J. (1972). *Can. J. Zool.*, **50**, 411-3
28. Arme, C. (1977). *Z. Parasitenkunde*, **51**, 261-3
29. Abbas, M. and Foor, W. E. (1978). *Exptl Parasitol.*, **45**, 263-73
30. Ash, A. S. F. and Tucker, J. F. (1967). *J. Pharm. Pharmacol.*, **19**, 240-5
31. Viglierchio, D. R. and Görtz, J. H. (1972). *Exptl Parasitol.*, **32**, 140-8
32. Fujimoto, D. (1975). *J. Biochem.*, **78**, 905-9
33. Harrington, W. F. *et al.* (1970). *Biochemistry*, **9**, 3714-24, 3725-33, 3734-45, 3745-54, 3754-63
34. Evans, H. J., Sullivan, C. E. and Piez, K. A. (1976). *Biochemistry*, **15**, 1435-9
35. Fujimoto, D. and Iizuka, K. (1972). *J. Biochem.*, **71**, 1089-91
36. Peczon, B. D., Venable, J. H., Beams, C. G. and Hudson, B. G. (1975). *Biochemistry*, **14**, 4069-75
37. Hung, C.-H., Ohno, M., Freytag, W. J. and Hudson, B. G. (1977). *J. Biol. Chem.*, **252**, 3995-4001
38. Peczon, B. D., Wegener, L. J., Hung, C.-H. and Hudson, B. G. (1977). *J. Biol. Chem.*, **252**, 4002-6
39. Fujimoto, D. and Kanaya, S. (1973). *Arch. Biochem. Biophys.*, **157**, 1-6
40. Fujimoto, D. (1975). *Compar. Biochem. Physiol.*, **51B**, 205-7
41. Anderson, S. O. (1974). *Nature*, **251**, 507-8
42. Haider, S. A. and Siddiqi, A. H. (1977). *J. Helminthol.*, **51**, 373-8
43. Fusco, A. C. (1978). *Exptl Parasitol.*, **44**, 155-60
44. Rose, J. E. and Kaplan, K. L. (1972). *J. Parasitol.*, **58**, 903-6
45. Tuchschmid, P. E., Kunz, P. A. and Wilson, K. J. (1978). *Europ. J. Biochem.*, **88**, 387-94
46. Wittenberg, B. A., Wittenberg, J. B. and Noble, R. W. (1972). *J. Biol. Chem.*, **247**, 4008-13
47. Viglierchio, D. R. and Görtz, J. H. (1972). *Exptl Parasitol.*, **32**, 211-6
48. Dedman, J. R. and Harris, B. G. (1975). *Biochem. Biophys. Res. Commun.*, **65**, 170-5
49. Langer, B. W., Smith, W. J. and Theodorides, V. J. (1972). *Biochem. J.*, **128**, 991-2
50. Yamaguchi, M., Nakamura, T., Oya, H. and Sekine, T. (1973). *Biochim. Biophys. Acta*, **317**, 312-5
51. Nakamura, T., Yanagisawa, T. and Yamaguchi, M. (1975). *Biochim. Biophys. Acta*, **412**, 229-40
52. Winkelman, L. (1976). *Compar. Biochem. Physiol.*, **55B**, 391-7
53. Swanson, C. J. (1971). *Nature, New Biol.*, **232**, 122-3
54. Zulauf, E. and Gut, C. (1978). *Europ. J. Biochem.*, **82**, 577-83
55. Pasternak, J. and Barrell, R. (1976). *J. Exptl Zool.*, **198**, 217-24
56. Kilejian, A. and MacInnis, A. J. (1976). *Rice Univ. Stud.*, **62**, 161-74
57. Schachat, F., O'Connor, D. J. and Epstein, H. F. (1978). *Biochim. Biophys. Acta*, **520**, 688-92
58. Searcy, D. G. and MacInnis, A. J. (1970). *Evolution*, **24**, 796-806
59. Simmons, J. E., Buteau, G. H., MacInnis, A. J. and Kilejian, A. (1972). *Int. J. Parasitol.*, **2**, 273-8

60. Child, C. M. (1941). *Patterns and Problems of Development*. Chicago; University of Chicago Press
61. Moritz, K. B. and Roth, G. E. (1976). *Nature,* **259**, 55–7
62. Tobler, H., Smith, K. D. and Ursprung, H. (1972). *Developm. Biol.,* **27**, 190–203
63. Goldstein, P. and Straus, N. A. (1978). *Exptl Cell Res.,* **116**, 462–6
64. Tobler, H., Zulauf, E. and Kuhn, O. (1974). *Developm. Biol.,* **41**, 218–23
65. Rodrick, G. E., Carter, C. E., Woodcock, C. L. F. and Fairbairn, D. (1977). *Exptl Parasitol.,* **42**, 150–6
66. Carter, C. E., Wells, J. R. and MacInnis, A. J. (1972). *Biochim. Biophys. Acta,* **262**, 135–44
67. Tobler, H. and Gut, C. (1974). *J. Cell Sci.,* **16**, 593–601
68. Ishikawa, H. (1977). *Compar. Biochem. Physiol.,* **56B**, 229–34
69. Ishikawa, H. (1977). *Compar. Biochem. Physiol.,* **58B**, 1–7
70. Willett, J. D. and Rahim, I. (1978). *Compar. Biochem. Physiol.,* **61B**, 243–6
71. Barrett, J. (1973). *Int. J. Parasitol.,* **3**, 393–400
72. Senft, A. W., Miech, R. P., Brown, P. R. and Senft, D. G. (1972). *Int. J. Parasitol.,* **2**, 249–60
73. Farland, W. H. and MacInnis, A. J. (1978). *Int. J. Parasitol.,* **8**, 177–86
74. Kuhn, O. and Tobler, H. (1978). *Biochim. Biophys. Acta,* **521**, 251–66
75. Schaefer, F. W., Weinstein, P. P. and Coggins, J. R. (1978). *Proc. Fourth Int. Congr. of Parasitology (Warsaw)* F, pp. 69–70
76. Mueller, J. F. (1974). *J. Parasitol.,* **60**, 3–14
77. Phares, C. K. and Carroll, R. M. (1978). *J. Parasitol.,* **64**, 401–5
78. Phares, C. K. and Cook, D. E. (1978). *J. Parasitol.,* **64**, 406–10
79. Czarnetzki, B. M. (1978). *Nature,* **271**, 553–4
80. Erasmus, D. A. and Davies, T. W. (1979). *Exptl Parasitol.,* **47**, 91–106
81. Perry, R. N. (1978). *ARC Res. Rev.,* **4**, 79–83
82. Hackett, C. J. and Chen, K.-C. (1978). *Anal. Biochem.,* **89**, 487–500
83. Hudson, B. G. (1978). In *Biology and Chemistry of Basement Membranes*, ed. N. A. Kefalides, pp. 253–263. New York; Academic Press
84. Stemberger, A. and Nordwig, A. (1974). *Hoppe-Seyler's Z. Physiol. Chem.,* **355**, 721–4
85. Lyons, K. M. (1966). *Parasitology,* **56**, 63–100
86. Nakamura, T., Yamaguchi, M. and Yanagisawa, T. (1979). *J. Biochem.,* **85**, 627–31
87. Lehman, W. and Szent-Györgyi, A. G. (1975). *J. Gen. Physiol.,* **66**, 1–30
88. Waller, P. J., Dash, K. M. and Major, G. W. (1979). *Int. J. Parasitol.,* **9**, 147–51
89. Lusier, P. E., Podesta, R. B. and Mettrick, D. F. (1978). *J. Parasitol.,* **64**, 1140–1

3 Catabolism and Energy Production

The main function of catabolic pathways is the production of energy. This energy, usually in the form of ATP, is required for mechanical, synthetic or osmotic work, and, in some systems, energy can also be dissipated as light or heat. As well as energy production, catabolic pathways have three other important functions; they generate reducing power for synthetic reactions, they produce intermediates for synthetic reactions and, finally, they provide a mechanism for the degradation of macromolecules as part of the constant turnover of cellular constituents.

Catabolic pathways tend to be convergent, the different pathways leading to the formation of a few key molecules. In mammals, catabolism can be divided into three phases. First, macromolecules are broken down by digestive enzymes or by intracellular enzymes to give monomers, amino acids, monosaccharides, fatty acids, etc. In the second phase, the monomers are broken down to simpler compounds—carbohydrate, for example, being broken down to acetyl-CoA. Amino acids and lipids are also broken down to acetyl-CoA and a few other products. These end-products are then completely degraded to carbon dioxide and water in the final stage of catabolism.

Catabolism in parasitic helminths differs from that in mammals in three important respects. First, the range of substrates that helminths can catabolise is limited and in most, if not all, species, carbohydrate is the only energy source in the parasitic stage. Secondly, acetyl-CoA does not occupy the same central role in metabolism in helminths as it does in mammals; instead, phosphoenolpyruvate appears to be the key metabolite. Finally, instead of degrading substrates completely to carbon dioxide and water, parasitic helminths characteristically excrete complex end-products, usually organic acids.

3.1. CARBOHYDRATE CATABOLISM

Carbohydrate is the main, and possibly the sole, energy reserve in the parasitic stages of helminths. The catabolism of carbohydrate by the parasitic adults of nematodes, digenetic trematodes, cestodes and acanthocephalans is characterised by the excretion of reduced end-products. In contrast, the monogenetic trematodes appear to be largely aerobic.

3.1.1. Carbohydrate Reserves

The main carbohydrate found in helminths is glycogen, but appreciable amounts of trehalose also occur in parasitic nematodes and acanthocephalans. The level of free glucose in parasitic helminths is extremely low (Section 2.2.1). Glycogen is broken down in helminths by phosphorylase to give glucose-1-phosphate and limit dextrins, complete hydrolysis of the dextrins requiring a second enzyme, amylo-1,6-glucosidase. So far, this enzyme has only been demonstrated in *H. diminuta.*

The use of trehalose by helminths is interesting. Some micro-organisms and protozoa are able to split trehalose by means of a trehalose phosphorylase:

$$\text{trehalose} + P_i \rightarrow \text{glucose} + \text{glucose-1-P}$$

This reaction, analogous to glycogen phosphorylase, conserves the bond energy. The enzyme has, however, not been found in helminths. Instead, in parasitic helminths, as in insects, trehalose is hydrolysed to glucose by trehalase, followed by phosphorylation to glucose-6-P via hexokinase. Trehalase is not an allosteric enzyme and so is not modulated by metabolites. This is in direct contrast to hexokinase and phosphorylase, the enzymes that control the catabolism of glucose and glycogen, both of which are regulatory enzymes (Section 5.1.3). Trehalase has an acid pH optimum and it has been suggested that it might be regulated by intracellular pH. In some insects, there is evidence that trehalase could be regulated by a protein modifier. The distribution of trehalase in parasite tissues has been studied in *A. lumbricoides.* Originally, it was thought that trehalase occurred only in the gut of *A. lumbricoides*, but it has since been demonstrated in the muscles and reproductive tissues as well[1]. It is possible that trehalose could be a tissue-specific metabolite acting as a specialised energy reserve for certain tissues only.

3.1.2. Pathways of Carbohydrate Catabolism

The outstanding feature of carbohydrate breakdown in parasitic helminths is, of course, the production of reduced organic end-products, and this persists even under aerobic conditions. The range of end-products produced by helminths is, however, considerably less than that found in micro-organisms. Nevertheless, when organic acid production by helminths was first described in the 1900s, there was considerable disbelief amongst biochemists that metazoa could produce organic end-products.

The pathways of carbohydrate catabolism have been investigated in detail in several parasitic helminths. Carbohydrate is broken down initially by glycolysis (*Figure 3.1*), the steps being similar to those in vertebrate tissue, at least as far as phosphoenolpyruvate. The glycolytic sequence has been demonstrated in a variety of helminths and, as in vertebrates, the glycolytic enzymes are soluble, although some of them, particularly hexokinase, may be weakly bound to the cell membranes. In some trypanosomes, the glycolytic enzymes appear to be sequestered in cell organelles called glycosomes. There is, as yet, no evidence for glycosomes in parasitic helminths. A number of glycolytic enzymes have been purified from helminths

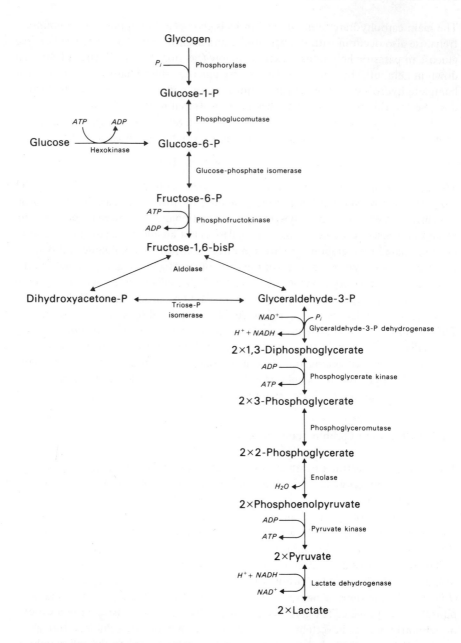

$$Sum: \quad \text{Glucose} + 2P_i + 2ADP \longrightarrow 2 \text{ Lactate} + 2ATP + 2H_2O$$

Figure 3.1 Glycolysis (cytoplasmic).

and their properties investigated, but no biologically significant differences between the glycolytic enzymes of helminths and the corresponding vertebrate enzymes have been reported. It is, however, in the fate of phosphoenolpyruvate that helminths differ from vertebrates. There are, in parasitic helminths, two major pathways for the catabolism of phosphoenolpyruvate. First, carbon dioxide fixation can take place into phosphoenolpyruvate via the enzyme phosphoenolpyruvate carboxykinase (GTP : oxaloacetate carboxylase, transphosphorylating), resulting in the formation of oxaloacetate. The oxaloacetate is then reduced to malate by a cytoplasmic malate dehydrogenase and malate enters the mitochondrion, where it is further catabolised. Phosphoenolpyruvate carboxykinase appears to be the only pathway of carbon dioxide fixation into C_3 compounds found in parasitic helminths. Pyruvate carboxylase, for example, seems to be absent in most helminths, although low levels may be present in *M. expansa*. The alternative fate for phosphoenolpyruvate is via pyruvate kinase to pyruvate, as in vertebrate tissue. The pyruvate is then reduced in the cytoplasm to lactate, or else enters the mitochondrion, where it is oxidatively decarboxylated to acetyl-CoA which is again further metabolised. The relative importance of these two pathways, pyruvate kinase or phosphoenolpyruvate carboxykinase, differs in different parasites and under different environmental conditions.

3.1.3. Carbohydrate Catabolism in *A. lumbricoides*

Carbohydrate breakdown has been most extensively studied in the muscle tissue of the parasitic nematode *A. lumbricoides* (*Figure 3.2*). Glycogen is broken down by glycolysis as far as phosphoenolpyruvate, the levels of pyruvate kinase in this tissue are low and oxaloacetate is formed by the action of a cytoplasmic phosphoenolpyruvate carboxykinase. The phosphoenolpyruvate carboxykinase of *A. lumbricoides* differs from the corresponding enzyme of vertebrates in that it is more active with IDP than GDP (ADP being inactive). The oxaloacetate is then reduced to malate by a cytoplasmic malate dehydrogenase and this reoxidises the NADH produced during glycolysis. Malate then enters the mitochondrion via a phosphate-dependent translocase and, inside the mitochondrion, a dismutation reaction takes place. Part of the malate is decarboxylated to pyruvate via a mitochondrial NAD-linked malic enzyme. This contrasts with the vertebrate, where the malic enzyme is cytoplasmic and NADP-linked. Malate is also in equilibrium with fumarate via fumarase (which in *A. lumbricoides* occurs in both the cytoplasm and mitochondrion) and the fumarate is reduced to succinate by a fumarate reductase complex. So, *A. lumbricoides* is using part of the tricarboxylic acid cycle (*Figure 3.3*) from succinate to oxaloacetate, but in the reverse direction, and has what may be described as a partial reversed tricarboxylic acid cycle.

The reduction of fumarate to succinate involves part of the cytochrome chain and results in a site I associated phosphorylation of ADP (Section 3.2.3). The ATP/malate ratio for this dismutation is thus 0.5.

In *A. lumbricoides* muscle, there are two systems for the reoxidation of NADH; in the cytoplasm, NADH formed during glycolysis from glyceraldehyde-3-phosphate

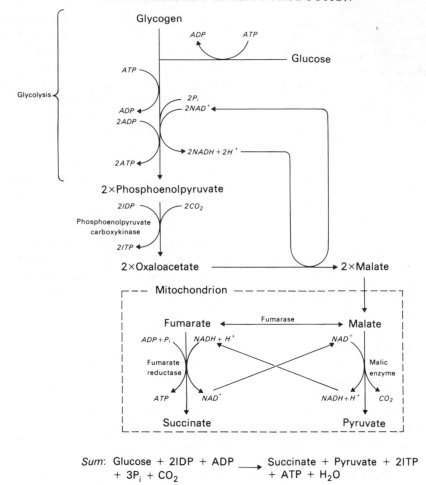

$$Sum: \text{Glucose} + 2IDP + ADP \longrightarrow \text{Succinate} + \text{Pyruvate} + 2ITP$$
$$+ 3P_i + CO_2 \qquad\qquad\qquad + ATP + H_2O$$

Figure 3.2 Carbohydrate catabolism in *Ascaris lumbricoides* muscle.

dehydrogenase is reoxidised by the reduction of oxaloacetate to malate; and in the mitochondrion, NADH formed by the malic enzyme is reoxidised by the reduction of fumarate to succinate. The catabolism of carbohydrate to succinate and pyruvate by *A. lumbricoides* muscle can then proceed entirely anaerobically, no oxygen being required for the reoxidation of NADH.

The Dismutation of Malate

In the mitochondria of *A. lumbricoides*, the dismutation of malate may not be quite so straightforward as this scheme suggests. It has been found that 80% of the mitochondrial fumarase activity and 60% of the mitochondrial malic enzyme activity are located, not in the matrix, but in the intermembrane space[2]. This means that during the dismutation of malate, both fumarate and NADH are pro-

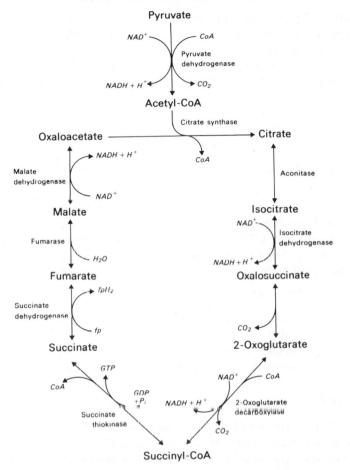

Figure 3.3 Tricarboxylic acid cycle (mitochondrial).

duced primarily in the intermembrane space, rather than in the matrix. There is, in the inner mitochondrial membrane of *A. lumbricoides*, a non-energy-linked $NAD^+/NADH$ transhydrogenase, which catalyses the exchange reaction:

$$*NADH + NAD^+ \rightleftharpoons *NAD^+ + NADH$$

This transhydrogenase is distinct from the cytochrome chain associated NADH dehydrogenase[3]. The function of the membrane-bound transhydrogenase in *A. lumbricoides* is probably the vectorial transport of hydride ions from the intermembrane space, across the inner membrane into the matrix. Reducing equivalents formed by the malic enzyme in the intermembrane space could, therefore, be transported into the matrix. However, the inner mitochondrial membrane of *A. lumbricoides* is said to be impermeable to fumarate[4]. This means that the fumarate reductase, which may be identical with the succinate dehydrogenase (Section 3.1.4), would have to be located on the outer surface of the inner membrane, in order to be accessible to the substrate (fumarate). If this were so, there would then seem little need to transport hydride ions into the matrix. The evidence, so far, suggests that the succinic dehydrogenase complex of *A. lumbricoides*, like the mammalian system, is located on the inner face of the inner membrane. A possibility might be that, in *A. lumbricoides*, the complex spans the membrane, the succinate dehydrogenase site being on the inside, the fumarate reductase site on the outside.

Nucleoside Triphosphate Metabolism

The proposed scheme for carbohydrate breakdown in *A. lumbricoides* muscle gives rise to 4 moles of nucleoside triphosphate for every hexose unit (C_6) catabolised (when glycogen is the substrate). Of these 4 moles of nucleoside triphosphate, 2 moles come from the phosphoenolpyruvate carboxykinase reaction, and so a large proportion of the nucleoside triphosphate produced by *A. lumbricoides* muscle will be in the form of ITP or GTP rather than ATP. However, there is an extremely active nucleoside-diphosphate kinase present in the muscles and this enzyme catalyses the rapid transfer of high-energy phosphate from GTP or ITP to ADP:

$$XTP + ADP \rightleftharpoons ATP + XDP$$

Despite the importance of the phosphoenolpyruvate carboxykinase reaction in the breakdown of carbohydrate by *A. lumbricoides*, inosine and guanosine nucleotides are present in only small amounts and the general pattern of organic phosphates in *A. lumbricoides* muscle resembles that found in vertebrate smooth muscle[5].

Volatile Acid Production

The initial end-products of carbohydrate catabolism in *A. lumbricoides* are pyruvate and succinate, and large amounts of succinate (up to 13.7 mM) occur in the haemolymph and tissues[6]. The main excretory products of carbohydrate catabolism in *A. lumbricoides* are, however, short chain fatty acids. Racemic mixtures of 2-methylvalerate and 2-methylbutyrate constitute 70–80% of the total acids produced; *n*-valeric, acetic, propionic, isobutyric, tiglic and *n*-caproic acids have also been found as minor components. Only 7–8% of the acids excreted by *A. lumbricoides* are non-volatile and lactate constitutes less than 0.04% of the total. 2-Methylbutyrate is formed by the condensation of one acetate and one propionate, and 2-methylvalerate by the condensation of two propionate molecules (*Figure 3.4*), acetate and propionate arising by the decarboxylation of pyruvate and succinate, respectively. The details of volatile fatty acid synthesis in *A. lumbricoides* are not completely clear. Possible pathways of 2-methylvalerate and 2-methylbutyrate synthesis are shown in *Figures 3.5* and *3.6*. The synthesis of these acids almost certainly involves CoA derivatives and two of the enzymes involved have been identified in *A. lumbricoides* muscle[7]. The first is an NAD-linked 2-methylacetoacetic reductase. This enzyme requires the CoA derivative of 2-methylacetoacetate or alternatively the ethyl ester:

2-methylacetoacetyl-CoA + NADH + H$^+$ $\rightleftharpoons$ 3-hydroxy-2-methylbutyryl-CoA + NAD$^+$

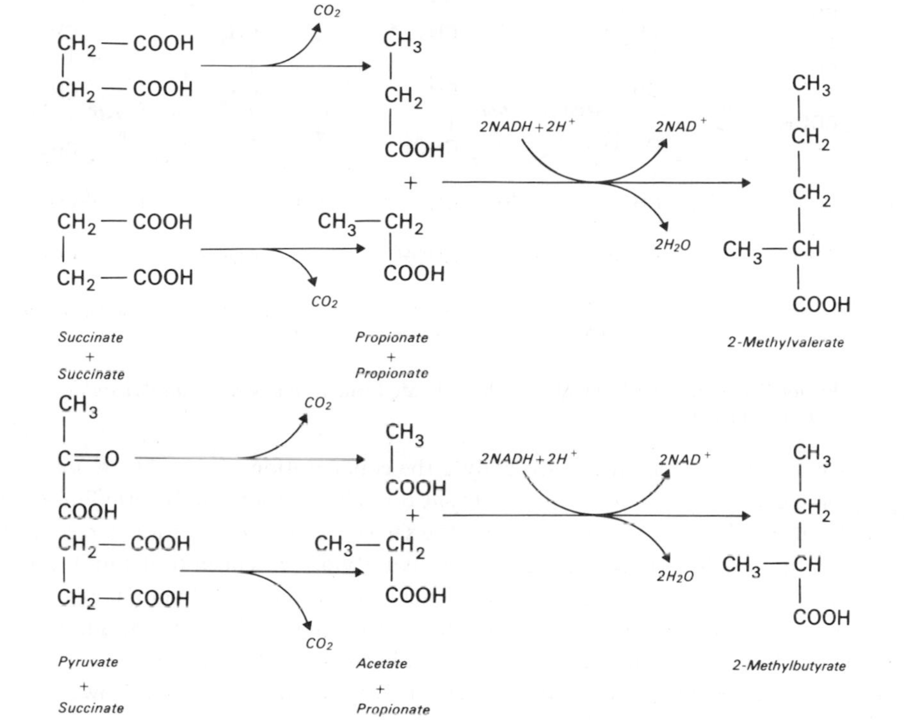

Figure 3.4 Formation of 2-methylvalerate and 2-methylbutyrate in *Ascaris lumbricoides*.

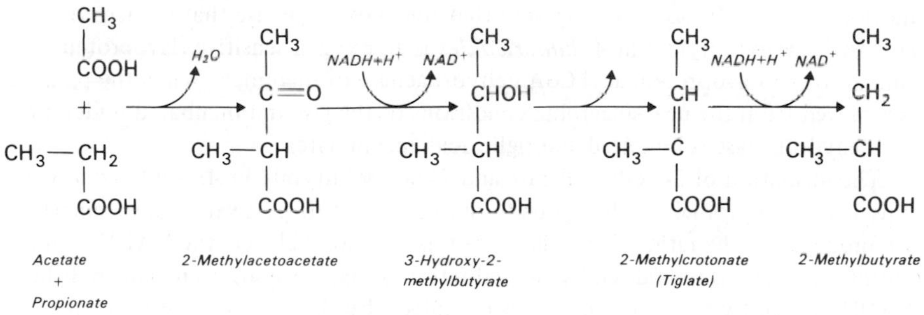

Figure 3.5 Possible pathway of 2-methylbutyrate formation in *Ascaris lumbricoides* (mitochondrial).

The 2-methylacetoacetate reductase will also reduce 3-keto-2-methylpentanoate. The second enzyme which has been found is a propionyl-CoA reductase (condensing enzyme):

$$2\text{propionyl-CoA} \rightarrow \text{3-keto-2-methylpentanoyl-CoA} + \text{CoA}$$

3-keto-2-methylpentanoyl-CoA + NADH + H^+ ⇌

$$\text{3-hydroxy-2-methylpentanoyl-CoA} + NAD^+$$

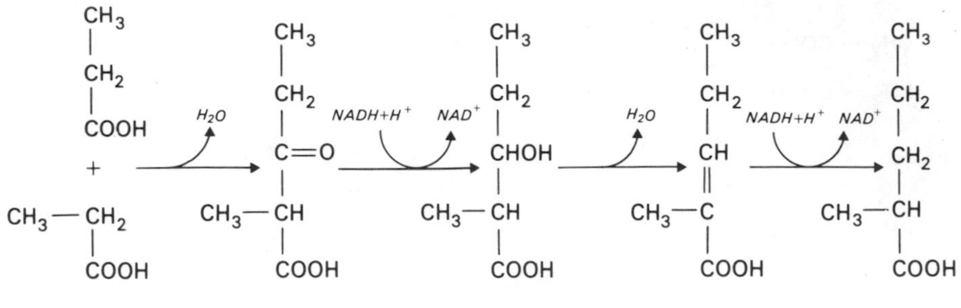

Figure 3.6 Possible pathway of 2-methylvalerate formation in *Ascaris lumbricoides* (mitochondrial).

Propionyl-CoA reductase may also catalyse the condensation of acetyl-CoA and propionyl-CoA to give 2-methylacetoacetyl-CoA. The synthesis of 2-methylbutyrate and 2-methylvalerate may, therefore, use the same enzymes. In addition, a racemase, active with both 2-methylvalerate and 2-methylbutyrate, has been found in *A. lumbricoides* muscle. The actual site of volatile acid formation, mitochondrial or cytoplasmic, is not certain, but it is probably mitochondrial. Intermediates in the synthesis of the branched chain acids have not been isolated, although these intermediates, like the intermediates of β-oxidation, may be enzyme-bound. However, tiglic (2-methylcrotonic) acid, which is a probable precursor of 2-methylbutyrate, does occur as a minor component in excretory acids. The levels of tiglic acid in the tissues of *A. lumbricoides* are normally low, but increase if the worms are kept *in vitro*. This could be due to the disruption of 2-methylbutyrate synthesis in the moribund worm. It has been suggested that the dehydrogenase that reduces tiglic acid to 2-methylbutyrate in *A. lumbricoides* is an oxygen-sensitive flavoprotein, similar to the flavoprotein acyl-CoA dehydrogenase of mammals. When the parasite is removed from the near-anaerobic conditions of the gut and incubated under air, the dehydrogenase is inhibited and tiglic acid accumulates.

The formation of 2-methylvalerate and 2-methylbutyrate in *A. lumbricoides* muscle poses a problem with regards to redox balance. If pyruvate and succinate are produced in the ratio of 1:1, the system is in redox balance, the NADH formed during glycolysis is reoxidised by the reduction of oxaloacetate to malate and the NADH formed by the malic enzyme is reoxidised by the reduction of fumarate to succinate. The formation of one 2-methylbutyrate or one 2-methylvalerate from propionate and acetate requires two additional NADH. The decarboxylation of pyruvate to acetate generates only one additional NADH (the decarboxylation of succinate does not yield NADH) and, therefore, extra reducing equivalents are needed for the synthesis of these acids. There is also an excess of pyruvate (or acetate) to be accounted for, since each mole of 2-methylvalerate produced uses up 2 moles of succinate and leaves 2 moles of pyruvate: the formation of 2-methylbutyrate requires one pyruvate and one succinate and so balances in this respect.

The dismutation of malate in the mitochondrion of *A. lumbricoides* need not, of course, necessarily result in the formation of equimolecular amounts of succinate and pyruvate. The ratio of these two end-products will depend on the prevailing redox conditions. If reducing equivalents are available, from sources other than the malic enzyme, more succinate would be produced. Alternatively, if NADH from the malic enzyme were being utilised by reactions, other than fumarate reductase, pyruvate production would predominate. Even so, it is not yet possible to draw up a balance sheet for the production of 2-methylvalerate and 2-methylbutyrate from succinate and pyruvate in *A. lumbricoides* muscle. The situation is further complicated by variations in the relative proportions of 2-methylvalerate and 2-methylbutyrate excreted by *A. lumbricoides*; some workers have reported 2-methylbutyrate to predominate, others 2-methylvalerate. It has also been suggested that 2-methylbutyrate and 2-methylvalerate are produced in equimolecular amounts by *A. lumbricoides* and that the changes in the relative proportions excreted may depend on a variety of factors, including the availability of oxygen. There is, almost certainly, selective excretion of acids by *A. lumbricoides*, since the fatty acid composition of the pseudocoelomic fluid differs from that of excreted acids. Succinate, in particular, accumulates in the tissues and pseudocoelomic fluid, and in the female a considerable proportion of the branched chain fatty acids are not excreted, but incorporated into the egg lipids (Section 2.3.2). The main route for volatile fatty acid excretion in *A. lumbricoides* is via the intestine, and there is some evidence for the selective reabsorption of acids from the gut lumen.

Origins of the Minor Excretory Acids

The origins of the minor fatty acids excreted by *A. lumbricoides* are not known. Some, such as acetic, propionic and tiglic, may be derived from intermediates in branched chain fatty acid synthesis. Other acids could be the result of condensations between acetyl-CoA and propionyl-CoA (*n*-valeric and *n*-caproic), or they may not be derived from carbohydrate breakdown at all, but come from the catabolism of amino acids (isoleucine, for example, could give rise to isobutyrate).

Only minute traces of lactate are excreted by *A. lumbricoides*, despite the presence of an active cytoplasmic lactate dehydrogenase. Since, in *A. lumbricoides*, pyruvate is formed mainly within the mitochondrion and not in the cytoplasm, there is no substrate available to the lactate dehydrogenase. Homogenates of *A. lumbricoides* muscle, in which this compartmentation has been destroyed, readily produce lactic acid. However, a more likely explanation for the absence of lactate production in intact *A. lumbricoides* is that the relatively high cytoplasmic free $[NAD^+]/[NADH]$ ratio maintains the lactate dehydrogenase equilibrium in favour of pyruvate production and pyruvate is being continuously removed by volatile fatty acid synthesis.

The Redox State in A. lumbricoides Muscle

The redox state of the free $[NAD^+]/[NADH]$ couple in the cytoplasm of *A. lumbricoides* muscle has been estimated as between 725:1 and 2214:1, a value that compares well with the free $[NAD^+]/[NADH]$ ratio in the cytoplasm of an aerobic tissue, such as rat liver, where the ratio is about 1000:1. So the coupling of the glyceraldehyde-3-phosphate dehydrogenase reaction with malate dehydrogenase in the cytoplasm of *A. lumbricoides* muscle enables the cytoplasm to stay in a relatively oxidised state, although carbohydrate catabolism is essentially anaerobic[8]. In the mitochondrion of *A. lumbricoides*, the free $[NAD^+]/[NADH]$ ratio has been estimated as about 0.1:1. This is considerably lower than comparable estimates of the redox state of the NAD couple in rat liver mitochondria, which is in the region of 10:1. Although the estimate for the free $[NAD^+]/[NADH]$ ratio in *A. lumbricoides* mitochondria is not very reliable, it does indicate that the ratio may be considerably lower than in vertebrate tissue. The low redox state in *A. lumbricoides* mitochondria may perhaps be correlated with the reduction of fumarate to succinate since, under the redox conditions in the vertebrate mitochondrion, succinate is being oxidised.

The only other helminth for which there are estimates of the free $[NAD^+]/[NADH]$ ratio is *F. hepatica*[9]. In the cytoplasm of *F. hepatica*, the free $[NAD^+]/[NADH]$ ratio has been estimated as 935:1, and in the mitochondrion as 1.3:1, the latter value being much more similar to the values reported in mammals. The free $[NADP^+]/[NADPH]$ ratio in *F. hepatica* was estimated as 2.4:1.

Neutral End-products

In addition to excreting acidic end-products, *A. lumbricoides* also produces small quantities of acetylmethylcarbinol (acetoin). This probably arises from a partial reaction of the pyruvate dehydrogenase complex, in which pyruvate condenses with 'active' aldehyde:

$$CH_3COCOOH + CH_3CHO \rightarrow CH_3 - \underset{\underset{OH}{|}}{CH} - \underset{\underset{O}{\|}}{C} - CH_3 + CO_2$$
$$\text{acetoin}$$

The tissues of *A. lumbricoides* can also synthesise 2-acetolactate by a similar condensation of two pyruvates:

$$2CH_3COCOOH \rightarrow CH_3 - \underset{\underset{}{\|}}{\overset{O}{C}} - \underset{\underset{COOH}{|}}{\overset{OH}{C}} - CH_3 + CO_2$$
$$\text{2-acetolactate}$$

In bacteria, 2-acetolactate can be decarboxylated to acetoin. However, no 2-acetolactate decarboxylase has been detected in *A. lumbricoides*. There have also been claims that *A. lumbricoides* can excrete significant amounts of ethanol.

3.1.4. Helminths that Rely Predominantly on Carbon Dioxide Fixation

The major pathway for carbohydrate catabolism in *A. lumbricoides* involves carbon dioxide fixation into phosphoenolpyruvate to give oxaloacetate which is reduced to

malate. The malate then undergoes a dismutation reaction, resulting in the formation of pyruvate and succinate. These initial end-products are then further metabolised to volatile fatty acids. Although this scheme for carbohydrate breakdown in

Table 3.1   End-products of carbohydrate breakdown in nematodes

Species	Aerobic	Anaerobic
Ancylostoma caninum	Acetate, propionate, traces of isobutyrate, 2-methylbutyrate	Similar to aerobic
Angiostrongylus cantonensis	Lactate	Similar to aerobic
Ascaridia galli	Lactate, acetate?, propionate	Similar to aerobic
Ascaris lumbricoides	2-Methylvalerate, 2-methylbuty-rate, traces of acetate, *n*-valerate, propionate, isobutyrate, tiglate, *n*-caproate, acetoin	Similar to aerobic
Brugia pahangi		
(adult)	Lactate	—
(microfilaria)	Lactate, acetate	Lactate
Chandlerella hawkingi	Lactate, traces of pyruvate	—
Dictyocaulus viviparus	Lactate, traces of pyruvate, propionate, acetate	—
Dipetalonema viteae	Lactate	—
Dirofilaria uniformis	Lactate	—
D. immitis	Lactate	Similar to aerobic
Dracunculus insignis	Lactate	Similar to aerobic
Haemonchus contortus	Similar to anaerobic	Acetate, propion-ate, propanol, traces of lactate, succinate, ethanol
Heterakis gallinae	Acetate, propionate, traces of lactate, pyruvate	Similar to aerobic
Litomosoides carinii	Lactate, acetate	More lactate, less acetate
Mecistocirrus digitatus	Lactate, butyrate	Lactate, acetate
Nippostrongylus brasiliensis	Lactate, traces of pyruvate	Lactate, succinate
Parascaris equorum	Lactate, propionate, 2-methylbutyrate	Similar to aerobic
Setaria cervi	Lactate	—
Trichinella spiralis		
(larva)	*n*-Valerate, acetate, propion-ate, traces of butyrate, caproate, lactate	Similar to aerobic larva
(adult)	—	*n*-Valerate, acetate, propionate, traces of caproate, buty-rate, formate
Trichostrongylus colubriformis	—	Acetate, propion-ate, traces of butyrate
Trichuris vulpis	Lactate, propionate, succinate, traces of acetate, *n*-valerate, butyrate, formate	—

Table 3.2   End-products of carbohydrate breakdown in cestodes

Species	Aerobic	Anaerobic
Diphyllobothrium dendriticum (adult and plerocercoid)	Succinate, lactate	Similar to aerobic
Echinococcus granulosus (adult)	Succinate, lactate, acetate	Similar to aerobic
(larva)	Lactate, pyruvate, acetate, succinate, ethanol	Similar to aerobic larva with more succinate, no pyruvate
Hymenolepis diminuta	Lactate, acetate, succinate	Similar to aerobic with more succinate
Ligula intestinalis (adult)	–	Lactate, some succinate, propionate, acetate, malate, pyruvate
(plerocercoid)	–	Similar to anaerobic adult
Mesocestoides corti (tetrathyridia)	Lactate, succinate, acetate	Similar to aerobic with more succinate
Moniezia expansa	Lactate, succinate	Similar to aerobic with more succinate
Schistocephalus solidus (plerocercoid)	Acetate, propionate (4:1)	Acetate, propionate (1:3)
Spirometra mansonoides (adult)	–	Acetate, propionate, traces of lactate, succinate
(larva)	–	Acetate, lactate, traces of propionate, succinate
Taenia taeniaeformis (adult)	Lactate, acetate, pyruvate, succinate, ethanol	Similar to aerobic adult with more succinate
(larva)	Similar to aerobic adult	Similar to aerobic adult

A. lumbricoides is now generally accepted, some of the details are still not completely understood. In particular, the dismutation of malate may be more complicated than first thought and the details of volatile fatty acid synthesis are still incomplete.

Parasitic helminths produce a bewildering array of end-products from carbohydrate breakdown (*Tables 3.1, 3.2, 3.3* and *3.4*). However, many of them appear similar to *A. lumbricoides*, in that they fix carbon dioxide, have a partial reverse tricarboxylic acid cycle and produce succinate and pyruvate or their derivatives as end-products of carbohydrate breakdown. Succinate is frequently a major excretory product of helminths. Pyruvate, on the other hand, is rarely excreted unchanged. Helminths that fix carbon dioxide often differ from *A. lumbricoides* in three respects. First, many of them have significant levels of pyruvate kinase. This means that pyruvate is formed from phosphoenolpyruvate, in the cytoplasm, and such

Table 3.3   End-products of carbohydrate breakdown in trematodes

Species	Aerobic	Anaerobic
Clinostomum complanatum (metacercaria)	Lactate, pyruvate, succinate	Lactate
Dicrocoelium dendriticum	Lactate?	Lactate, acetate, propionate, succinate
Echinostoma liei	*n*-Valerate, traces of *n*-hexanoate, propionate, butyrate, acetate, 2-methylbutyrate, lactate, succinate	Similar to aerobic
Fasciola gigantica	Lactate	—
F. hepatica	Acetate, propionate, traces of lactate, isobutyrate, isovalerate, 2-methylbutyrate, succinate	Similar to aerobic
Paragonimus westermani	Lactate?	—
Schistosoma mansoni	Lactate	Lactate

Table 3.4   End-products of carbohydrate breakdown in acanthocephalans

Species	Aerobic	Anaerobic
Echinorhynchus gadi	Lactate	Lactate, succinate
Moniliformis dubius	Ethanol, traces of lactate, succinate, acetate, butyrate, and possibly formate	Similar to aerobic
Neoechinorhynchus emydis	Lactate	—
N. pseudemydis	Lactate	—
Polymorphis minutus	—	Lactate, succinate (1:1)

parasites often produce appreciable quantities of lactate. Secondly, in many of these helminths, the mitochondrial reducing power required for the reduction of fumarate to succinate may come from sources other than the malic enzyme. Thirdly, in some helminths, at least, a significant proportion of the NADH produced by carbohydrate breakdown is reoxidised by oxygen and not by coupling to the reduction of an organic substrate.

Apart from *A. lumbricoides*, only three other parasites, *P. equorum, T. spiralis* (both nematodes) and the trematode *Echinostoma liei*[10], produce C_5 and C_6 acids as major end-products. The excretory acids of *P. equorum* are similar to those of *A. lumbricoides*, but include appreciable amounts of lactate. The adults and muscle larvae of *T. spiralis* produce mainly *n*-valerate, with small amounts of formate, acetate, propionate, butyrate, caproate and lactate. *n*-Valerate is probably formed by the condensation of acetate and propionate, the latter coming from the decarboxylation of pyruvate and succinate, respectively. The larvae of *T. spiralis* also resemble *A. lumbricoides* in that the intact worm produces little lactate, whilst homogenates do.

One way of looking at the array of end-products produced by parasitic helminths is to consider the redox couples involved. With this in mind, helminths that predominantly fix carbon dioxide as their major pathway for carbohydrate breakdown can be divided broadly into three groups: (i) the acetate and propionate producers, (ii) the acetate, lactate and propionate (or succinate) producers and, finally, (iii) the succinate and lactate producers.

Acetate and Propionate Producers

These are parasites such as *F. hepatica, S. solidus, A. caninum* and *Trichostrongylus colubriformis* that excrete acetate and propionate. Both *F. hepatica* and *A. caninum* also excrete small amounts of volatile fatty acids, but these are derived from the breakdown of amino acids and not from carbohydrate catabolism. The ratios of acetate and propionate produced by these parasites vary, but in *A. caninum* and *F. hepatica* the ratio approaches 1:2. One problem, of course, is that variable amounts of excretory acids are retained in the tissues. Assuming that the pathways in these parasites are similar to *A. lumbricoides*, if pyruvate and succinate are produced in equimolecular amounts from glucose, this balances with respect to oxidations and reductions. The formation of acetate from pyruvate generates a further mole of NADH, which could be reoxidised by the reduction of an extra fumarate to succinate. So, for every acetate produced, 2 moles of fumarate would be reduced to succinate, which on decarboxylation yields propionate. This then gives an acetate/propionate ratio of 1:2. If acetate and propionate (or acetate and succinate) are produced in the ratio of 1:2, this maintains the mitochondrial redox balance. Variations from this ratio can be explained either by extra reducing equivalents being available from sources other than the dismutation of malate or by reducing equivalents being used by reactions other than the reduction of fumarate. The former would lead to an increase in the proportions of propionate, the latter to an increase in acetate.

The Pathways of Acetate and Propionate Production in F. hepatica

Acetate and propionate are formed by the decarboxylation of pyruvate and succinate, respectively. However, it is so far only in *F. hepatica* that the actual pathways of acetate and propionate formation have been studied[11,12]. In this parasite, pyruvate is oxidatively decarboxylated via pyruvate dehydrogenase to acetyl-CoA which is then cleaved to give acetate. Propionate production in *F. hepatica* follows the same pathway as in mammalian liver, succinate being metabolised via succinic thiokinase, methylmalonyl-CoA mutase, methylmalonyl-CoA racemase and propionyl-CoA carboxylase to propionyl-CoA (*Figure 3.7*). The cleavage of acetyl-CoA and propionyl-CoA to acetate and propionate can take place either via a carnitine-dependent hydrolase or via CoA transferase. The latter requires a suitable cosubstrate and it is possible to propose cyclic mechanisms involving CoA transferase which lead to a net production of ATP from the cleavage of acetyl-CoA or propionyl-CoA (Section 3.1.9).

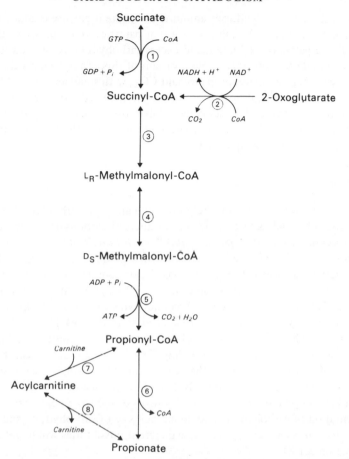

Figure 3 7 The pathway of propionate formation in *Fasciola hepatica*: 1, succinate thiokinase or CoA transferase; 2, 2-oxoglutarate decarboxylase (a minor source of succinyl-CoA); 3, methylmalonyl-CoA mutase; 4, methylmalonyl-CoA racemase; 5, propionyl-CoA carboxylase; 6, CoA transferase; 7, carnitine acyltransferase; 8, acylcarnitine hydrolase.

Two of the enzymes of the propionate pathway, methylmalonyl-CoA mutase and propionyl-CoA carboxylase, have also been found in the larvae and adults of the cestode *Spirometra mansonoides*[13].

Acetate, Lactate and Propionate (or Succinate) Producers

The second group of parasites are those such as *E. granulosus, H. diminuta, T. taeniaeformis, L. intestinalis, D. dendriticum* and *Heterakis gallinae* that, in addition to excreting acetate and propionate or acetate and succinate, also excrete significant quantities of lactic acid. Lactic acid production, like anaerobic glycolysis in vertebrate muscle, balances with respect to oxidations and reductions and, since lactate is formed in the cytoplasm, it can be considered as a cytoplasmic end-product. Both *S. solidus* and *F. hepatica*, which are primarily acetate and propionate producers, also excrete significant amounts of lactate if glucose is added to the incubation medium. Possibly, in this group of parasites, the capacity of the carbon dioxide fixing pathways is limited, and excess carbohydrate is diverted to lactate.

The nematode *H. contortus* shows a variant of this system and breaks glucose down to acetate, propionate, propanol and CO_2, with small amounts of lactate, succinate and ethanol[14]. Propanol production in helminths appears, so far, to be unique to *H. contortus* and presumably involves the reduction of propionaldehyde produced as an intermediate in propionic acid formation. Propanol production does, of course, utilise reducing equivalents.

Succinate and Lactate Producers

The third group of helminths that rely predominantly on carbon dioxide fixation produce succinate and lactate as the end-products of carbohydrate breakdown. These parasites, such as *M. expansa, Diphyllobothrium dendriticum, P. minutus* and *Echinorhynchus gadi*, pose a problem with regard to redox balance. The formation of lactate balances with respect to oxidations and reductions; the catabolism of carbohydrates, as far as malate, also balances the cytoplasmic $[NAD^+]/[NADH]$ couple (the NADH produced by the glyceraldehyde-3-phosphate dehydrogenase being reoxidised by the reduction of oxaloacetate to malate). However, the further catabolism of malate to succinate requires extra reducing equivalents. The source of the extra reducing power in these helminths is at present unknown. It could come, as in *A. lumbricoides*, from the dismutation of malate, but with the resulting pyruvate being metabolised completely to carbon dioxide or to some, as yet, unidentified compound. Other potential sources of reducing power are from the cofermentation of carbohydrate and amino acids or of carbohydrate and lipids or from the tricarboxylic acid cycle. These different possibilities will be returned to later (Section 3.1.8).

Transhydrogenases

In *H. diminuta*, the malic enzyme is NADP-linked, the fumarate reductase reaction, on the other hand, being NAD-linked. There exists in the mitochondrion of *H. diminuta* a non-energy-linked transhydrogenase, which catalyses the reaction:

$$NADPH + NAD^+ + H^+ \rightleftharpoons NADP^+ + NADH + H^+$$

This transhydrogenase couples the malic enzyme with the fumarate reductase. NAD/NADP transhydrogenases are also found in mammals, but these are usually energy-linked. In addition, the mitochondrion of *H. diminuta* also possesses an NAD/NADH transhydrogenase similar to that described in the mitochondria of *A. lumbricoides*[15]. In *Spirometra mansonoides*, the mitochondria have also been found to contain both NADH/NAD and NADPH/NAD transhydrogenases, the latter being inhibited by AMP[16]. The fumarate reductase of *S. mansonoides* appears to be unique in that it can be either NADH- or NADPH-linked.

Alternative Pathways

It has been assumed that since all of the helminths described so far produce end-products similar, or related, to those found in *A. lumbricoides*, they all use similar pathways. That is to say, they all fix carbon dioxide and have a partial reverse tricarboxylic acid cycle. Whilst, at present, there is no evidence to indicate that this is not so, it is only in *A. lumbricoides* that the pathways of acid production have been studied in detail. Of the key enzymes involved in the *A. lumbricoides* type of pathway, phosphoenolpyruvate carboxykinase and fumarate reductase have been demonstrated in *Strongyluris brevicaudata*[17], *H. contortus, D. dendriticum, F. hepatica, M. expansa, H. diminuta* and in the plerocercoids of *S. solidus* and *L. intestinalis*. Phosphoenolpyruvate carboxykinase has also been shown in *T. spiralis* larvae, in *M. dubius* and in the cestodes *Bothriocephalus gowkongensis, Khawia sinensis, Triaenophorus crassus* and *E. granulosus*. The malic enzyme has been found in *H. contortus, T. spiralis* larvae, *S. brevicaudata, D. dendriticum, F. hepatica, S. mansonoides* and *H. diminuta*. Only low levels of malic enzyme are found in *M. expansa* and *S. solidus*. In *M. dubius*, low levels of malic enzyme occur in the cystacanths, but there are conflicting reports of its presence in the adult. A number of these helminths (*S. solidus, M. expansa, H. diminuta* and *F. hepatica*) also possess an active nucleoside-diphosphate kinase, another enzyme that is possibly associated with the phosphoenolpyruvate carboxykinase pathway[18]. A number of helminths that are primarily homolactic fermenters, rather than carbon dioxide fixers, also show phosphoenolpyruvate carboxykinase, fumarate reductase and malic enzyme activity, and these are described in Section 3.1.6.

Nevertheless, excretory acids could be produced by a number of alternative pathways. Some acids, such as 2-methylbutyrate, propionate, pyruvate, succinate and acetate, can be derived from the breakdown of amino acids. Another possible source of acetate is the cleavage of citrate. There is no citrate lyase in *F. hepatica* or *A. lumbricoides*, but the enzyme has been detected in *Metastrongylus apri*. Propionate can also be formed by the direct reduction of lactate:

$$\text{lactate} \xrightarrow{\text{H}_2\text{O}} \text{acrylate} \xrightarrow{\text{NADH}} \text{propionate}$$

This occurs in micro-organisms and has been suggested as the pathway of propionate formation in the scoleces of *E. granulosus*. However, propionate is not a major end-product in this parasite and the acrylate pathway has not been confirmed. In addition, propionate can be derived from the oxidation of odd-numbered fatty acids and succinate can be formed by carbon dioxide fixation into phosphoenolpyruvate or propionate or from the tricarboxylic acid cycle. Until other helminths have been investigated in detail, the possible alternatives to the *A. lumbricoides* pathway cannot be entirely dismissed.

Pathways in Free-living Invertebrates

There are a number of similarities between the end-products of carbohydrate break-down in parasitic helminths and those of free-living annelids and molluscs produced under anaerobic conditions. Acetate and propionate are excreted under anaerobic conditions by a variety of annelids (*Nereis, Arenicola, Tubifex*), whilst propionate and succinate are excreted by *Lumbricus terrestris*. The oligochaete *Alma emini* excretes the volatile fatty acids methylbutyrate and butyrate as well as acetate and propionate. Bivalves also produce succinate, propionate and acetate. In addition, most of these invertebrates produce a certain amount of lactate as well as quite large amounts of alanine (Section 3.1.9); and in the insects, Chironomid larvae accumulate alanine, lactate, succinate and ethanol under anaerobic conditions. The pathways these invertebrates use involve phosphoenolpyruvate carboxykinase and fumarate reductase. However, in contrast to *A. lumbricoides*, in bivalves, at least, the malic enzyme does not seem to be involved.

3.1.5. The Reduction of Fumarate to Succinate

In parasites that fix carbon dioxide, the reduction of fumarate to succinate is an important step in the pathway. Succinic dehydrogenases isolated from different sources differ greatly in their properties. The enzyme from aerobic organisms, such as mammals or plants, has a high rate of succinate oxidation relative to fumarate reduction—in mammals the ratio (succinate → fumarate)/(fumarate → succinate) is about 60. The aerobic enzyme has a high affinity for succinate, fumarate is only a weak inhibitor and the enzyme is activated by substrate. In addition, the succinate dehydrogenase from aerobes is always membrane-bound and contains a covalently linked flavin nucleotide. On the other hand, the succinate dehydrogenase from obligate anaerobes, such as the micro-organism *Micrococcus lactyliticus*, has a high affinity for fumarate, a low affinity for succinate and the succinate oxidase/fumarate reductase ratio is one-thousandth of that of the aerobic enzyme (0.03 in *M. lactyliticus*). In the extreme case of the cytoplasmic, anaerobic dehydrogenases from yeast, no succinate oxidation can be detected and they function only as fumarate reductases. The fumarate reductases of anaerobes are not activated by substrate and the flavin is not covalently bound. Facultative anaerobes such as *Escherichia coli* and yeast have both types of succinic dehydrogenase and the relative proportions of the two types is under genetic and environmental control. However, the facultative anaerobe *Propionibacterium* has a succinic dehydrogenase with properties intermediate between those of the aerobic and anaerobic enzymes. The enzyme from *Propionibacterium* has a succinate oxidase/fumarate reductase ratio of about 3, and the affinity of the enzyme for succinate and fumarate is intermediate between the aerobic and anaerobic types.

　　The succinate dehydrogenase from helminths that reduce fumarate to succinate resembles the aerobic-type enzyme in being membrane-bound and, at least in *F. hepatica* and *H. diminuta*, the enzyme can exist in active and inactive forms[19]. The succinic oxidase/fumarate reductase ratio of helminth succinate dehydrogenases is in the range·0.3–5, similar to those of facultative anaerobes. Unfortunately, however, there are no data on the K_m of parasite succinic dehydrogenases for fumarate or succinate. It is not at all clear in helminths whether there is a single reversible succinic dehydrogenase (of the *Propionibacterium* type) or whether there are two separate enzymes, the fumarate reductase being a distinct enzyme from the succin-oxidase. Work so far on *A. lumbricoides* suggests that there may be a single reversible enzyme. However, in *H. contortus*, fumarate reductase activity is inhibited by thia-bendazole whilst succinoxidase is not, suggesting that there are two separate enzymes.

The reduction of fumarate to succinate in helminths is accompanied by the phosphorylation of ADP, one ATP being produced for each fumarate reduced. This phosphorylation involves the cytochrome chain and is described in Section 3.2.3.

3.1.6. Helminths that Rely Predominantly on Glycolysis

In contrast to *A. lumbricoides* and other carbon dioxide fixing helminths, a number of animal parasites primarily produce lactate as the major end-product of carbohy-drate catabolism. The adults and schistosomulae of *S. mansoni* are essentially homolactic fermenters, as are the cercariae of *S. mansoni* under anaerobic con-ditions. Lactate is also the major end-product of the nematodes *A. galli*, *Angio-strongylus cantonensis* and *Dictyocaulus viviparus* and of the filarial worms *Brugia pahangi*, *Chandlerella hawkingi*, *Dipetalonema viteae*, *Dirofilaria uniformis* and *S. cervi*. In another filarial worm, *L. carinii*, 80% of the glucose is catabolised to lactate, acetate and carbon dioxide and 20% to acetoin. The proportions of lactate and acetate produced depend on the availability of oxygen. Under anaerobic conditions more lactate is formed, and more acetate under aerobic conditions. The microfilariae of *B. pahangi* similarly produce lactate under anaerobic conditions and acetate under aerobic[20]. In both *L. carinii* and in the microfilariae of *B. pahangi*, acetate is derived from the direct decarboxylation of pyruvate, probably via pyruvate dehydrogenase. Acetoin could then be formed in *L. carinii* as a side reaction of the pyruvate dehydrogenase complex, as was suggested earlier for *A. lumbricoides* (Section 3.1.3). Under aerobic conditions, *L. carinii* appear able to catabolise exogenous acetoin[65]. The filarial worm *S. cervi* also excretes some acetoin.

The situation in *N. brasiliensis* may be typical of many of the smaller gastro-intestinal nematodes. Aerobically, *N. brasiliensis* produces lactate and some pyru-vate whilst, anaerobically, lactate and succinate are formed. Volatile fatty acids occur in the free fatty acid pool of *N. brasiliensis* but they are not excreted. There is an active phosphoenolpyruvate carboxykinase in *N. brasiliensis* and possibly, under anaerobic conditions, succinate is formed by a pathway similar to that in *A. lumbricoides*. The whip worm *Trichuris vulpis* resembles *N. brasiliensis*, half of the carbohydrate catabolised by *T. vulpis* is converted to lactate, carbon dioxide and propionate, 15% to succinate, with smaller amounts of volatile acids, and again there is evidence for carbon dioxide fixation. The trematode *S. mansoni* and the filarial worms *L. carinii*, *C. hawkingi* and *S. cervi*, all of which are predominantly lactic acid producers, have an active phosphoenolpyruvate carboxykinase and both this enzyme and fumarate reductase have been reported in *D. viviparus*. In this last nematode, isotope experiments indicate that carbon dioxide fixation takes place but there is no malic enzyme. In addition to lactate, *D. viviparus* does produce small amounts of succinate, propionate and acetate.

A number of other species of parasitic nematode have been shown to have appreciable phosphoenolpyruvate carboxykinase levels: *Hyostrongylus rubidus, Rhabdias bufonis, Syphacia muris* and the larvae and adults of *O. cuniculi* and *S. ratti*. In addition, *S. muris* and *R. bufonis* show fumarate reductase activity. Unfortunately, nothing is known of the end-products of carbohydrate catabolism in these nematodes. Phosphoenolpyruvate carboxykinase can, of course, be involved in gluconeogenesis as well as carbon dioxide fixation (Section 4.2.1).

The division of parasitic helminths into carbon dioxide fixers and glycolytic fermenters is obviously not absolute, since many carbon dioxide fixers also excrete some lactate and many lactate producers can also fix carbon dioxide. In reality, there is a continuous spectrum from succinate producers to lactate producers.

Ethanol Production

The acanthocephalan *M. dubius* shows a variant of the glycolytic scheme, the main end-product being ethanol, with small amounts of lactate, succinate and volatile acids. Ethanol production by *M. dubius* appears to parallel the alcoholic fermentation of yeast. Glycogen is broken down by glycolysis to pyruvate, which is decarboxylated to acetaldehyde. The acetaldehyde is reduced to ethanol and this reoxidises the glycolytic NADH. However, the alcohol dehydrogenase of *M. dubius* differs from the enzyme of yeast or mammalian liver in being NADP- rather than NAD-linked. This means that the glyceraldehyde-3-phosphate dehydrogenase reaction, which is NAD-linked, cannot be directly coupled with the reduction of acetaldehyde to ethanol. There may be some form of transhydrogenase, similar to that found in *H. diminuta* (Section 3.1.4) or there could be some alternative form of coupling. A possible alternative scheme for *M. dubius* is shown in *Figure 3.8*. In this scheme, carbon dioxide fixation takes place into phosphoenolpyruvate to give oxaloacetate which is reduced to malate, thus reoxidising the glycolytic NADH. The oxidative decarboxylation of malate to pyruvate by the malic enzyme could then generate NADPH for the alcohol dehydrogenase step. There are high levels of phosphoenolpyruvate carboxykinase in *M. dubius*, but whether malic enzyme also occurs in this parasite is not clear.

Alcohol dehydrogenase is extremely active in the larvae of the nematode *Anisakis* and is also present in *S. brevicaudata*, so it is probable that ethanol is a major product of these parasites as well.

3.1.7. The Pyruvate Kinase/Phosphoenolpyruvate Carboxykinase Ratio

Parasitic helminths can be divided into two broad types, those which fix carbon dioxide and have a partial reversed tricarboxylic acid cycle and those which rely

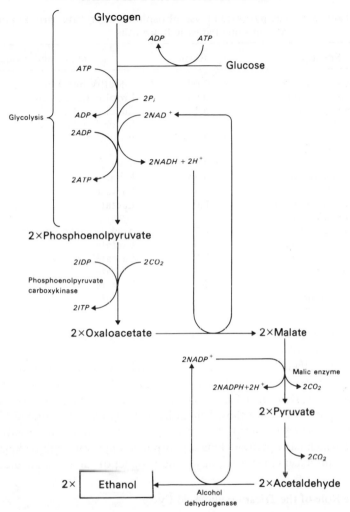

Figure 3.8 Alternative pathway for ethanol production in *Moniliformis dubius* (cytoplasmic).

predominantly on glycolysis. These divisions are not absolute and there is considerable overlap between the two types. There is no correlation between phylogeny and type of metabolism in parasitic helminths, although none of the cestodes are homolactic fermenters. Nor is there any obvious correlation between site of parasitism and type of metabolism, although most intestinal parasites fix carbon dioxide, whilst the majority of homolactic fermenters are blood or tissue parasites.

Most parasitic helminths seem to have the ability both to fix carbon dioxide and to produce lactate. The pyruvate kinase/phosphoenolpyruvate carboxykinase ratio in the different helminths may give an indication as to which is the major pathway *in vivo*, providing both enzymes have been assayed under optimal conditions. Pyruvate kinase and phosphoenolpyruvate carboxykinase are potential regulatory sites (Section 5.1.4), so there may be a switch at the level of phosphoenolpyruvate,

Table 3.5 The pyruvate kinase/phosphoenolpyruvate carboxykinase
ratio in some parasitic helminths

Species	Ratio	Major end-product
Ascaris lumbricoides	0.04	2-Methylbutyrate, 2-methylvalerate
Dicrocoelium dendriticum	0.05	Propionate, acetate
Moniezia expansa	0.1	Succinate, lactate
Hymenolepis diminuta	0.2	Succinate, lactate
Fasciola hepatica	0.25–0.4	Propionate, acetate
Trichinella spiralis		
(larva)	0.3	*n*-Valerate
Moniliformis dubius	0.34	Ethanol
Setaria cervi	0.4	Lactate
Dictyocaulus viviparus	1.0	Lactate
Schistocephalus solidus		
(plerocercoid)	1.7	Acetate, propionate
Nippostrongylus brasiliensis	2.0	Lactate
Litomosoides carinii	2.8	Lactate, acetate
Chandlerella hawkingi	8.5	Lactate
Schistosoma mansoni	5–10	Lactate
Dirofilaria immitis	10.6	Lactate

the relative flux through the alternative pathways depending upon the environment-al and metabolic conditions.

Nevertheless, there is quite a good correlation between the major end-products of carbohydrate metabolism and the pyruvate kinase/phosphoenolpyruvate carboxykinase ratio (*Table 3.5*). Parasites that rely primarily on glycolysis have a ratio in the region of 2–10, whilst those helminths that rely on carbon dioxide fixation have a ratio in the region of 0.1–0.05. An apparent exception is the acanthocephalan *M. dubius*, which has a pyruvate kinase/phosphoenolpyruvate carboxykinase ratio of 0.34, yet produces ethanol as a major end-product of carbohydrate breakdown.

3.1.8. The Role of the Tricarboxylic Acid Cycle

The metabolic pathways so far described in helminths do not involve a classical tricarboxylic acid cycle. Yet all helminths that have been investigated in detail have been found to have a complete sequence of tricarboxylic acid cycle enzymes. However, the levels of aconitase and isocitrate dehydrogenase in parasitic helminths are frequently extremely low. In particular, NAD-linked isocitrate dehydrogenase can often not be detected at all. In mammals, the tricarboxylic acid cycle flux is thought to proceed entirely via the NAD-linked isocitrate dehydrogenase. However, in invertebrates, this may not necessarily be the case, and the NADP-linked dehydrogenase may be involved in the cycle. In parasitic helminths, there is always considerably more NADP-linked isocitrate dehydrogenase than NAD-linked. *Table 3.6* shows the relative activities of the tricarboxylic acid cycle enzymes in *F. hepatica* and *A. lumbricoides* muscle. A similar pattern of enzyme activities occurs in other helminths that are primarily carbon dioxide fixers (*H. diminuta, S. solidus, L. intestinalis, M.*

Table 3.6. The comparative activities of the tricarboxylic acid cycle enzymes
in *Fasciola hepatica* and *Ascaris lumbricoides*

Enzyme	Activity (nmoles/min/mg protein) (at 30 °C)		
	A. lumbricoides	*F. hepatica*	Rat liver
Pyruvate dehydrogenase	32	18	23
Citrate synthase	10	15	25
Aconitase	0.8	5	80
Isocitrate dehydrogenase (NAD$^+$)	0.4	0	1.0
Isocitrate dehydrogenase (NADP$^+$)	5	17	263
2-Oxoglutarate decarboxylase	4	22	18
Succinate dehydrogenase	215	28	21
Fumarase	225	100	432
Malate dehydrogenase	7650	2180	3100

dubius, D. immitis). It is interesting that aconitase and isocitrate dehydrogenase, the
two enzymes that have a very low activity in these helminths, are inducible enzymes
in yeast during the anaerobic/aerobic transition.

The low activity of the enzymes at the beginning of the tricarboxylic acid cycle
in helminths such as *A. lumbricoides* and *F. hepatica* would severely restrict the
capacity of the cycle in these parasites. Studies with labelled glucose and with
metabolic inhibitors indicate that the tricarboxylic acid cycle is not an important
pathway of carbohydrate breakdown in such helminths.

Why, then, is the tricarboxylic acid cycle retained if it is no longer a significant
pathway for carbohydrate catabolism? The reason may lie in the function of the
tricarboxylic acid cycle in providing intermediates for other pathways. In *A. lumbricoides*, for example, reasonable levels of all the tricarboxylic acid cycle intermediates can be detected[21]. So, although it may not function to any significant
extent in carbohydrate catabolism, the tricarboxylic acid cycle in helminths may
still be able to bring about the interconversion of carbon skeletons.

Enzyme Distribution

The intracellular distribution of the tricarboxylic acid cycle enzymes in helminths
is frequently different from that found in rat liver. The significance of these differences is not known, and not enough comparative work has been done with helminths
or other invertebrates for any conclusions to be drawn.

The low levels of aconitase or isocitrate dehydrogenase in many helminths poses
the question as to whether these enzymes are evenly distributed throughout the
tissues. Most enzyme assays involve the use of whole homogenates, so it is not clear
whether there is a low activity throughout the parasite or whether the enzymes are
restricted to specialised tissues, for example nervous tissue, where the levels may
be locally high and a functional cycle possible. Frequently, parasite biochemists
are making conclusions based on the subcellular distribution of an enzyme, when
the gross distribution is not known.

Functional Tricarboxylic Acid Cycles

There has recently been increasing evidence that, under aerobic conditions, some helminths, at least, can catabolise significant amounts of carbohydrates via a functional tricarboxylic acid cycle. The plerocercoids of *S. solidus*[22] may do this, as may the adults of *H. contortus*, and there is some evidence for a functional tricarboxylic acid cycle in three other species of nematode, *A. galli, Neoaplectana glaseri* and *Nematodirus* sp. In the cestode *M. expansa*, Bryant[23] has suggested that there could be separate aerobic and anaerobic mitochondria—the anaerobic mitochondria primarily concerned with the reduction of fumarate, the aerobic ones having a classical tricarboxylic acid cycle. A precedent for this occurs in molluscs, where the cytosomes are thought to be specialised anaerobic mitochondria. The aerobic and anaerobic mitochondria could occur in the same tissue or they might be found in different tissues of the same parasite. The morphological variation in helminth mitochondria has similarly led to the suggestion that there might be specialised carbon dioxide fixing mitochondria in the gut of *A. lumbricoides*.

Tricarboxylic Acid Cycle as a Source of Reducing Power

The tricarboxylic acid cycle could also provide a source of mitochondrial reducing power for the reduction of fumarate to succinate. One way of achieving this (*Figure 3.9*) is by having the first part of the cycle, from pyruvate to succinate, working in the forward direction and the last part of the cycle working in reverse (oxaloacetate to succinate). The oxaloacetate for both sides of the cycle could be derived from the phosphoenolpyruvate carboxykinase reaction and the NADH formed by pyruvate, isocitrate and 2-oxoglutarate dehydrogenase would be re-oxidised by the reduction of fumarate to succinate. Succinate would then be the end-product of both sides of the cycle. In this scheme, oxaloacetate would be produced in the cytoplasm (phosphoenolpyruvate carboxykinase is mostly cytoplasmic in helminths), and so there would have to be some system to transport oxaloacetate into the mitochondrion (probably as malate). There is some evidence that this type of coupling, involving all of the tricarboxylic acid cycle enzymes, can occur in molluscs under anaerobic conditions. However, there is no evidence, as yet, that this system functions in helminths and, in the majority of parasitic helminths that reduce fumarate to succinate, the mitochondrial reducing power is derived from the malic enzyme or possibly the pyruvate dehydrogenase complex.

Relative Importance of the Cycle in Different Helminths

At the moment, it seems that in helminths such as *F. hepatica, M. dubius* and *A. lumbricoides*, which are carbon dioxide fixers, the tricarboxylic acid cycle is not involved in carbohydrate catabolism. The only function of the cycle enzymes in these helminths may be the interconversion of carbon skeletons. In other helminths, such as the plerocercoids of *S. solidus*, adult *H. contortus* and possibly *M. expansa*, there is now increasing evidence that under aerobic conditions some carbohydrate (as much as 75% in *S. solidus*) may be catabolised by a functional tricarboxylic

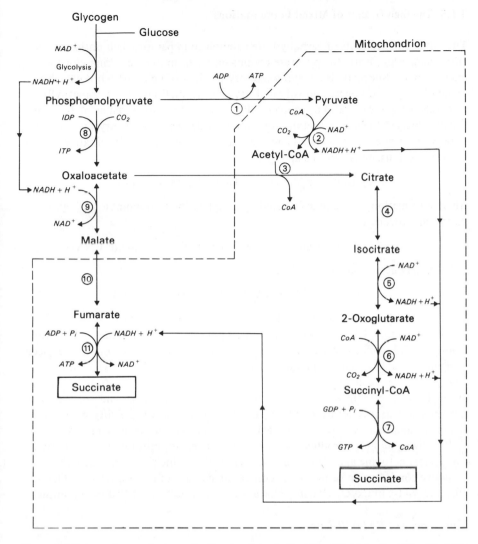

Figure 3.9 Scheme for succinate production involving both sides of the tricarboxylic acid cycle: 1, pyruvate kinase; 2, pyruvate dehydrogenase; 3, citrate synthase; 4, aconitase; 5, isocitrate dehydrogenase; 6, 2-oxoglutarate decarboxylase; 7, succinate thiokinase; 8, phosphoenolpyruvate carboxykinase; 9, malate dehydrogenase; 10, fumarase; 11, fumarate reductase. A variant of this scheme would be to have pyruvate formed from malate via the malic enzyme rather than via pyruvate kinase.

acid cycle. The situation in helminths that rely primarily on glycolysis is less clear. There is no functional tricarboxylic acid cycle in the filarial worms *L. carinii* and *B. pahangi*, but there is some evidence for a functional cycle in the trematode *S. mansoni*. In general, with one or two exceptions, the status of the tricarboxylic acid cycle in parasitic helminths has not been clearly established, and there appear to be considerable differences in the relative importance of the cycle in the overall energy production of different helminths.

3.1.9. The Significance of Mixed Fermentations

The initial end-products of carbohydrate catabolism in parasitic helminths are succinate and/or pyruvate, the pyruvate coming either from pyruvate kinase or the malic enzyme. Succinate is a major excretory product of helminths, but can also be metabolised to propionate and volatile fatty acids (2-methylvalerate, 2-methylbutyrate, valerate and caproate) or propanol. Pyruvate is rarely excreted as such and is usually changed to lactate, acetate, formate, volatile fatty acids (butyrate, caproate, 2-methylbutyrate), acetoin or ethanol. In many invertebrates, an alternative fate for pyruvate is transamination to alanine:

$$\text{pyruvate} + \text{glutamate} \rightleftharpoons \text{alanine} + \text{2-oxoglutarate}$$

Alanine formation can be redox-related by coupling the transaminase with glutamate dehydrogenase:

$$\text{2-oxoglutarate} + NH_3 + NADH + H^+ \rightleftharpoons \text{glutamate} + NAD^+$$

or there may be an alanine dehydrogenase:

$$\text{pyruvate} + NH_3 + NADH + H^+ \rightleftharpoons \text{alanine} + NAD^+$$

The reductive formation of alanine has been described in *A. lumbricoides* and *H. diminuta* (Section 4.4.1). However, alanine is not a major end-product in parasitic helminths, although some alanine is produced by adult *S. mansoni* and it does occur in significant amounts in trematode sporocysts (Section 3.1.13). In view of the wide occurrence of alanine as an anaerobic end-product of carbohydrate breakdown in free-living invertebrates (it occurs in insects, annelids, molluscs and crustacea), it is surprising that it is not excreted by parasitic helminths. A possibility is that alanine production has not, in fact, been extensively looked for in parasites.

Free-living molluscs produce two other derivatives of pyruvate under anaerobic conditions: octopine and N-(1-carboxyethyl)alanine, which are formed by the reductive condensation of pyruvate with arginine and alanine, respectively. Octopine and N-(1-carboxyethyl)alanine have, so far, not been identified in helminths.

Maintenance of Redox Balance

The production, by parasitic helminths, of reduced end-products can be correlated with the need to maintain a suitable redox state within the tissues. The NADH formed during glycolysis is coupled to the reduction of pyruvate to lactate or of oxaloacetate to malate. In helminths that fix carbon dioxide, the oxidation, within the mitochondrion, of malate to pyruvate or of pyruvate to acetate is coupled with the reduction of fumarate to succinate. In addition to these major catabolic pathways, there are other metabolic processes which either produce or utilise reducing equivalents. The synthesis of the branched chain fatty acids 2-methylbutyrate and 2-methylvalerate requires extra reducing equivalents, as does the formation of alcohols. The catabolism of amino acids, in general, generates reducing equivalents, as does the pentose phosphate pathway and (if present) the tricarboxylic acid cycle.

In the presence of oxygen, many, if not all, parasitic helminths may be able to oxidise at least part of their NADH via their cytochrome chains (Section 3.2). In addition, synthetic reactions both require and produce reducing equivalents, the overall balance being towards a net production of reducing power. The parasitic helminth must be able to accommodate these changes in the production and utilisation of reducing equivalents due to changes in the internal and external conditions. This can be done, most easily, by quantitatively and qualitatively altering the nature of the end-products produced from the breakdown of carbohydrate. When synthetic activity is high, or oxygen not available, the proportions of the more reduced end-products could be increased; when synthetic activity was low, or oxygen available, more oxidised end-products would predominate.

Different catabolic end-products are formed in different cellular compartments; lactate and ethanol are cytoplasmic end-products, succinate and volatile fatty acids are mitochondrial end-products. Differences in the redox needs between the cytoplasm and the mitochondria will also be reflected in differences in the proportions of the cytoplasmic and mitochondrial end-products.

The need to maintain a favourable redox balance in the tissues under various conditions may explain why the end-products of carbohydrate catabolism produced by parasitic helminths vary so much. There are almost always differences between the aerobic and anaerobic end-products, and varying physiological conditions would account for many of the discrepancies found in the literature.

In certain helminths (*F. hepatica, S. solidus, E. granulosus*), the addition of glucose to the incubation medium causes an increase in lactate production. This may represent an 'overflow metabolism'. These helminths all fix carbon dioxide and the phosphoenolpyruvate carboxykinase step may be rate-limiting. When excess glucose is present, phosphoenolpyruvate would tend to accumulate and so 'overflow' into lactate production. Similarly, acetate excretion by parasites could provide a means of relieving 'acetate pressure', acetyl-CoA tending to accumulate because of the high glycolytic capacity of helminths compared with the limited tricarboxylic acid cycle capacity. So, altering the excretory acids may not only help to balance the redox couples in helminth tissues, it may also help to balance the fluxes through the different catabolic pathways.

Minor Excretory Acids

As well as the major excretory acids, most helminths excrete a variety of minor products. These may represent intermediates from the synthesis of the major excretory acids or they may be the result of side reactions of these intermediates. Minor excretory acids can also, at least in some cases, result from the breakdown of amino acids or, alternatively, they may represent end-products of metabolism from certain specialised tissues.

Neutral End-products

Analysis of end-products in helminths has tended to concentrate on the acidic end-products, and neutral compounds, such as alcohols, have not been extensively investigated. Acetoin is excreted by *L. carinii*, *S. cervi* and *A. lumbricoides*. Ethanol is a major end-product in the acanthocephalan *M. dubius* and, possibly, in larval *Anisakis*. Propanol is an important end-product in *H. contortus* and mixtures of 3-pentanol and 3-pentanone have been found in *Terranova decipiens*[24]. Small amounts of ethanol are also produced by *H. contortus* and ethanol is found as a minor excretory component of several cestodes. In the free-living nematodes *Aphelenchus avenae* and *Caenorhabditis elegans*, ethanol is the major end-product of glycolysis under anaerobic conditions, and in the free-living nematode *Panagrellus redivivus* the alcohol metabolising pathway appears to be inducible. When incubated with acetate, the free-living nematode *Caenorhabditis briggsae* excretes a variety of acidic and neutral end-products, including glycerol, but there is no evidence that glycerol is a normal excretory product.

The pathways of alcohol production in helminths have not been investigated in detail, but the production of alcohols rather than acids by helminths would reoxidise more NADH.

Advantages of Organic Acid Production

In addition to giving the parasite an increased flexibility in balancing its redox couples, the production of organic acids by helminths may have a number of other advantages.

First, parasites that fix carbon dioxide utilise part of the tricarboxylic acid cycle. The retention of at least part of the cycle may be significant since, as mentioned earlier (Section 3.1.8), in addition to its role in energy metabolism, the cycle is also involved in the interconversion of carbon skeletons.

Another advantage of volatile fatty acid production is that fatty acids have a lower dissociation constant than lactate or succinate:

lactate, $K_a = 1.4 \times 10^{-4}$ 2-methylvalerate, $K_a = 1 \times 10^{-5}$

succinate, $K_{a_1} = 6.6 \times 10^{-5}$ 2-methylbutyrate, $K_a = 1 \times 10^{-5}$

The volatile acids are weaker acids and, therefore, much less irritating to the tissues of the host (and the parasite) than lactate or succinate. Interestingly, parasites that produce primarily acetate and lactate are usually blood or tissue parasites, these being the regions where lactate accumulation occurs naturally so the host is better able to cope.

The production of large amounts of organic acids by helminths nevertheless poses pH problems for the parasite. Although fatty acids have a lower K_a than lactate or succinate, high concentrations of fatty acids disrupt mitochondrial function. The production of alcohols avoids the pH problem, but high concentrations of alcohols also disrupt cell membranes. It is not really known how helminths cope with the problem of the toxicity of the end-products that they produce. Calcareous corpuscles (Section 2.1) have been implicated in pH buffering, but there are no data as to whether helminth tissues have an exceptionally high buffering capacity or not (Section 3.2.10). Probably a major factor is the rapid removal and detoxification of helminth end-products by the host.

Under anaerobic conditions, free-living organisms tend to store their metabolic end-products, and when oxygen is again available either catabolise their end-products completely or else resynthesise them. There is then, usually, a post-anaerobic increase in oxygen consumption (oxygen debt) in free-living organisms, whilst the accumulated end-products are being metabolised. In contrast, parasitic helminths excrete the end-products of carbohydrate breakdown and in this way avoid accumu-lating an appreciable oxygen debt. Also, by excreting the end-products of carbohy-drate breakdown, helminths may be able to produce a wider range of end-products. Free-living organisms have to be able to metabolise their anaerobic end-products when oxygen once more becomes available. These animals must then avoid meta-bolic 'dead ends', that is, end-products which cannot be further metabolised. Helminths, which excrete their end-products, do not have this restriction. Many of the end-products of carbohydrate metabolism produced by parasitic helminths can, of course, be absorbed by the host and further metabolised, giving rise to a complex host/parasite system.

Production of ATP

A final advantage of organic acid production in parasitic helminths is that it may increase the yield of ATP per mole of glucose catabolised. Glycolysis (homolactic fermentation or ethanol production) gives a net production of 2 moles of ATP per mole of glucose (4 moles of ATP are actually produced, but two are used up, one in the hexokinase reaction, the other in the phosphofructokinase step). If glycogen is the substrate for glycolysis, the yield is 3 moles of ATP per hexose unit, no ATP being needed for the phosphorylase step. In parasitic helminths, the reduction of fumarate to succinate is an energy-yielding step. So, in parasites such as *A. lumbri coides* that fix carbon dioxide, the ATP yield per mole of glucose is increased to 3 (4 per hexose unit if glycogen is the substrate). The helminth system involving carbon dioxide fixation and a partial reversed tricarboxylic acid cycle is more efficient in terms of ATP per hexose unit catabolised than vertebrate muscle under anaerobic conditions (anaerobically vertebrate muscle produces lactate). Although the ATP yield of the helminth system per mole of hexose is very small when compared to the complete oxidation of glucose via glycolysis and the tricar-boxylic acid cycle, which gives 39 moles of ATP per hexose unit (with glycogen as the substrate). However, if efficiency is defined as energy trapped as ATP per free-energy change (i.e. difference in free energy between substrates and products), the different pathways, i.e. glycolysis, tricarboxylic acid cycle, and succinate produc-tion, are all about 40% efficient.

The decarboxylation of succinate and pyruvate in parasitic helminths are also potential energy-yielding steps, since the products of decarboxylation, i.e. propionyl-CoA and acetyl-CoA, are both high-energy compounds. In bacteria, the cleavage of CoA compounds is coupled to ATP production via phosphotrans-acetylase and acetate kinase:

$$\text{acetyl-CoA} + P_i \rightleftharpoons \text{acetyl} \sim P + \text{CoA} \qquad phosphotransacetylase$$

$$\text{acetyl} \sim P + \text{ADP} \rightarrow \text{acetate} + \text{ATP} \qquad acetate\ kinase$$

This system has, however, not been demonstrated in helminths. So far, the only helminth in which acetate and propionate production has been studied is *F. hepatica* (Section 3.1.4) and here the cleavage of acetyl-CoA or propionyl-CoA involves either a carnitine-dependent hydrolase:

$$\text{acetyl-CoA} + \text{carnitine} \rightleftharpoons \text{acetylcarnitine} + \text{CoA}$$

$$\text{acetylcarnitine} + H_2O \rightarrow \text{carnitine} + \text{acetate}$$

or a CoA transferase:

$$\text{acetyl-CoA} + \text{acceptor} \rightleftharpoons \text{acceptor-CoA} + \text{acetate}$$

Neither of these two mechanisms results in ATP production. The decarboxylation of succinate to propionyl-CoA does result in ATP production (from the propionyl-CoA carboxylase reaction, *Figure 3.7*), but this is not a net synthesis since ATP or GTP is required to synthesise succinyl-CoA from succinate at the start of the pathway. However, it is possible to get a net production of ATP from the cleavage of acetyl-CoA or propionyl-CoA by coupling the CoA transferase reaction with the synthesis of succinyl-CoA:

$$\text{acetyl-CoA} + \text{succinate} \rightleftharpoons \text{succinyl-CoA} + \text{acetate}$$

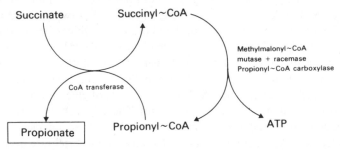

Figure 3.10 Propionate-CoA transferase system in *Fasciola hepatica*.

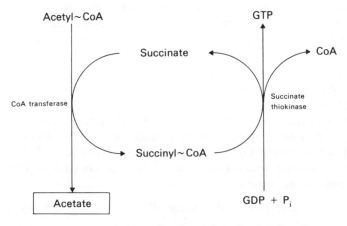

Figure 3.11 Acetate-CoA transferase system in *Fasciola hepatica*.

'There are two ways in which this could be done. The first (*Figure 3.10*) gives a cyclic system for the conversion of succinate to propionate and there is a net production of ATP from the propionyl-CoA carboxylase step. In the second scheme (*Figure 3.11*), CoA transferase is linked to succinate to give succinyl-CoA and GTP is formed by the reversal of succinic thiokinase. There is evidence that both of these systems occur in *F. hepatica*[11,12,13,66].

Tissue Differences in End-product Formation

The pattern of end-products from carbohydrate breakdown in helminths may be complicated by different tissues of the parasite producing different end-products. Different regions of the cestode *H. diminuta* produce lactate, succinate and acetate in different proportions[25], and in the nematode *A. lumbricoides* it has been shown that, whilst the muscle tissue produces volatile fatty acids, the reproductive tissue does not. One reason why helminths continue to produce organic acids even when they are under aerobic conditions could be because the deeper tissues remain anaerobic.

In free-living invertebrates, under anaerobic conditions, the nature of the end-products has been found to vary with the length of the incubation time and with the age and sex of the individual. The same factors probably also apply to helminths and in *A. galli*, for instance, acetate is produced by young adults and propionate by older adults[26].

In almost all biochemical studies with parasitic helminths, analysis of end-products or carbon balance studies have been performed on entire animals and enzyme assays have used whole homogenates. It is only in the case of the few very large helminths, such as *A. lumbricoides*, that isolated tissues have been used. Studies using whole parasites or whole homogenates measure the total metabolic capabilities of the parasite, but such methods do not show the differences in metabolism between different tissues, nor do they show how the different tissues interrelate. All parasitic helminths have some sort of circulatory system, either in the form of a pseudocoelom or excretory canals. It is quite probable that, in helminths, not only do different tissues produce different end-products (indicating differences in metabolism) but that the end-products of one tissue can be metabolised by another. In *A. lumbricoides*, for example, succinate produced by the reproductive organs may be metabolised to volatile fatty acids by the muscle tissue; and, in *M. expansa*, it has been postulated that malate may act as an intermediate between tissues[23]. Like mammals where, for example, lactate produced in the muscles is resynthesised to carbohydrate in the liver, so in helminths (and invertebrates generally) there is biochemical specialisation of tissues. So, when considering the overall metabolism of helminths, it must be remembered that this is the overall result of the integrated activities of biochemically heterogeneous tissues.

3.1.10. Catabolism of Hexoses Other than Glucose

Helminths are usually able to phosphorylate a variety of hexoses. In many helminths, the hexokinase, like the hexokinase of mammals, is relatively non-specific. In *A*.

lumbricoides and *H. contortus*, the hexokinase phosphorylates both glucose and fructose. In addition to these two sugars, the enzyme from *D. immitis* phosphorylates mannose and glucosamine, whilst the enzyme from *L. carinii* and *C. hawkingi* can also phosphorylate mannose and galactose. In *F. hepatica*, the hexokinase will phosphorylate glucose, fructose, galactose, mannose and glucosamine. In contrast, in *S. mansoni* and in *E. granulosus* (scoleces), there appear to be separate kinases for glucose, fructose, mannose and glucosamine, these kinases phosphorylating the sugars in the 6 position. There may also be a separate glucokinase, mannokinase and galactokinase in *A. galli*. In *H. diminuta*, the hexokinase can phosphorylate glucose, fructose and mannose, and there is a specific galactokinase which phosphorylates galactose in the 1 position:

$$galactose + ATP \rightarrow galactose\text{-}1\text{-}P + ADP$$

Entry into Glycolysis

Fructose-6-phosphate can enter the glycolytic sequence directly (*Figure 3.1*). The fructokinase of mammalian liver, unlike the fructokinases of *S. mansoni* and *E. granulosus*, phosphorylates fructose in the 1 position, and mammals have a special fructose-1-P aldolase which splits fructose-1-P into D-glyceraldehyde and dihydroxyacetone phosphate.

Mannose-6-phosphate can be converted to fructose-6-phosphate by mannose-phosphate isomerase:

$$mannose\text{-}6\text{-}P \rightleftharpoons fructose\text{-}6\text{-}P$$

and this enzyme has been shown in *A. lumbricoides, A. galli* and *H. contortus*. The conversion of galactose-1-phosphate to glucose-1-phosphate involves initially the formation of UDP-galactose. In mammals, there are two pathways for UDP-galactose formation. In adults it involves UTP: galactose-1-phosphate uridylyl transferase:

$$galactose\text{-}1\text{-}P + UTP \rightleftharpoons UDP\text{-}galactose + PP_i$$

The second pathway, which is found in infants, uses the enzyme UDP-glucose: galactose-1-phosphate uridylyl transferase:

$$galactose\text{-}1\text{-}P + UDP\text{-}glucose \rightleftharpoons UDP\text{-}galactose + glucose\text{-}1\text{-}P$$

The UDP-galactose is then converted to UDP-glucose by UDP-glucose-4-epimerase, an enzyme which has an absolute requirement for NAD:

$$UDP\text{-}galactose \underset{}{\overset{NAD}{\rightleftharpoons}} UDP\text{-}glucose$$

UDP-glucose can be used directly for synthetic reactions or be converted to glucose-1-P and so enter glycolysis. All of the enzymes necessary to convert galactose to glucose via the second pathway (galactokinase, UDP-glucose : galactose-1-phosphate uridylyl transferase, UDP-glucose-4-epimerase) are present in *H. diminuta*[27]. The activities of these enzymes in *H. diminuta* are relatively low and this probably accounts for the inability of galactose completely to replace glucose as an energy source in this tapeworm. In addition to *H. diminuta*, there is indirect evidence that *T. taeniaeformis*, *F. hepatica* and *A. galli* can all convert galactose to glucose.

Sorbitol Metabolism

The sorbitol pathway converts glucose to fructose:

$$\text{glucose} + \text{NADPH} + \text{H}^+ \rightleftharpoons \text{sorbitol} + \text{NADP}^+ \qquad \textit{sorbitol dehydrogenase}$$

$$\text{sorbitol} + \text{NAD}^+ \rightleftharpoons \text{fructose} + \text{NADH} + \text{H}^+ \qquad \textit{aldose reductase}$$

In mammals, sorbitol is a tissue-specific metabolite for sperm and, possibly, also for the foetus. Sorbitol dehydrogenase has been detected in larval *P. decipiens* and low levels of both sorbitol dehydrogenase and aldose reductase occur in *A. lumbricoides* muscle[28,29], although the possible functions of the pathway in parasites are obscure.

3.1.11. Rate of Carbohydrate Catabolism in Parasitic Helminths

The glycolytic capacity of parasitic helminths is surprisingly high. The maximum glycolytic capacity of *A. lumbricoides* muscle is of the order of 10 μmoles of C_6 unit per minute per gram of fresh tissue[30], which is similar to values reported for cephalopod and crustacean muscles and to the glycolytic capacity of mammalian red muscle. The high glycolytic capacity of helminths may be related to the low ATP production per mole of hexose catabolised, the low efficiency being compensated for by a high flux rate.

The observed rates of carbohydrate utilisation in helminths (obtained from *in vitro* incubations) are usually much lower than the maximum capacity of the glycolytic enzymes. In *A. lumbricoides*, the observed rate of glycogen utilisation for the whole parasite is only about 0.05 μmoles of C_6 unit/min/g fresh weight. How far the *in vitro* rates apply *in vivo* is, however, open to question.

3.1.12. The Pentose Phosphate Pathway

The pentose phosphate pathway (*Figure 3.12*) can carry out the complete oxidation of glucose, according to the equation:

$$\text{glucose-6-P} + 12\text{NADP}^+ + 7\text{H}_2\text{O} \rightarrow 6\text{CO}_2 + 12\text{NADPH} + 12\text{H}^+ + \text{P}_i$$

The pentose phosphate pathway is not a major pathway for obtaining energy from glucose; it is a multifunctional sequence whose main role is to provide NADPH and pentoses (in particular, D-ribose-5-phosphate) for synthetic reactions. The pentose phosphate pathway also functions in the degradation of pentoses by converting them to hexoses, which can then enter the glycolytic pathway.

A complete sequence of pentose phosphate pathway enzymes has been demonstrated in *A. lumbricoides*, *E. granulosus* and the acanthocephalans *M. hirudinaceus* and *Neoechinorhynchus* sp.[31,32]; the first two enzymes of the cycle, glucose-6-

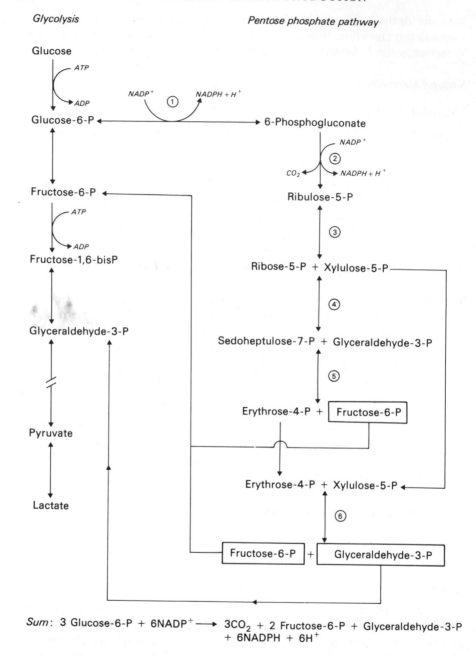

Sum: 3 Glucose-6-P + 6NADP$^+$ ⟶ 3CO$_2$ + 2 Fructose-6-P + Glyceraldehyde-3-P
                                                        + 6NADPH + 6H$^+$

Figure 3.12 Simplified diagram of the pentose phosphate pathway: 1, glucose-6-phosphate dehydrogenase; 2, 6-phosphogluconate dehydrogenase; 3, ribose-5-phosphate ketoisomerase + ribulose-5-phosphate epimerase; 4, transketolase; 5, transaldolase; 6, transketolase.

phosphate dehydrogenase and 6-phosphogluconate dehydrogenase have been demonstrated in a wide variety of adult and larval helminths.

The relative importance of the pentose phosphate pathway in a tissue can be assessed by measuring the differing rates of $^{14}CO_2$ production when the tissue is incubated with glucose-1-^{14}C and glucose-6-^{14}C. This has been done in *A. lumbricoides* and *F. hepatica*, and in both cases only about 10% of the carbohydrate catabolised goes via the pentose phosphate pathway. Experiments with $^{14}CO_2$ fixation in *H. diminuta* and *E. granulosus* also suggest that the pentose phosphate pathway plays only a minor role in carbohydrate breakdown. These results are similar to those obtained with mammalian tissues where, again, the pentose phosphate pathway only accounts for about 10% of the carbohydrate catabolised.

The presence of glucose-6-phosphate dehydrogenase and 6-phosphogluconate dehydrogenase in helminths is usually taken as evidence for a functional pentose phosphate pathway. However, in mammalian tissue, during active nucleic acid synthesis the pentose phosphate pathway can end at this point:

$$\text{glucose-6-P} + 2NADP^+ + 2H_2O \rightarrow \text{D-ribose-5-P} + 2NADPH + 2H^+ + CO_2$$

D-ribose-5-phosphate being used for nucleic acid synthesis. So the presence of the two starting enzymes of the pentose phosphate pathway in helminths does not necessarily mean that there is a complete cycle.

3.1.13. Carbohydrate Catabolism in the Free-living and Intermediate Stages of Helminths

In contrast to the adult, the metabolism of the free-living and intermediate stages of helminths has been little investigated.

Nematodes

The free-living larvae of nematodes appear to be aerobic and have a normal glycolytic sequence and functional tricarboxylic acid cycle.

The developing eggs of *A. lumbricoides* also have a complete glycolytic sequence and functional tricarboxylic acid cycle. Both trehalose and glycogen are extensively used during the early stages of development of *A. lumbricoides* eggs. Lipid metabolism then becomes more important and carbohydrate utilisation almost ceases (*Figure 3.13*). As the larva develops in the egg, the carbohydrate reserves which were being depleted during the first ten days of development are resynthesised from triacylglycerol (Section 4.2.1). The fully developed egg of *A. lumbricoides* is dormant, and so infection of the final host also involves activation of the dormant stage (Section 5.2.6).

The enzyme profile in the fully developed infective nematode larva often differs from that of the earlier free-living stages and may, to a limited extent, resemble the enzyme pattern of the adult. The infective larva of *H. contortus*, for example, has a functional tricarboxylic acid cycle, but can fix carbon dioxide and has a fumarate

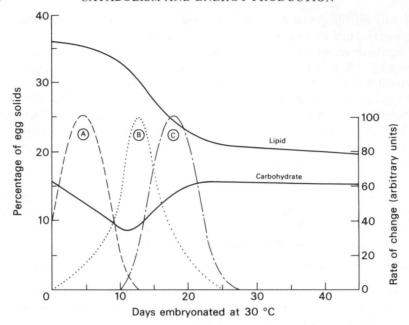

Figure 3.13 Lipid and carbohydrate changes in developing *Ascaris lumbricoides* eggs: A, rate of carbohydrate utilisation; B, rate of lipid utilisation; C, rate of carbohydrate resynthesis.

reductase. So the infective stages of nematodes may be able to carry out at least some of the anaerobic fermentations found in the adult parasite.

Trematodes

The free-living miracidia and cercariae of trematodes appear to be largely aerobic, although they may be able to survive anaerobically for varying periods of time. There is evidence for a glycolytic sequence and a functional tricarboxylic acid cycle and cytochrome chain in the miracidia and cercariae of *F. hepatica* and *S. mansoni*. Anaerobically, the cercariae of *S. mansoni* are homolactic fermenters, like the adult.

The metabolism of the intramolluscan stages of trematodes (sporocysts and rediae) may be different from that of the free-living stages and to a certain extent resembles that of adult trematodes. The sporocysts of *S. mansoni* use oxygen, but produce lactate; the sporocysts of *Microphallus similis* have a glycolytic sequence and tricarboxylic acid cycle, but are facultative anaerobes, producing lactate, alanine and succinate.

Cestodes

The larval stages of cestodes are found in a variety of environments, some stages are free-living, whilst others occur in arthropods or in the tissues of warm- and cold-blooded vertebrates. Larval cestodes from vertebrates (plerocercoids, cysticerci, tetrathyridia) have metabolic pathways similar to those of adult tapeworms and are described above. The free-swimming coracidia of Pseudophyllideans appear, like trematode miracidia, to be essentially aerobic and use glycogen as their energy source, although there are reports that coracidia use glycolysis only. The cysticercoids and onchospheres of the Cyclophyllidean tapeworm *H. diminuta* also contain glycogen and are probably aerobic.

Acanthocephalans

There has been very little work on the intermediary metabolism of larval acanthocephalans. Glycogen is the main energy reserve in larval acanthocephalans, and in the cystacanths of *M. dubius* carbon dioxide fixation seems to play a significant role.

3.2. TERMINAL OXIDATION

Despite the major pathways of carbohydrate catabolism being essentially anaerobic in parasitic helminths, all of the species so far studied use oxygen when it is available; that is, at least *in vitro*, they have a measurable oxygen consumption. Furthermore, the presence of oxygen usually leads to quantitative and qualitative changes in the end-products of carbohydrate catabolism (Section 3.1). Part of the oxygen uptake in helminths may, of course, be related to synthetic reactions and not be concerned with energy metabolism at all. However, the fact that the presence of oxygen frequently alters the nature of the end-products of carbohydrate breakdown indicates that oxygen does, in fact, affect the metabolic balance of the parasite.

The problem can be posed in three parts. First, what is the mechanism of oxygen uptake in parasitic helminths? Secondly, is the uptake of oxygen accompanied by the formation of ATP? And, finally, if oxidative phosphorylation does occur in parasitic helminths, what is its contribution to the overall energy balance of the parasite?

Looking first at the most extensively studied helminths, such as *A. lumbricoides*, *F. hepatica* and *M. expansa*, it is found that the uptake of oxygen by these parasites shows a number of peculiar characteristics. They are all oxygen conformers, that is, the rate of oxygen uptake is dependent on the partial pressure. In *A. lumbricoides*, the intact worm, muscle minces and subcellular fractions are all oxygen conformers, suggesting that the oxygen dependency is due to the nature of the terminal oxidase, rather than to the limitations of oxygen diffusion. Flavine oxidases (such as glucose oxidase and the yellow enzyme) have a low affinity for oxygen and show oxygen dependency. The low affinity of flavine oxidases for oxygen, however, makes it unlikely that they will act as terminal oxidases. The oxygen dependency of helminths can be interpreted as showing that it is the rate of oxidation of the terminal oxidase that is rate-limiting, rather than the rate of reduction of the terminal oxidase. The second peculiarity of these helminths is that oxygen uptake is largely cyanide-insensitive and in some helminths (*A. lumbricoides*, *H. contortus*, the larvae of *D. viviparus*, *F. hepatica*, *Paramphistomum cervi* and *M. expansa*) cyanide may even stimulate oxygen uptake. Finally, when substrates are oxidised by these helminths, hydrogen peroxide is formed.

3.2.1. Cytochrome Chains

The three characteristics, i.e. oxygen dependency, lack of inhibition by cyanide and hydrogen peroxide production, would suggest the presence of flavoprotein oxidases. However, the work of Cheah[33,34] has shown that these large intestinal helminths all possess a functional cytochrome system and that the cytochromes can account for the observed rates of oxygen consumption. The cytochrome chains of these parasites, however, differ from those of mammals (*Figure 3.14*) in that there are multiple terminal oxidases.

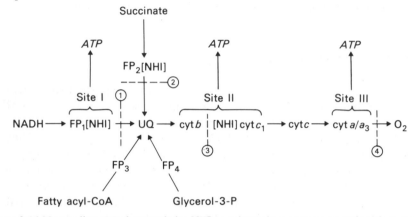

Figure 3.14 Mammalian cytochrome chain: NHI, non-haem iron centres, exact location uncertain; FP, flavoproteins; UQ, ubiquinone; cyt b, there are two b cytochromes in the mammalian chain, $b_{K'}$ and $b_{T'}$, and the relationship of these two cytochromes to one another is uncertain. A b-type cytochrome was at one time thought to be associated with the succinate dehydrogenase complex (FP_2), but this is now thought not to be the case. 1, rotenone, amytal (barbiturate), piericidin A; 2, thenoyltrifluoroacetone; 3, antimycin A; 4, cyanide, azide, CO, H_2S.

Branched Cytochrome Chains

In *A. lumbricoides* (*Figure 3.15*), the cytochrome chain has two branches. One branch is similar to the classical mammalian system involving cytochromes b, c_1, c and with cytochrome a/a_3 as the terminal oxidase. The alternative pathway branches at the level of the quinone/cytochrome b complex, and the terminal oxidase for this branch is an o-type cytochrome. Cytochrome o is an autoxidisable b-type cytochrome which is also found in micro-organisms, rumen protozoa and plants. Quantitatively, the alternative pathway to cytochrome o is the major pathway in *A. lumbricoides*, whilst the classical part of the chain only contributes about 30% of the oxidase activity. The concentration of cytochrome a/a_3 in *A. lumbricoides* muscle mitochondria is about one-tenth of that in ox neck muscle mitochondria, whilst the total cytochrome concentration in *A. lumbricoides* muscle mitochondria is approximately one-half of that of ox neck muscle mitochondria. So, the concentration of cytochromes in *A. lumbricoides* muscle mitochondria is considerably less than in mammalian muscle mitochondria and the cytochrome concentration expressed per gram of muscle is probably less again.

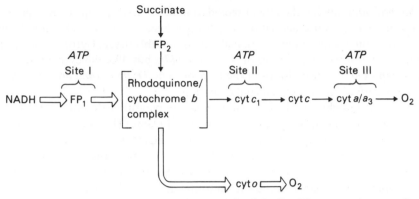

Figure 3.15 Proposed cytochrome system in *Ascaris lumbricoides*. There are at least two flavo-protein components associated with the chain and cytochrome b_{560} is now thought to be part of the chain.

The details of the branch point in the *A. lumbricoides* cytochrome chain are not clear. There is, probably, at least one *b* cytochrome associated with the branch to cytochrome *o*, but whether the branch connects to the quinone or the *b* cytochrome of the classical chain is unknown. The most likely branch point is at the level of the quinone. In *A. lumbricoides*, the alternative pathway to cytochrome *o* is specifically inhibited by *O*-hydroxydiphenyl but is insensitive to low concentrations of anti-mycin A or cyanide.

The cytochrome chains of *M. expansa* mitochondria are very similar to those of *A. lumbricoides*. In *M. expansa*, there is again a branched chain, one of which is a classical chain with cytochrome a/a_3 as the terminal oxidase, the other chain having cytochrome *o*. The classical chain constitutes about 20% of the oxidase capacity and, as in *A. lumbricoides*, cytochrome *o* is quantitatively the major oxidase. The alternative chain in *M. expansa* branches from the classical chain at the level of the quinone/cytochrome *b* complex. In both *M. expansa* and *A. lumbricoides*, the quinone component of the cytochrome chain is not ubiquinone (CoQ) as in mam-mals but rhodoquinone (Section 2.3.7). Rhodoquinone has been found in a number of other helminths; it is the only quinone in adult *Stephanurus dentatus* and *Ascaridia dissimilis* and both rhodoquinone and ubiquinone occur in the larvae of *H. contortus, S. dentatus, Trichostrongylus axei, T. spiralis* and in the adults of *Oesophagostomum radiatum, H. gallinae, H. contortus* and *S. trachea*. Rhodoquin-one has also been isolated from *H. diminuta*.

In addition to *A. lumbricoides* and *M. expansa*, there is evidence for branched cytochrome chains in *F. hepatica, H. contortus, M. apri, A. caninum, T. hydatigena, T. taeniaeformis* and *M. dubius*. In *F. hepatica*, there is a classical cytochrome chain and a branch with cytochrome *o* as the terminal oxidase[35]. There are at least two *b*-type cytochromes involved and the concentration of cytochromes in *F. hepatica* mitochondria is very similar to that in *A. lumbricoides*.

In helminths with branched cytochrome chains, there may be other terminal oxidases in addition to cytochromes *o* and a/a_3, and the possibility of terminal flavoprotein oxidases also being present cannot be entirely ruled out. However, in

A. lumbricoides muscle, the rate of reoxidation of reduced flavoprotein is about a thousand times slower than that of cytochromes *b* and *c*, so this makes it unlikely that flavoproteins are acting as terminal oxidases in this tissue. Cytochrome a_1 has been found in some preparations of *A. lumbricoides* but, like the cytochrome *d* (a_2) reported in culture forms of the trypanosome *Trypanosoma brucei*, it is probably derived from bacterial contamination.

Branched cytochrome chains are not unique to parasitic helminths but occur widely in micro-organisms, parasitic protozoa and plants. The development of multiple terminal oxidases in bacteria is often associated with low partial pressures of oxygen. Whether the multiple terminal oxidases in helminths are likewise related to the low environmental oxygen levels and whether the different terminal oxidases in helminths are inducible, as they are in bacteria, are not known.

Hydrogen Peroxide Formation

When cytochrome *o* reacts with oxygen, hydrogen peroxide is formed, although this may not be the only product (water may be formed as well). So, cytochrome *o* rather than flavoprotein oxidases may be the source of hydrogen peroxide in helminths. The production of hydrogen peroxide by parasitic helminths such as *A. lumbricoides* and *F. hepatica* might also be an artefact of the assay systems used. Under hyperbaric conditions, mammalian mitochondria produce hydrogen peroxide during substrate oxidation, the site of hydrogen peroxide formation being at the level of the *b* cytochromes. Oxygen uptake experiments on helminth mitochondria are usually performed in air, where the partial pressure of oxygen is much higher than *in vivo*; a situation for the helminth mitochondria analogous to hyperbaric conditions for mammalian mitochondria. So, whether significant quantities of hydrogen peroxide are produced *in vivo* by *A. lumbricoides* and other helminths, which live in low oxygen environments, has yet to be shown.

The cestode *T. taeniaeformis* differs from *A. lumbricoides*, *F. hepatica* and *M. expansa* in that the oxidation of substrate (glycerol-3-phosphate) does not result in hydrogen peroxide formation. The failure to detect hydrogen peroxide in this helminth could be due to an active catalase or perhaps, less likely, to the presence of a different terminal oxidase system.

Cyanide-insensitive Respiration

Cytochrome *o* binds cyanide much less strongly than cytochrome a/a_3 and so it is tempting to equate cyanide-insensitive respiration with the alternative pathway. Cyanide-insensitive respiration is also found in some protozoa, plants and micro-organisms and these also contain *o*-type cytochromes. However, in plants and micro-organisms there is growing evidence that cyanide-insensitive respiration is mediated via a non-haem iron component and not via the *o*-type cytochrome.

There is also, at present, no satisfactory explanation for the stimulation of oxygen uptake in certain helminths by cyanide. The alternative branch of the cytochrome chain may well be the cyanide-insensitive pathway, but whether cytochrome *o* or a non-haem iron component is the cyanide-insensitive oxidase is not certain. Cyanide stimulation may be due to the removal of inhibition of the flavoprotein enzymes by virtue of cyanide's carbonyl-combining or metal-chelating properties, or the cyanochromagens may have a more favourable redox potential for oxidation. In mammalian systems, cyanide has been found to stabilise succinic dehydrogenase in its active configuration. Another possible explanation for the action of cyanide, analogous to the stimulation of glycolysis by cyanide, is that if the classical cytochrome chain is blocked, ATP production will be reduced, and so, to compensate for this, the flux through the alternative oxidase will be increased.

Cyanide-stimulated respiration could also be, in part, an artefact. Catalase is inhibited by cyanide, and this would stop hydrogen peroxide breakdown and so prevent oxygen being returned to the system. The overall rate of oxygen uptake would, therefore, appear to increase. However, helminths normally contain very little catalase (Section 3.2.8).

Non-haem Iron Components

Evidence for the involvement of non-haem iron components in the cytochrome chains of helminths comes from inhibitor and electron paramagnetic resonance studies on *T. taeniaeformis, H. microstoma* and *H. diminuta* and, to a lesser extent, from spectroscopic studies on *M. expansa*. The location of the non-haem iron components within the cytochrome chains of helminths is, at present, not known.

Parallel Cytochrome Chains

The cytochrome chains in intestinal helminths have been described as being branched, but the results obtained could equally well be explained by two parallel cytochrome chains, one the classical chain, the other with cytochrome *o* as the terminal oxidase. These two chains might or might not be functionally linked (for example, at the level of the quinone). At present, it has not been possible experimentally to distinguish between the two possibilities, i.e. branched chains or parallel chains, although opinion tends to favour the branched chain model. The possibility of parallel chains would, however, become important if the two different chains were in fact spatially separated in different mitochondria.

Unbranched Cytochrome Chains

Not all parasitic helminths have a branched cytochrome chain and the adults of *S. mansoni* and *Metastrongylus elongatus* have an unbranched mammalian-type chain. The larvae of *T. spiralis* are similarly thought to have a mammalian-type cytochrome chain, but *o*-type cytochromes have also been reported to be present[36,67]. In *T. spiralis* larvae, oxygen uptake is independent of the partial pressure, and there is also an unconfirmed report that carbon monoxide, instead of inhibiting the respiration of *T. spiralis* larvae, stimulates it. This stimulation of respiration may be analogous to the stimulation of respiration by cyanide which occurs in several helminths, or it may be due to the conversion of carbon monoxide to carbon dioxide. The inhibition of respiration by carbon monoxide is, however, often difficult to demonstrate and may give rise to spurious results.

A cytochrome system of some form is indicated by the demonstration of cytochrome *c* or cytochrome oxidase in *M. apri, T. vulpis, N. brasiliensis, S. muris, C. trispinosus* and in the infective larvae of *Necator americanus, H. contortus, Strongyloides papillosus* and *S. ratti*.

A number of nematodes, *D. viviparus, B. pahangi, D. viteae* and *L. carinii* appear to have no detectable cytochromes or cytochrome oxidase. The nematode *L. carinii*, despite the absence of any apparent cytochrome system, requires oxygen for its survival and motility, and oxygen uptake is cyanide-sensitive. Oxygen uptake in *L. carinii* is also inhibited by cyanine dyes such as dithiazanine. Under aerobic conditions, *L. carinii* produces acetate (anaerobically, lactate predominates) and presumably oxidation of reducing equivalents produced during acetate formation is coupled to ATP synthesis. However, the nature of the terminal oxidase is unknown.

Ascaris Eggs

Another interesting situation occurs in *A. lumbricoides* eggs, where the nature of the terminal oxidase appears to change during development. Cytochrome *c* oxidase cannot be detected in unembryonated eggs but, as the eggs develop, cytochrome oxidase activity steadily increases. This increase in cytochrome oxidase activity is paralleled by an increase in cyanide sensitivity. Cytochrome *c* oxidase activity also increases if the eggs are stored anaerobically, even though under these conditions the eggs do not divide. So, one has biochemical development without morphological development. Flavin adenine nucleotide has been detected in unembryonated eggs and it has been proposed that, in the unembryonated egg and in the early stages of development, terminal oxidation is mediated by flavoproteins and that cytochrome oxidase becomes increasingly important as development proceeds. However, the changes in catalase activity in developing *A. lumbricoides* eggs do not parallel the proposed changes in the flavoprotein oxidase, and there is no evidence for a terminal oxidase other than cytochrome oxidase in the fully embryonated eggs. After infection of the final host, cytochrome oxidase is present in the third-stage larvae of *A. lumbricoides* recovered from the lungs, but has disappeared by the fourth stage.

So, with the exception of some nematodes (*L. carinii, D. viteae, B. pahangi, D. viviparus*), where the nature of the terminal oxidase has not yet been elucidated, all of the helminths so far studied have a cytochrome chain, which in many cases is branched. The presence of cytochrome chains in helminths does not, of course, mean that there is necessarily a functional tricarboxylic acid cycle. The reducing equivalents oxidised by the electron transport systems could come from modification of the anaerobic pathways and, as discussed earlier, this would lead to a change in the nature of the metabolic end-products.

3.2.2. Oxidative Phosphorylation

There is unequivocal evidence for oxidative phosphorylation and respiratory control in *A. lumbricoides* mitochondria, and the presence of the classical coupling sites I, II and III has been demonstrated. Oxidative phosphorylation has also been shown in another nematode (*A. caninum*), in cestodes (*M. expansa, H. diminuta*) and in trematodes (*F. hepatica, S. mansoni*). There is no other information on oxidative phosphorylation in parasitic helminths, although the classical uncoupler of oxidative phosphorylation, 2,4-dinitrophenol, stimulates oxygen uptake in *D. dendriticum*, the tetrathyridia of *Mesocestoides corti* and in the larval stages of *E. ignotus, N. americanus* and *A. lumbricoides.* The eggs of *A. lumbricoides* also have an ATPase similar to that of mammalian mitochondria, suggesting a partial reaction of oxidative phosphorylation.

It seems reasonable to assume that the mammalian-type part of the cytochrome chain in parasitic helminths is capable of oxidative phosphorylation and possesses the classical coupling sites I, II and III. However, in helminths with branched cytochrome chains, there is no evidence for oxidative phosphorylation occurring on the branch from the quinone/b complex to cytochrome o. So, in these helminths, the oxidation of NADH via the classical part of the chain and cytochrome a/a_3 would be expected to give a P:O (phosphorylation:oxygen uptake) ratio of 3, whilst oxidation of NADH via the alternative pathway and cytochrome o would only give a P:O ratio of 1 (coupling site I being common to both chains). It is not known if there is any regulatory mechanism which channels electron flow through one or other of the two branches. If no regulatory system is present, a branched cytochrome chain would appear less efficient than the unbranched mammalian chain, since, if part of the electron flow takes place through cytochrome o, the P:O ratio will always be less than 3. Cytochrome oxidase has a higher affinity for oxygen than does cytochrome o, so the classical part of the chain will function at low partial pressures of oxygen, whilst the alternative pathway will become active at higher oxygen levels. So, as the oxygen tension alters, there may be changes in the relative importance of the two oxidases. Since the alternative pathway is not subject to respiratory control, it would also allow substrate oxidation to proceed when ADP or P_i was limiting. Another possible function of cytochrome o, at least in some plants, may be the production of heat by essentially short-circuiting the cytochrome chain.

3.2.3. Reduction of Fumarate

In helminths such as *A. lumbricoides, F. hepatica* and *M. expansa* that fix carbon dioxide, the electron transport systems are also involved in the reduction of fumarate to succinate. Aerobically, these helminths can oxidise succinate via succinate dehydrogenase and the branched cytochrome chain. Anaerobically, mitochondrial

CATABOLISM AND ENERGY PRODUCTION

NADH is reoxidised by the reduction of fumarate to succinate. The NADH-linked fumarate reductase reaction results in a site I electron transport associated phosphorylation of ADP (*Figure 3.16*).

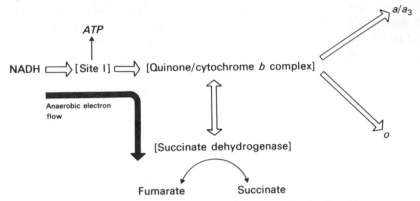

Figure 3.16 Anaerobic electron flow in helminth mitochondria.

Anaerobic phosphorylation coupled to fumarate reduction has been demonstrated in *A. lumbricoides*, *F. hepatica*, *S. mansonoides* and *H. diminuta*. In these helminths, oxygen or fumarate can act as alternative electron acceptors. There is no evidence that any other organic molecules can act as electron acceptors in helminth cytochrome systems, but it should be theoretically possible (the crotonyl-CoA/butyryl-CoA couple, for example, has a lower redox potential than the fumarate/succinate couple).

Several workers have found that, in helminth systems, under anaerobic conditions, reduced cytochrome *o* is reoxidised by the addition of fumarate. Since the redox potential of helminth cytochrome *o* is not known, it is difficult to know where it stands in relation to the flavoproteins and to the other *b* group cytochromes. Nor is it known if cytochrome *o* is situated on the inner or outer face of the inner mitochondrial membrane. It is possible that cytochrome *o*, the other *b* cytochromes and fumarate reductase (succinate dehydrogenase) are all linked by the quinone/hydroquinone system in a modified Q cycle. So, when fumarate is added, cytochrome *o* becomes oxidised by reverse electron flow. The occurrence of rhodoquinone rather than ubiquinone in many parasitic helminths could be related to the reduction of fumarate to succinate. Alternatively, cytochrome *o* might be an intimate part of the fumarate reductase system and be the link between the enzyme and the rest of the chain. This would then explain the widespread occurrence and importance of cytochrome *o* in helminths.

3.2.4. NADH Shuttle System

Like vertebrate mitochondria, the mitochondria from helminths are impermeable to NADH, and this impermeability appears to reside in the inner mitochondrial membrane. In mammalian mitochondria, there are two shuttle mechanisms known for

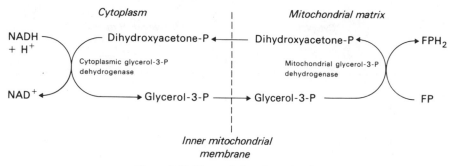

Figure 3.17 Glycerol phosphate shuttle.

the transfer of NADH from the cytoplasm into the mitochondrion, namely the glycerol-phosphate shuttle and the malate:aspartate shuttle.

In the glycerol-phosphate shuttle (*Figure 3.17*), cytoplasmic NADH reduces dihydroxyacetone phosphate (from glycolysis) to glycerol-3-phosphate. The glycerol-3-phosphate then enters the mitochondrion where it is reoxidised to di-hydroxyacetone phosphate. In mammals, the mitochondrial glycerol-3-phosphate dehydrogenase is a flavoprotein dehydrogenase which, like succinate dehydrogenase, passes its electrons directly to the cytochrome chain at the level of the quinone (i.e. after coupling site I). In the bloodstream forms of the trypanosome *Trypanosoma brucei*, the glycerol-3-phosphate shuttle forms the terminal oxidase: instead of a cytochrome chain linked dehydrogenase, glycerol-3-phosphate is reoxidised by a specific glycerol-phosphate oxidase.

Parasitic helminths probably have an active glycerol-phosphate shuttle, since glycerol-3-phosphate is readily oxidised by mitochondria isolated from *A. lumbricoides, M. expansa, H. diminuta* and *T. taeniaeformis*. The mitochondria of *T. taeniaeformis* have a particularly high rate of glycerol-phosphate oxidation; this helminth preferentially uses glycerol as a substrate and possesses a mitochondrial glycerolkinase:

$$\text{glycerol} + \text{ATP} \rightarrow \text{glycerol-3-phosphate} + \text{ADP}$$

In all the helminths looked at, the mitochondrial glycerol-3-phosphate dehydrogenase is associated with the cytochrome chain and there is no evidence for a trypanosome-type glycerol-phosphate oxidase.

The malate:aspartate shuttle (*Figure 3.18*) is more complex and involves malate dehydrogenase and aspartate:glutamate transaminase. The enzymes of the malate: aspartate shuttle occur in helminths, but whether the shuttle is operative is not known. The glycerol-3-phosphate shuttle is unidirectional, transporting NADH from the cytoplasm to the matrix. The malate : aspartate shuttle is bidirectional. However, there is some evidence that aspartate efflux may be energy-linked, in which case the shuttle would become unidirectional. An alternative NADH shuttle, analogous to the malate : aspartate shuttle, has been proposed in mammalian sperm and involves branched chain hydroxy acids and branched chain amino acids.

A number of helminths (*A. lumbricoides, H. diminuta, S. mansonoides*) that

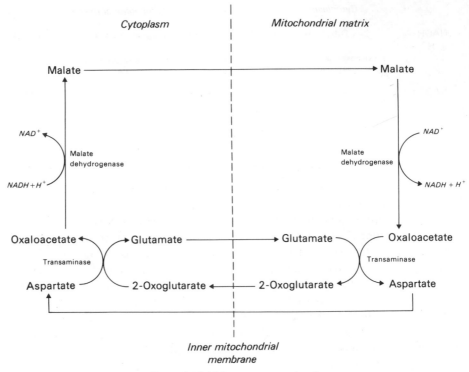

Figure 3.18 Malate : aspartate shuttle.

reduce fumarate to succinate possess a membrane-bound NAD/NADH transhydrogenase (Section 3.1.4). The function of this enzyme, which is located in the inner
mitochondrial membrane, is probably the vectorial transport of NADH into the
mitochondrion from the intermembrane space. This may represent a specialisation
associated with the reduction of fumarate to succinate, and it is possible that there
is a functional relationship between the transhydrogenase and the fumarate
reductase complex.

The transport of NADPH across the mitochondrial membrane is probably in the
form of isocitrate, and mitochondrial and cytoplasmic NADP-linked isocitrate
dehydrogenases are widely distributed in helminths.

3.2.5. Metabolite Transport Systems

The inner mitochondrial membrane has specific transport mechanisms for certain
metabolites. These transport mechanisms, or translocases, promote the reversible
equimolecular exchange of metabolites between the mitochondrial matrix and the
intermembrane space. The major metabolite translocases found in rat liver are the
ATP : ADP translocase, phosphate translocase, monocarboxylic acid translocase,
dicarboxylic acid translocase, tricarboxylic acid translocase, aspartate : glutamate
translocase and the 2-oxoglutarate : malate translocase. Different organisms may,

however, have different translocases; insect flight muscle mitochondria, for example, appear to lack both the di- and tricarboxylic acid transport systems. The only helminth system that has been looked at is *A. lumbricoides*, where the mitochondria have been shown to possess an ATP : ADP translocase, a phosphate translocase and a dicarboxylic acid translocase (the other translocases have not been studied). The ATP : ADP translocase of *A. lumbricoides* is very similar to that of mammals; however, the dicarboxylate translocase will transport succinate and malate, but not fumarate[4]. The mammalian system, in contrast, transports all three dicarboxylic acids. Helminth mitochondria, like mammalian mitochondria, will also accumulate inorganic ions[37].

3.2.6. Microsomal and Other Cytochrome Systems

In mammalian tissues, there are two non-phosphorylating cytochrome systems associated with the endoplasmic reticulum, one containing cytochrome P_{450}, the other cytochrome b_5. These systems are involved in microsomal hydroxylation and desaturation reactions and are particularly important in the detoxification of drugs. Microsomal cytochrome systems have not been investigated in detail in parasitic helminths, despite their possible relevance to chemotherapy (Section 4.8). Crude particulate preparations of parasitic helminths could, however, contain microsomal cytochromes and these may have been confused with the mitochondrial cytochromes.

A rotenone- and barbiturate-insensitive NADH/cytochrome *c* reductase is present in the outer membrane of *A. lumbricoides* mitochondria. A similar barbiturate-insensitive cytochrome *c* reductase has been found in the outer membrane of mammalian liver mitochondria. The biochemical role of this system is unknown, but in mammals it may be associated with the microsomal cytochromes or with heat production.

3.2.7. Utilisation of Oxygen by Oxidases and Oxygenases

Although most of the oxygen uptake in parasitic helminths can be attributed to the cytochrome chains, there are two classes of enzymes, the oxidases and the oxygenases, which also utilise molecular oxygen. Flavoprotein oxidases catalyse the direct oxidation of the substrate and this is usually accompanied by the formation of hydrogen peroxide. Two flavoprotein oxidases, L-amino acid oxidase and monoamine oxidase, have been found in low levels in helminths (*A. lumbricoides, H. diminuta* and *S. mansoni*) and two other oxidases, xanthine oxidase and urate oxidase (uricase), are presumed to be involved in purine catabolism (Section 3.5.2). In mammals, the flavoprotein oxidases that produce hydrogen peroxide are usually found, together with catalase (Section 3.2.8), sequestered in subcellular organelles called peroxisomes. Peroxisomes have not, however, been found in parasitic helminths.

Oxygenases catalyse the insertion of oxygen into the substrate to form hydroxyl groups. There are two classes of oxygenase—the dioxygenases, such as tryptophan oxygenase which catalyses the insertion of both atoms of the oxygen molecule into the substrate, and the mono-oxygenases (hydroxylases) which insert only one atom. Several of the mono-oxygenases (fatty acid mono-oxygenase, squalene oxidocyclase) are microsomal and function, in conjunction with the microsomal cytochromes, in short non-phosphorylating cytochrome chains. Other mono-oxygenases, such as proline-4-mono-oxygenase, are much simpler and are not associated with the endoplasmic reticulum. Mono-oxygenases require a second substrate to donate electrons, in order to reduce the second atom of oxygen to water, and are often called mixed-function oxidases:

$$AH + XH_2 + O_2 \rightarrow A\text{–}OH + H_2O + X$$

A number of important synthetic reactions are catalysed by mono-oxygenases. Of these, fatty acid mono-oxygenase, which is involved in the desaturation of fatty acids, and squalene oxidocyclase, which converts squalene to lanosterol in steroid synthesis, appear to be absent in parasitic helminths (Section 4.3). Coproporphyrinogen oxidase which converts the propionyl side chain of coproporphyrinogen III to the vinyl side chain of protoporphyrin IX, is present at only very low levels in adult A. *lumbricoides* (Section 4.4.2). However, two oxygenases have been found in appreciable amounts in helminths, proline-4-mono-oxygenase and phenolase. Proline-4-mono-oxygenase has been demonstrated in A. *lumbricoides* and is the enzyme that converts the proline in protocollagen to hydroxyproline (Section 4.4.1). Phenolase oxidises monophenols first to the diphenol, then to the highly reactive quinone.

Quinone-tanned proteins are found in trematodes, cestodes and nematodes (Section 2.5.1). Histochemically, phenolases have been detected in the vitellaria of several species of trematode and some pseudophyllidean cestodes. The phenolases of F. *hepatica, Clonorchis sinensis* and S. *mansoni* have been isolated and their properties are similar to the enzyme from mushrooms. As in insects, the phenolases of trematodes appear to be present in the tissues as inactive prophenolases[38,39].

Another product of phenolase activity on tyrosine, phenylalanine or tryptophan are melanins, which are formed by polymerisation of the corresponding quinones. Melanin-like pigments are found in the eye spots of cercariae and possibly in the egg shells of trematodes, but they have not been identified with any certainty. Eumelanin (indolic melanin) occurs in some nematode eyespots[68].

In plants, there are NAD-linked enzymes (dehydroquinone reductases) which can reduce quinones back to diphenols. These enzymes, together with phenol oxidase, could form a terminal oxidase, independent of the cytochrome chain. Such a terminal oxidase involving phenolase has been suggested to account for the oxygen uptake of *F. hepatica,* but there is no evidence that this type of system is present in trematodes.

A number of mixed-function oxidases require tetrahydrobiopterin as a coenzyme and reduced biopterin has been isolated from *A. lumbricoides.*

3.2.8. Superoxide Dismutase, Catalase and Peroxidase

During electron transport, partial reduction products of oxygen may be formed, of which the superoxide anion $O_2^{-\cdot}$ is the most important. Aerobic tissues contain an enzyme, superoxide dismutase, which converts superoxide radicals into hydrogen peroxide and oxygen:

$$2O_2^{-\cdot} + 2H^+ \rightarrow H_2O_2 + O_2$$

Superoxide dismutase is often absent from the tissues of obligate anaerobes. Preliminary studies indicate that superoxide dismutase is present in helminth tissues at levels comparable with those found in free-living organisms[40].

Another toxic product produced during electron transport is hydrogen peroxide. In helminths, this is probably formed primarily by cytochrome *o*, but it could also arise at the level of the other *b* group cytochromes or from flavoprotein oxidases (Section 3.2.1). In vertebrate tissues, hydrogen peroxide is decomposed by catalase:

$$2H_2O_2 \rightarrow 2H_2O + O_2$$

Despite considerable hydrogen peroxide production by helminths *in vitro,* catalase appears to be either absent, or present in very low amounts. Catalase has been detected in *A. galli, A. lumbricoides* (adults and eggs), *D. viviparus, T. vulpis, H. gallinae, Mecistocirrus digitatus, T. taeniaeformis* and *Taenia pisiformis* and there are conflicting reports of its presence in *F. hepatica.* Adult *A. lumbricoides* die in about one hour in pure oxygen and considerable amounts of hydrogen peroxide can be shown to have accumulated. Peroxidase activity has been described in *H. diminuta, M. expansa, F. hepatica, A. galli,* in the tissues and pseudocoel of *A. lumbricoides* and in the plant parasitic nematode *Meloidogyne.* Peroxidases occur primarily in plant tissues and catalyse the reaction:

$$AH_2 + H_2O_2 \rightarrow A + 2H_2O$$

The substrate AH_2 is frequently a phenol, but a wide variety of compounds can act as electron donors. An extremely active cytochrome *c* peroxidase occurs in the mitochondria of *A. lumbricoides, H. diminuta, M. expansa* and probably of *F. hepatica* as well[40,41]. The relationship of cytochrome *c* peroxidase to the mitochondrial cytochromes in these helminths is, however, not known.

Haem compounds including haemoglobin and myoglobin can catalyse the decomposition of hydrogen peroxide in the presence of a suitable substrate, in what is usually described as a pseudoperoxidase reaction. Tissue haemoglobins of helminths may likewise function as pseudoperoxidases to remove accumulated hydrogen peroxide (Section 2.5.2).

3.2.9. The Role of Oxidative Processes in Parasitic Helminths

Helminth parasites are all capable of oxidative phosphorylation and use oxygen when it is available. The relative contribution of oxidative phosphorylation to the overall energy balance of parasites is, however, difficult to assess. The amount of oxygen available to a parasite is, of course, very variable. Some helminths occupy unambiguously aerobic sites in the body, such as the bloodstream and the lungs, but others which live in the lumen of the intestine and in the bile ducts have an oxygen-poor environment. Even in the intestine, there may be an appreciable oxygen tension at the surface of the mucosa, so all parasitic helminths probably have at least some oxygen available to them (Section 1.1.1).

The fact that parasitic helminths produce reduced end-products, even under aerobic conditions, indicates that oxidative phosphorylation cannot supply all of the energy requirements of the parasite. The occurrence of anaerobic glycolysis under aerobic conditions is not restricted to parasites and occurs in a number of mammalian tissues, such as red blood cells and the retina of the eye.

The persistence of anaerobic metabolism in parasitic helminths under aerobic conditions could be due, not to the inadequacies of oxidative phosphorylation, but to peculiarities in the regulatory mechanisms of their metabolic pathways. The parasite may not, in fact, be able to reduce the flux through the glycolytic system during aerobic periods, or there may be a dominant Crabtree effect. The Crabtree effect is the inhibition of oxygen uptake by cells caused by the addition of glucose, and it is thought to be due to glycolysis using up the available ADP and P_i, resulting in a state 3 (respiratory chain limiting) to a state 4 (ADP limiting) transition in the cytochrome chain. Since parasitic helminths have a very high glycolytic capacity, this is a distinct possibility, and a Crabtree effect has been demonstrated in isolated *A. lumbricoides* intestines and in the cercariae of *S. mansoni*[42,43]. Alternatively, synthetic processes may be removing metabolic intermediates at such a rate that there are none left to fuel the tricarboxylic acid cycle. Another possibility is that helminths may be limited in their ability to transport reducing equivalents across the inner mitochondrial membrane, so that anaerobic coupling persists in the cytoplasm even when oxygen is available. So, the presence of anaerobic metabolism under aerobic conditions in helminths does not necessarily mean that oxidative phosphorylation makes a negligible contribution to the overall energy balance of the parasite. Also, when a helminth is transferred from an oxygen-poor environment (such as the intestine) to air, the sudden increase in the partial pressure of oxygen may result in metabolic disruptions analogous to those that occur when aerobic organisms are subjected to hyperbaric oxygen.

In some parasitic helminths, oxygen is necessary for motility (*N. brasiliensis, D. viviparus, L. carinii, T. spiralis* larvae), whilst in others it is not. In those helminths that require oxygen for movement, aerobic metabolism may supply the additional energy required either for muscular activity or for nervous coordination. Alternatively, the presence of oxygen may stimulate the parasites into activity and not be involved in energy metabolism at all. Similarly, some parasites require oxygen for survival, whilst others such as *S. mansoni* and *H. contortus* require it for reproduction. Again, it is not known if oxidative phosphorylation provides the additional energy required or if the oxygen is used for degradative or synthetic reactions. In the majority of helminths studied, the presence of oxygen increases the *in vitro* survival time. However, the partial pressure of carbon dioxide may be a critical factor in survival, and in many of the older studies this was not controlled. In the cestodes, some species can be successfully cultured under fairly strict anaerobic conditions (*S. mansonoides, Hymenolepis nana, H. diminuta*), whereas others thrive best under air (*H. microstoma, T. crassiceps, E. granulosus, M. corti*). The trematode *S. mansoni* can be successfully cultured in air, but can also be maintained for long periods under anaerobic, or at least near-anaerobic, conditions.

Different species of helminths show considerable differences in the *in vitro* effects of oxygen on such things as survival, motility, reproduction and development. How far these *in vitro* effects apply *in vivo* is open to question.

Pasteur Effect and Oxygen Debt

The presence or absence of a Pasteur effect should also give some indication of the contribution of oxidative phosphorylation towards the energy requirements of the parasite. As before, some parasites show a marked Pasteur effect (*L. carinii, A. galli, A. caninum, N. brasiliensis, A. lumbricoides, H. contortus*, the larvae of *E. ignotus*, and the cercariae of *S. mansoni*), and in these helminths oxidative phosphorylation may be relatively important. Other parasitic helminths show no Pasteur effect and anaerobic processes may be able to supply all of the energy requirements of these species. However, energy requirements under aerobic and anaerobic conditions are almost certainly different and so any contribution by oxidative phosphorylation may well be obscured. The ability of helminths to accumulate an oxygen debt is also very variable and is in no way correlated with the presence of a Pasteur effect. The nematode *A. lumbricoides*, for example, shows no Pasteur effect but does show an increase in post-anaerobic respiration, whilst *L. carinii* shows a marked Pasteur effect but no oxygen debt. The ability to incur an oxygen debt is dependent on the accumulation in the tissues of anaerobic end-products which can serve as substrates for the increased oxygen consumption.

Rate of Oxygen Uptake

The importance of oxidative processes in the energy balance of parasitic helminths clearly differs in different parasites and may also vary between the tissues of the same parasite. All parasitic helminths use oxygen when it is available, but can probably all survive under anaerobic conditions for varying lengths of time. However, many, if not all, helminths seem to require at least some oxygen for normal sustained activity. The actual rates of oxygen uptake by parasitic helminths in air are extremely high, considering the anaerobic nature of most of their catabolic pathways. In *A. lumbricoides*, for example, the oxygen uptake is 0.08 ml/g fresh weight/h. This compares with 0.03 ml/g fresh weight/h for the annelid *Arenicola*, which is of a comparable size, and 0.2 ml/g fresh weight/h for resting man. The QO_2

of adult helminths is usually in the range 2–6 $\mu l/mg$ dry weight and, as in free-living organisms, the QO_2 depends on the sex, age and size of the parasite, as well as on the conditions of incubation (pO_2, temperature, pH, ions). Again, how far these *in vitro* measurements apply to the *in vivo* situation is questionable. However, it has been estimated that the respiratory rate of the intestinal nematodes *N. brasiliensis* and *N. dubius* may reach 80% and 40%, respectively, of the *in vitro* rate, when measured at the oxygen tensions which prevail in these parasites' normal sites in their host (small intestine).

Free-living and Intermediate Stages

The free-living, infective larvae of nematodes, unlike the adult parasites, are highly aerobic and die fairly rapidly under anaerobic conditions. Free-living miracidia and cercariae are also primarily aerobic, whereas the intramolluscan stages (sporocyst and rediae) are facultative anaerobes like the adults. Although the free-living stages of trematodes and nematodes are primarily aerobic, they too can all survive anaerobically for limited periods. The eggs of helminths are also able to survive anaerobiosis, often for considerable lengths of time. However, most, if not all, helminth eggs require at least some oxygen for complete development. Again, the degree of anaerobic development differs in different parasites; in *A. lumbricoides*, oxygen is required for the first cell division whereas, in *Oxyuris equi* and *Enterobius vermicularis*, the eggs will develop anaerobically to the gastrula and tadpole stages, respectively. Egg hatching, however, does not necessarily need oxygen, and the eggs of *A. lumbricoides*, *A. galli*, *Toxocara mystax* and *F. hepatica* can all hatch anaerobically. The exsheathment of the infective larvae of *H. contortus* and *T. axei* can also take place anaerobically. The evagination of some cestode larvae, however, requires oxygen. So, as in the adult parasite, there is great variation in the oxygen requirements of larval helminths and this must reflect differences in the underlying metabolic pathways.

3.2.10. Carbon Dioxide Transport

Parasitic helminths, in general, live in high carbon dioxide environments (Section 1.1.2), but little is known of the mechanisms by which they eliminate metabolic carbon dioxide. The amount of carbon dioxide present in the body fluids of animals always exceeds the amount in simple solution. The difference between carbon dioxide dissolved and carbon dioxide contained is due to the combination of carbon dioxide, largely in the form of bicarbonate, with cations from various buffer systems. The only helminth which has so far been studied is *A. lumbricoides*[44]: the pCO_2 of fresh pseudocoelomic fluid is high, 158 mmHg, and the main buffer systems are bicarbonate and phosphate, proteins making little contribution. The pCO_2 in the protonephridial fluid of *H. diminuta* is also high, around 120 mmHg.

Carbonic anhydrase has been found in the tissues of a number of helminths, *M. expansa*, *Anoplocephala magna*, *F. hepatica*, *A. lumbricoides* and *P. equorum*. This enzyme catalyses the reversible hydration of carbon dioxide:

$$CO_2 + H_2O \underset{\text{\textit{anhydrase}}}{\overset{\text{\textit{carbonic}}}{\rightleftharpoons}} H_2CO_3 \rightleftharpoons H^+ + HCO_3^-$$

and is probably involved in carbon dioxide transport.

Many helminths fix carbon dioxide and for them it is an important metabolite (Section 3.1.4). Anaerobic catabolism and carbon dioxide fixation make RQ (QCO_2/QO_2) determinations on parasitic helminths misleading, and often low values are reported (less than 1) even though carbohydrate is the only substrate.

3.3. LIPID CATABOLISM

Parasitic helminths often contain appreciable quantities of lipid, but there is, how-ever, no good evidence that any adult parasitic helminth can catabolise its lipid stores.

3.3.1. Fatty Acid Catabolism

In mammals, the rate of fatty acid breakdown is controlled by the rate of supply of free fatty acids. The hydrolysis of triacylglycerols is catalysed by triacylglycerol lipase which exists in two interconvertible forms, an active phosphorylated state and an inactive dephosphorylated state. This aspect of lipid catabolism has not been studied in helminths.

β-oxidation

In aerobic organisms, fatty acids are broken down by β-oxidation (*Figure 3.19*) to give acetyl-CoA, NADH and reduced flavoprotein. All parasitic helminths so far investigated possess some, if not all, of the enzymes of the β-oxidation sequence. In the muscle tissue of *A. lumbricoides*, the β-oxidation enzymes are all present at relatively high activities (about 10% of the levels found in mammal kidney). A com-plete sequence of β-oxidation enzymes has also been found in *F. hepatica* and in the plerocercoids of *S. solidus*; and a partial sequence of enzymes occurs in *H. diminuta*, *M. dubius*, the plerocercoids of *L. intestinalis* and the parasitic females of *S. ratti*. In all of these helminths, however, there are only low levels of the β-oxidation enzymes, and acyl-CoA dehydrogenase and 3-hydroxyacyl-CoA dehydrogenase, in particular, have only very low activities. No GTP-dependent long chain fatty acyl-CoA synthetase has yet been found in helminths[45,46,47].

The intracellular distribution of the β-oxidation enzymes has been studied in the plerocercoids of *S. solidus*[46]. The fatty acyl-CoA synthetases occur in both the cytoplasmic and particulate fractions. In vertebrate tissues with an active β-oxida-tion pathway, the synthetases are primarily mitochondrial. The remainder of the β-oxidation enzymes in *S. solidus* are mitochondrial, as they are in mammalian tissues. Fatty acids are transported into the mammalian mitochondria in the form of carnitine esters. A similar carnitine-dependent mechanism seems to be present in helminths.

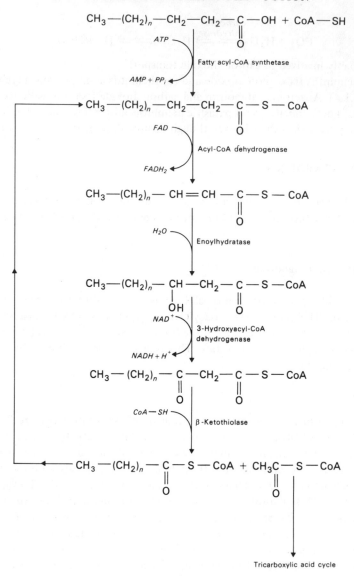

Figure 3.19 The β-oxidation sequence.

α- and ω-oxidation

A small amount of radioactive carbon dioxide is produced when helminths are incubated with universally labelled palmitate. There is some evidence that this arises from the decarboxylation of the long chain fatty acids (α-oxidation).

In ω-oxidation, carbon atoms are removed from the C terminal end of the fatty acid. This involves the microsomal cytochrome systems and has not been demonstrated in helminths.

Ketone Bodies

The metabolism of ketone bodies (3-(OH)-butyrate, acetoacetate) has not been investigated in helminths.

3.3.2. Role of the β-oxidation Sequence in Helminths

Lipid catabolism in helminths poses two interesting problems. First, if the β-oxidation enzymes are all present, why is the pathway not active? And, secondly, if the β-oxidation enzymes are not involved in fatty acid catabolism, what is their function?

The absence of a functional β-oxidation sequence in parasitic helminths, despite the presence of the β-oxidation enzymes, could be related either to the relative unimportance of the tricarboxylic acid cycle in these parasites (Section 3.1.8) or to the low environmental pO_2. The absence of a classical tricarboxylic acid cycle would severely limit the further catabolism of the acetyl-CoA produced by β-oxidation. The large amounts of NADH and reduced flavoprotein formed during β-oxidation require reoxidation via an oxidase system. The β-oxidation pathway cannot, therefore, function anaerobically and anaerobic bacteria, for example, do not catabolise fatty acids.

Cofermentation of Lipid and Carbohydrate

It is possible to postulate a scheme for the cofermentation of lipid and carbohydrate. The reducing equivalents formed during β-oxidation could be reoxidised by coupling with the reduction of fumarate to succinate, the acetyl-CoA could be cleaved and acetate excreted to relieve the acetate pressure. There is no evidence from carbon balance studies in helminths for the cofermentation of lipid and carbohydrate, although attempts to balance excretory acids with redox couples in helminths (Section 3.1.4) suggest that some mitochondrial reducing power must come from a source other than the breakdown of carbohydrate.

Function of the β-oxidation Enzymes

The function of the β-oxidation enzymes in parasitic helminths is not clear. The enzymes could, of course, be associated primarily with the developing eggs in readiness for the free-living stages, which are aerobic (Section 3.3.4). In A. lumbricoides, it had been suggested that the β-oxidation enzymes might be involved in the production of the C_5 and C_6 branched chain excretory acids. However, this now seems unlikely (Section 3.1.3).

A possible role for the β-oxidation enzymes in helminths could be the malonyl-CoA independent elongation of fatty acids (Section 4.3.1). This is a mitochondrial system, which is also found in mammals. In it, an acetyl-CoA molecule is condensed with a long chain fatty acyl-CoA and the system requires two NADPH (or equivalent) for each acetyl-CoA (C_2) added. The condensation appears to take place by the reversal of the steps of β-oxidation. In the mammal, the synthetic route differs from the degradative pathway in that the 3-(OH)-acyl-CoA dehydrogenase and the acyl-CoA dehydrogenase of the synthetic route are both NADP-linked. In β-oxidation, the 3-(OH)-acyl-CoA dehydrogenase is NAD-linked and acyl-CoA dehydrogenase is a flavoprotein enzyme. So far, neither NADP-linked 3-(OH)-acyl-CoA dehydrogenase nor NADP-linked acyl-CoA dehydrogenase have been demonstrated in parasitic helminths.

The chain lengthening system can, in theory, be coupled to carbohydrate catabolism. The breakdown of one glucose to two acetyl-CoA gives a net production of two ATP and four NADH; the condensation of two acetyl-CoA molecules with a long chain fatty acyl-CoA would utilise four NADH (or equivalents) and so there would be a net production of 2 ATP per mole of glucose. The equivalent of two ATP would be required for the initial activation of the long chain fatty acid (fatty acyl-CoA synthetase uses both high-energy phosphate bonds of ATP, yielding AMP rather than ADP). This scheme would require reducing equivalents to be transported across the inner mitochondrial membrane, since the glycolytic NADH is formed in the cytoplasm, whilst malonyl-CoA independent fatty acid synthesis occurs in the mitochondrion. In terms of ATP produced per mole of glucose catabolised, this system has no advantage over glycolysis. However, it could be useful if the excretion of organic acids was, for some reason, restricted. Long chain fatty acids have been shown to be synthesised by terrestrial gastropods under anaerobic conditions[48] and it is possible that this might involve a malonyl-CoA independent pathway. There is no evidence, however, that this occurs in helminths.

Finally, the catabolism of the aliphatic amino acids, valine, leucine and isoleucine, involves steps analogous to those of β-oxidation. In mammals, different enzymes are utilised in amino acid breakdown and fatty acid oxidation, and the same is almost certainly true of helminths.

3.3.3. Excretion and Accumulation of Lipids

It has been suggested, especially in trematodes, that lipid might be the end-product of carbohydrate catabolism in parasitic helminths. Trematodes, in particular, excrete lipid droplets via the excretory canal (and possibly the intestine), and in *F. hepatica* lipid excretion can amount to as much as 2% of the wet weight per 24 h. However, cholesterol, cholesterol esters, triacylglycerols, free fatty acids and phospholipids are all excreted by *F. hepatica*, indicating that this may be a general loss of lipid, rather than the excretion of a specialised end-product. There is also no evidence, either from carbon balance or isotope studies, that long chain fatty acids act as terminal acceptors for NADH and acetyl-CoA in parasitic helminths.

The lipids excreted by the adults and metacercariae of several other trematode species (*Cotylurus* sp., *E. revolutum, L. constantiae*) have been analysed. Again, a variety of lipid classes are excreted, including phospholipids, free fatty acids and triacylglycerols with sterols and sterol esters predominating[49-52]. Since there is no breakdown of fatty acids in adult helminths, the only way that there can be any turnover of tissue lipids is by excretion. This may be one reason why trematodes excrete lipids.

The absence of lipid catabolism in parasitic helminths also raises the question of why these animals accumulate lipid if they are unable to catabolise it. In females, at least part of the lipid may be destined for incorporation into the eggs. Alternatively, the adult parasite may have to take in large amounts of lipid in order to get enough of a particular fatty acid or fat-soluble vitamin, and the excess lipid is stored rather than excreted again. Finally, in a number of gastrointestinal nematodes, the accumulation of lipid can be correlated with the onset of the host's immune response. The significance of this apparent relationship between immunology and lipid metabolism is unknown. Possibly, lipid accumulation is related to the retention of potentially immunogenic compounds.

3.3.4. Free-living and Intermediate Stages

The free-living stages of parasitic nematodes rely heavily on lipid for their energy metabolism, and there have been numerous studies showing lipid utilisation, particularly by infective nematode larvae. In a number of infective nematode larvae, the loss of stored lipid correlates with loss of activity and loss of infectivity. In addition, an active β-oxidation sequence has been shown in the free-living adults and larvae of *S. ratti* and in the developing eggs of *A. lumbricoides*.

In the trematodes, lipid has been demonstrated in the miracidia of several species as well as in sporocysts and rediae. However, it has not been shown if miracidia can actually catabolise their lipid stores, although there is indirect evidence that sporocysts do metabolise lipids[53]. The occurrence of lipid in cercariae is rather variable; the cercariae of *S. mansoni* contain little lipid, whilst other species of cercariae, such as *Glypthelmins pennsylvaniensis*, contain relatively large amounts of free fatty acids. Lipid utilisation has been demonstrated in a number of free-swimming cercariae, and it has been suggested that, with cercariae, there may be a correlation between lipid utilisation and activity. Cercariae which are very active utilise lipid, whilst cercariae that are relatively immobile do not. Alternatively, the presence or absence of lipid in the free-living stages of parasites may be related to their life-spans, long-lived larvae such as nematodes using lipid, whilst short-lived larvae such as miracidia and many cercariae rely mainly on glycogen. Lipid could also be functioning as a flotation agent in the aquatic stages of these helminths.

Lipid catabolism in the larval stages of cestodes and acanthocephalans has been little investigated. There is some histochemical evidence that lipid may be catabolised by the free-swimming coracidia of Pseudophyllidean cestodes, but there is no β-oxidation in the plerocercoids of *S. solidus* or *L. intestinalis* (Section 3.3.1). In the cyclophyllidean tapeworms, there is no β-oxidation in the cysticercoid of *H. diminuta* and, in the acanthocephalans, β-oxidation could not be detected in the cystacanths of *M. dubius*.

3.4. AMINO ACID CATABOLISM

Amino acids do not appear to be an important energy source in parasitic helminths. Only trematode sporocysts and some plant parasitic nematodes have been shown appreciably to catabolise amino acids. In organisms that are heavily committed to synthesis, such as dividing bacteria, growing plants and possibly parasitic helminths as well, the degradation of amino acids is not a prominent process. On the other hand, vertebrates actively oxidise both exogenous and endogenous amino acids. A problem with using amino acids as a major energy source is that, with the possible exception of insects and Mermithid nematodes, there does not seem to be a specific storage protein for amino acids in adult animals.

During catabolism, amino acids lose their α-amino nitrogen and the remaining carbon skeletons are converted to glycolytic or tricarboxylic acid cycle intermediates. These intermediates can then either be completely degraded or else resynthesised into glucose. In vertebrates, there are some twenty multienzyme sequences for the degradation of the twenty different amino acids. The fates of the carbon skeletons of the amino acids of vertebrates are summarised in *Table 3.7*. The pathways of amino acid catabolism can be very complex and the various intermediates are often important precursors for other pathways.

Table 3.7 End-products of amino acid breakdown in mammals

Amino acid	End-products
Alanine, cysteine, glycine, hydroxyproline, serine	Pyruvate
Arginine, glutamate, glutamine, histidine, proline	2-Oxoglutarate
Aspartate, asparagine	Oxaloacetate
Methionine, valine	Succinyl-CoA
Threonine	Acetyl-CoA (minor pathway to propionyl-CoA)
Isoleucine	Acetyl-CoA, succinyl-CoA
Leucine, tryptophan	Acetyl-CoA, acetoacyl-CoA
Lysine	Acetoacyl-CoA
Phenylalanine, tyrosine	Acetoacyl-CoA, fumarate

3.4.1. Removal of the Amino Group

The first step in amino acid catabolism is the removal of the α-amino nitrogen. There are two main pathways for this, transamination or oxidative deamination. In addition, there are a number of specific, non-oxidative deaminases.

Transamination

The amino group is transferred from the amino acid to a 2-keto acid (usually 2-oxoglutarate):

L-aspartate + 2-oxoglutarate ⇌ oxaloacetate + L-glutamate

This reaction requires pyridoxal phosphate as a cofactor. Most transaminases use 2-oxoglutarate as one of the amino group acceptors, but they are somewhat less specific towards the other amino donor. In vertebrates, the major 2-oxoglutarate linked transaminases are aspartate transaminase, alanine transaminase, leucine transaminase and tyrosine transaminase. 2-Oxoglutarate linked transaminases are widely distributed in parasitic helminths. Aspartate:2-oxoglutarate transaminase and alanine:2-oxoglutarate transaminase have been found in virtually every helminth investigated. In addition, 2-oxoglutarate transaminases active with a variety of amino acids (arginine, glycine, leucine, isoleucine, methionine, phenylalanine, serine, tyrosine, valine, proline, ornithine, 4-aminobutyrate) have been described from different species (*Table 3.8*).

Table 3.8 2-Oxoglutarate linked transaminases in parasitic helminths

Species	Donor amino acids
Nematodes	
Ascaris lumbricoides	Alanine, arginine, aspartate, glycine, methionine, phenylalanine, serine, 4-aminobutyrate
Ascaridia galli	Alanine, aspartate
Stephanurus dentatus	Alanine, aspartate
Trematodes	
Fasciola hepatica	Alanine, arginine, aspartate, leucine, isoleucine, methionine, phenylalanine, proline, tyrosine, valine, ornithine
Schistosoma japonicum	Alanine, arginine, aspartate
Cryptocotyle lingua (rediae)	Alanine, aspartate
Cercaria emasculans (sporocyst)	Alanine, aspartate
Microphallus pygmaeus (sporocyst)	Alanine, aspartate
Gyrocotyle fimbriata	Alanine
Cestodes	
Hymenolepis diminuta	Alanine, aspartate, asparagine
Hymenolepis citelli	Alanine, aspartate, asparagine
Hymenolepis nana	Asparagine, aspartate
Taenia taeniaeformis	Aspartate
Moniezia expansa	Alanine, aspartate, 4-aminobutyrate
Acanthocephalans	
Moniliformis dubius	4-Aminobutyrate

An aspartate:pyruvate transaminase system has also been detected in several helminths (*H. diminuta, A. lumbricoides, F. hepatica,* larval trematodes). Other amino acids that can act as donors in the pyruvate transaminase reaction are ornithine (*F. hepatica*) and glycine and serine (*A. lumbricoides*). However, compared with vertebrates, relatively few amino acids seem to be able to act as cosubstrates for transaminase reactions in parasitic helminths.

The amino groups from the different amino acids are collected, via transaminase reactions, into one acid (glutamate), which can then act as a donor for the formation of the different nitrogenous end-products (Section 3.6).

Oxidative Deamination

Glutamate dehydrogenase catalyses the oxidative deamination of glutamate:

L-glutamate + H_2O + $NAD^+(NADP^+)$ $\rightleftharpoons$ 2-oxoglutarate + NH_4^+ + NADH(NADPH)

The amino groups, collected into glutamate via transaminase reactions, are released as ammonia. Glutamate dehydrogenase can use either NAD or NADP, although NAD is the preferred cofactor. Mammalian glutamate dehydrogenase is an allosteric enzyme, being activated by ADP, GDP and certain amino acids, and being inhibited by ATP, GTP and NADH. In mammals, its activity is also modified by hormones. Glutamate dehydrogenase plays a major role in deamination since, in most organisms, glutamate is the only amino acid for which there is an active dehydrogenase. Glutamate dehydrogenase is widely distributed in helminths, but its regulatory properties have not been studied in any detail. The enzyme from *H. contortus* is said to be inhibited by AMP, ADP, ATP, aspartate and thyroxine. The cytoplasmic glutamate dehydrogenase from *H. diminuta*, on the other hand, was not appreciably affected by AMP, ADP, ATP, GDP, GTP, amino acids or glycolytic intermediates[54]. In addition to glutamate dehydrogenase, a specific alanine dehydrogenase has been described in *A. lumbricoides* and *H. diminuta* (Section 4.4.1).

A minor pathway for the oxidative deamination of amino acids is via the flavin linked L-amino acid oxidase:

$$L\text{-amino acid} + H_2O + FMN \rightarrow 2\text{-oxoacid} + NH_3 + FMNH_2$$

$$FMNH_2 + O_2 \rightarrow FMN + H_2O_2$$

L-amino acid oxidases have been demonstrated in *H. diminuta, A. galli, Nematodirus* sp. and in the muscles and intestine of *A. lumbricoides*. The corresponding D-amino acid oxidases have not been investigated in helminths.

Specific Deaminases

A number of amino acids, arginine, aspartate, histidine, serine, threonine and glutamine, can be non-oxidatively deaminated by specific deaminases. Some of these enzymes have been found in parasitic helminths. Arginase cleaves arginine into ornithine and urea:

$$\text{arginine} + H_2O \rightarrow \text{ornithine} + \text{urea}$$

This enzyme is widely distributed in parasitic helminths (Section 3.6). L-serine dehydratase has been found in *Gyrocotyle fimbriata*[55]:

$$\text{serine} \rightarrow \text{pyruvate} + NH_3$$

The first enzyme in the catabolism of histidine, i.e. histidase, has been found in *G. fimbriata, F. hepatica, A. galli* and *A. lumbricoides*:

$$\text{histidine} \rightarrow \text{urocanic acid} + NH_3$$

Finally, glutaminase has been found in the free-living nematode *P. redivivus*:

$$\text{glutamine} + H_2O \rightarrow \text{glutamic acid} + NH_3$$

3.4.2. Metabolism of Carbon Skeletons

In vertebrates, the carbon skeletons of amino acids are ultimately converted into glycolytic or tricarboxylic acid cycle intermediates. In parasitic helminths, the pathways of amino acid breakdown have only been studied in a few isolated cases.

Arginine and Proline

A number of monogeneans and digeneans contain relatively large amounts of proline in their free amino acid pools (Section 2.4.1), and some of the enzymes of proline metabolism have been investigated in *F. hepatica*[56,57]. Ornithine is converted to proline in *F. hepatica* via Δ^1-pyrroline-5'-carboxylic acid (*Figure 3.20*). Glutamate

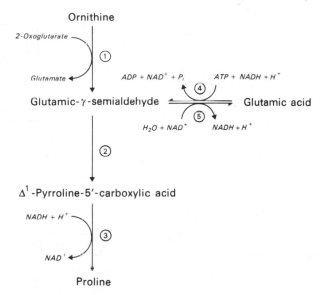

Figure 3.20 Proline metabolism in *Fasciola hepatica*: 1, ornithine transaminase; 2, spontaneous; 3, pyrroline-5'-carboxylate reductase; 4, glutamate kinase + dehydrogenase; 5, Δ^1-pyrroline-5'-carboxylate dehydrogenase.

does not appear to be a source of glutamic-γ-semialdehyde and the absence of Δ^1-pyrroline-5'-carboxylate dehydrogenase activity in *F. hepatica* means that glutamate is not formed from ornithine (or proline). In *F. hepatica*, ornithine is probably derived primarily from the cleavage of arginine by arginase. Proline oxidase, which in vertebrates is the first step in the catabolism of proline:

$$\text{proline} + \tfrac{1}{2}O_2 \rightarrow \Delta^1\text{-pyrroline-5'-carboxylate} + H_2O$$

is not present in *F. hepatica*. So, in this parasite, proline appears to be the endproduct of arginine catabolism. In vertebrates, both arginine and proline are converted to glutamate. The production of proline from arginine utilises NADH, and may provide an additional mechanism for the reoxidation of reducing equivalents produced during carbohydrate breakdown. A possible advantage of proline production over acid production is that, as a neutral compound, proline can readily penetrate the mitochondrion.

Adult *F. hepatica* excrete significant amounts of proline (50 mg/100 g wet weight/h *in vitro*) and there is a 10 000 fold increase in bile proline in infected animals due to proline excretion by the flukes. There is also some evidence that proline may be responsible for bile duct hyperplasia[58,69].

The production of proline as an end-product in *F. hepatica* contrasts strongly with certain insects, such as the tsetse fly and the cockchafer, and with some haemoflagellates (*Leishmania tarentolae* and the culture forms of *Trypanosoma rhodesiense*) where proline is metabolised via glutamate to 2-oxoglutarate and so enters the tricarboxylic acid cycle (*Figure 3.21*). It should perhaps be noted that, in these animals, glutamate is converted to 2-oxoglutarate by transamination, rather than via glutamate dehydrogenase.

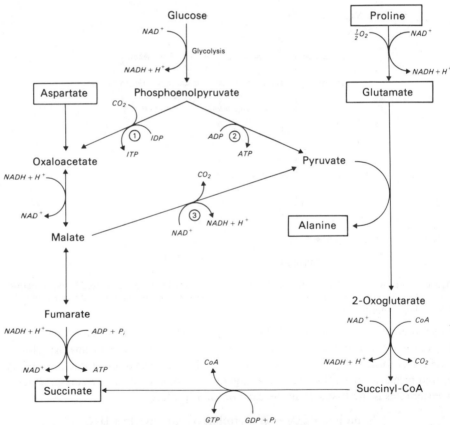

Figure 3.21 Possible pathways for the cofermentation of carbohydrate and amino acids: 1, phosphoenolpyruvate carboxykinase; 2, pyruvate kinase; 3, malic enzyme.

Valine, Leucine and Isoleucine

Not all of the volatile fatty acids produced by parasitic helminths come from the breakdown of carbohydrate, some being derived from amino acid catabolism

(Section 3.1.4). In *F. hepatica* and *A. caninum*, valine and leucine are converted to isobutyrate and isovalerate, respectively. Isoleucine can also be converted to 2-methylbutyrate by *F. hepatica*, and the tapeworm *Calliobothrium verticillatum* converts valine to 2-ketoisovalerate. The probable pathways of these conversions are summarised in *Figure 3.22* and are identical with the initial steps of valine, leucine and isoleucine degradation in mammals.

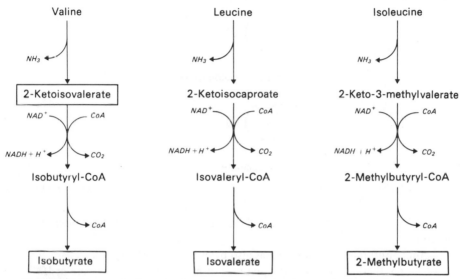

Figure 3.22 The metabolism of valine, leucine and isoleucine to volatile acids by parasitic helminths.

Histidine

The initial enzyme of histidine catabolism, histidase, occurs in several helminths (Section 3.4.1). There is some evidence that, in *A. lumbricoides, A. galli* and *F. hepatica*, the breakdown of histidine may be similar to that in mammals, the imidazole ring of urocanic acid being cleaved to yield, ultimately, glutamate.

Tryptophan

In mammals, the first step in tryptophan catabolism is oxidation to L-formyl-kynurenine via L-tryptophan oxygenase. This enzyme could not be detected in *S. mansoni*[59].

The 4-Aminobutyrate Bypass

A 4-aminobutyrate bypass may be present in *A. lumbricoides* muscle, since appreciable amounts of glutamate decarboxylase and 4-aminobutyrate transaminase activity have been found. This pathway (*Figure 3.23*), which occurs in the vertebrate brain and in some plants and micro-organisms, provides a route for the conversion of glutamate to succinate without the involvement of 2-oxoglutarate decarboxylase.

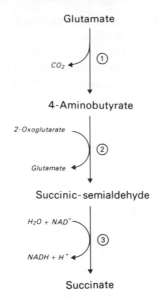

Figure 3.23 The 4-aminobutyrate bypass: 1, glutamate decarboxylase; 2, 4-aminobutyrate transaminase; 3, succinate-semialdehyde dehydrogenase.

The significance of this pathway, if it does, in fact, operate in *A. lumbricoides*, is obscure.

4-Aminobutyrate transaminase has also been found in *M. expansa*. There are, however, conflicting reports of the presence of glutamate decarboxylase in *M. expansa*, and isotope studies provide no evidence for the presence of a functional 4-aminobutyrate bypass in this parasite[60].

3.4.3. Decarboxylation of Amino Acids

Amino acids can be decarboxylated to give the corresponding amines, many of which are physiologically active. Adult *A. lumbricoides* can decarboxylate arginine, glutamate, histidine, lysine and ornithine to give agmatin, 4-aminobutyrate, histamine, cadaverine and putrescine, respectively. Lysine and arginine decarboxylases have been described in *A. galli* and *M. expansa*, whilst glutamate decarboxylase has been found in *A. galli* and *Taenia solium*, but there are conflicting reports of its presence in *M. expansa*[60]. A histidine decarboxylase has also been identified in the trematodes *Mesocoelium monodi* and *F. hepatica*.

A number of larval cestodes and larval and adult nematodes excrete a wide variety of amines (Section 3.6.4). The mode of formation of these amines is not known, but many of them are presumably formed by decarboxylation of the corresponding amino acids.

The cestode *H. diminuta* liberates carbon dioxide in the presence of aspartate. This is not, however, due to aspartate-4-decarboxylase activity but to the decarboxylation of oxaloacetate formed by transamination *(Figure 3.24)*[61].

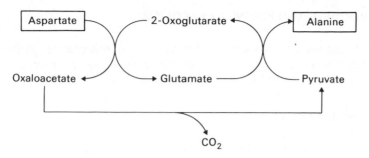

Figure 3.24 Proposed pathway for the apparent decarboxylation of aspartate by *Hymenolepis diminuta*[61].

Monoamine Oxidase

This enzyme catalyses the oxidative deamination of a wide variety of monoamines:

$$R' - CH_2NH_2 + O_2 + H_2O \rightarrow R' - C\!\!\begin{array}{c} {}^{\displaystyle H} \\[-2pt] {}_{\displaystyle O} \end{array} + NH_3 + H_2O_2$$

The resulting aldehydes are either oxidised to acids or reduced to alcohols depending on the organism. Low levels of monoamine oxidase have been shown in *S. mansoni* and *H. diminuta* and histochemically in *Aspiculuris tetraptera* and *F. gigantica*. Aldehyde reductases have also been found in parasitic helminths[62]. The function of monoamine oxidase is the removal of biologically active amines, such as released monoamine neurotransmitters, and also the detoxification of exogenous amines present in the host's diet.

Diamine oxidase, a similar enzyme which acts on diamines, has not been found in helminths.

3.4.4. Cofermentation of Amino Acids and Carbohydrate

In bivalve molluscs, under anaerobic conditions, there is evidence for the cofermentation of carbohydrate and amino acids. Bivalves, like many helminths, produce succinate as a major end-product of carbohydrate breakdown under anaerobic conditions (Section 3.1.4). It has been claimed that at least some of this succinate is derived from the catabolism of amino acids (*Figure 3.21*). Glutamate can be converted to 2-oxoglutarate and hence via succinyl-CoA to succinate. The degradation of aspartate can provide oxaloacetate, and the redox systems can be coupled in a variety of ways. There is, so far, no evidence in parasitic helminths for any significant cofermentation of amino acids and carbohydrate. The mechanism of amino acid breakdown in trematode sporocysts has, however, yet to be investigated.

3.5. PYRIMIDINE AND PURINE CATABOLISM

Nucleotides derived from nucleic acids by the action of nucleases are hydrolysed enzymatically to yield free pyrimidine and purine bases. The free bases are then either salvaged and re-used (Section 4.6) or further degraded.

3.5.1. Pyrimidine Catabolism

In mammals, pyrimidines are broken down initially to β-alanine or β-aminoisobutyric acid (*Figure 3.25*). β-Alanine and β-aminoisobutyrate can be further catabolised to malonic-semialdehyde or methylmalonyl-semialdehyde, respectively, both of which are intermediates in propionate metabolism. Pyrimidines can thus be completely broken down to carbon dioxide and ammonia. Some micro-organisms may be able to catabolise pyrimidines via isobarbituric acid to urea; this pathway was

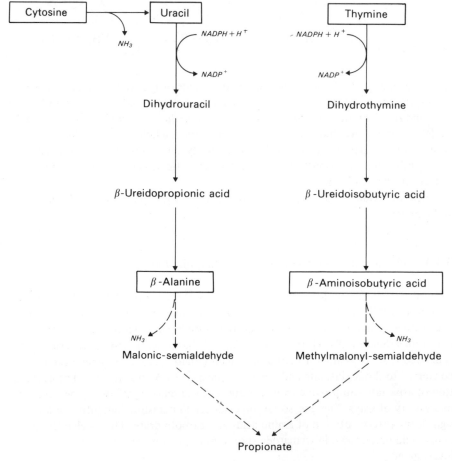

Figure 3.25 Pyrimidine catabolism.

once thought to operate in mammals, but this is now thought not to be the case. The pathways of pyrimidine breakdown in parasitic helminths are probably the same as in the mammal. The principal end-products of pyrimidine catabolism, β-alanine and β-aminoisobutyrate, have been found in several cestodes, in the nematode *A. galli* and in some, but not all, trematodes studied. In *H. diminuta*, pyrimidine catabolism has been investigated in more detail and here it has been shown that uracil is degraded via dihydrouracil and β-ureidopropionic acid to β-alanine as outlined in *Figure 3.25*. Pyrimidine catabolism in nematodes does not seem to have been studied. However, since pyrimidines have not been found in the excretory products of nematodes, they are presumably completely degraded to ammonia and carbon dioxide.

3.5.2. Purine Catabolism

The catabolism of purines by animals can lead to a variety of end-products, since degradation stops at different points in different organisms (*Figure 3.26*). The major purines, i.e. adenine and guanine, are first converted to xanthine, which is then oxidised to uric acid. In mammals, this is brought about by a flavoprotein xanthine oxidase, but in insects there may be an NAD-linked enzyme instead.

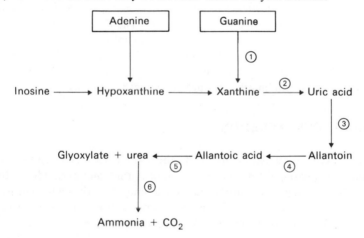

Figure 3.26 Purine catabolism: 1, guanine deaminase; 2, xanthine oxidase; 3, uricase; 4, allantoinase; 5, allantoicase; 6, urease.

Small amounts of uric acid are excreted by some cestodes and trematodes. Uric acid and xanthine are found in the eggs of *A. lumbricoides*, whilst in *Rhabditis strongyloides*, xanthine occurs in the 'rhabditin' inclusions found in the intestine. It is, however, probable that most helminths degrade uric acid further to urea and/or ammonia. In *A. galli* and *A. lumbricoides*, AMP, adenine, xanthine, uric acid and allantoin are broken down to ammonia and urea; guanine, however, was not catabolised. The ability to degrade purines was more marked in young specimens of *A. galli* and *A. lumbricoides* than in old ones. The reason for this is not known. The pathway of purine catabolism in these two nematodes is probably as shown in

Figure 3.26. The only enzyme of this sequence so far identified in parasitic nematodes is urease, although adenosine, adenine and guanine deaminases, xanthine oxidase and uricase have been found in the free-living nematode *Panagrellus redivivus*. The inability of *A. galli* and *A. lumbricoides* to catabolise guanine is presumably due to the absence of guanine deaminase (guanase). Whether the absence of guanine deaminase is going to be a general feature of parasitic nematodes is not known. Guanine deaminase has a rather sporadic distribution in animals. It is, for example, present in the free-living nematode *P. redivivus*, but probably does not occur in chelicerates where guanine is a major end-product, and in mammals the enzyme is absent from pigs.

AMP deaminase activity has been found in *A. galli*, so the catabolism of AMP could involve initial conversion to inosine:

$$AMP \xrightarrow[NH_3]{} IMP \xrightarrow[P_i]{} inosine \xrightarrow[ribose]{} hypoxanthine$$

There are, however, conflicting reports of AMP deaminase activity in *A. lumbricoides*[5]. The purine nucleotide cycle is discussed in Section 4.6.1.

Almost all of the information on purine catabolism in parasites comes from nematodes, and the only other helminths for which any information at all is available are the trematodes *S. mansoni* and *F. hepatica*. Adenosine and guanine deaminase have both been reported from *S. mansoni*. The liver fluke *F. hepatica* does not excrete uric acid, but workers have been unable to detect allantoinase, allantoicase or urease in this parasite. From these observations, it would appear that *F. hepatica* does not degrade purines and it is possible that in *F. hepatica*, as in some free-living platyhelminths, purines are excreted unchanged.

3.6. NITROGENOUS EXCRETION

Some 90% of excreted nitrogen comes from the α-amino nitrogen of amino acids, the remainder originating from the breakdown of purines and pyrimidines. In parasitic helminths, the major excretory product is ammonia, with small quantities of urea, uric acid, amino acids and, in some cases, amines. It has also been suggested that, in nematodes, moulting could be a method for getting rid of nitrogenous wastes.

3.6.1. Ammonia Production

Ammonia usually constitutes about 80% of the total excretory nitrogen in helminths. This is a toxic compound and is, characteristically, an end-product of aquatic organisms. Quite a lot of ammonia is salvaged in living organisms by reversal of the glutamate dehydrogenase reaction (Section 3.4.1) and so is never excreted.

The major source of ammonia in parasitic helminths is probably the oxidative deamination of glutamate and, possibly, alanine (Section 3.4.1). The amino acid oxidases may also make a minor contribution. Another source of ammonia is from the cleavage of urea by the enzyme, urease:

$$NH_2CONH_2 + H_2O \rightarrow 2NH_3 + CO_2$$

Urease does not occur in vertebrates and is found only sporadically in invertebrates. Amongst parasitic helminths, urease has a restricted distribution, being found in nematodes (*Contracaecum aduvicum, Nematodirus* sp., *A. galli, H. contortus, A. lumbricoides*), but not in trematodes (*F. hepatica*). Amongst the cestodes, no urease could be detected in the Cyclophyllidea (*Moniezia benedeni, T. pisiformis*) nor in the Tetraphyllidea (seven species), it did occur in two species of Trypanorhyncha but was absent in a third. The presence of urease in two species of Trypanorhyncha (*Lacistorhynchus tenuis, Pterobothrium lintoni*) is of interest since these tapeworms live in the intestines of sharks and are exposed to a high urea level in the environment (approximately 0.2–0.5 M). Not only homogenates, but also whole worms, cleave exogenous urea. The urease reaction is exergonic, but no mechanism is known whereby it can be coupled to ATP synthesis. An interesting possibility would be if urea cleavage could be linked with carbamoyl phosphate formation, since helminths seem either to lack, or only to have low levels of, carbamoyl-phosphate synthetase (Section 4.6.2). The only other urea-cleaving system known apart from urease is urea amidolyase, and this requires ATP, rather than producing it. The other possibility is that *L. tenuis* and *P. lintoni* require the ammonia or the carbon dioxide for synthetic reactions.

Interestingly, in larval tetraphyllideans (the adults of which are also found in sharks), urea is an important developmental stimulus.

3.6.2. Urea Production

In parasitic helminths, some 2–10% of the total nitrogenous end-products is urea. The mechanism of urea formation by helminths is, however, uncertain. In vertebrates, urea is produced by the urea cycle (*Figure 3.27*), but it is very doubtful if there is a complete urea cycle in parasitic helminths. One of the enzymes of the cycle, arginase, is widely distributed in trematodes, cestodes and nematodes, but carbamoyl-phosphate synthetase is either absent or present in only very low amounts in helminths (Section 4.6.2). Ornithine transcarbamoyltransferase is also now thought to be absent in helminths, despite earlier reports of its presence[63]. So, none of the helminths so far studied seems to possess a complete sequence of urea cycle enzymes. However, the rates of urea production found in helminths would only require very low activities of the enzymes. Low activities of all of the urea cycle enzymes are found in the free-living nematode *Panagrellus silusiae*.

The urea excreted by helminths probably comes from the cleavage of dietary arginine by arginase. A final possible source of urea could be the cleavage of allantoic acid, the latter being derived from the breakdown of purines (Section 3.5.2).

It is not known to what extent changes in the environment lead to changes in the pattern of the excretory products in helminths. It was, at one time, thought that *A. lumbricoides* could modify its excretory products, depending on the availability

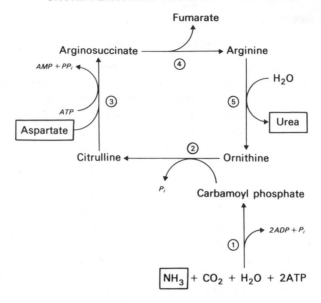

Figure 3.27 The urea cycle: 1, carbamoyl-phosphate synthetase; 2, ornithine transcarbamoylase; 3, arginosuccinate synthetase; 4, arginosuccinate lyase; 5, arginase.

of water. If water was restricted, urea production increased, whilst ammonia production decreased. So *A. lumbricoides* was classed with the select group of animals, such as lung fish and crocodiles, that can modify their end-products of nitrogenous metabolism to suit the environmental conditions. However, more recent work has failed to show any change in the excretory products of *A. lumbricoides* under different conditions of water availability. It is possible that the changes in the proportions of ammonia and urea production found in the original experiments were due, not to the availability of water, but to metabolic disruption caused by long *in vitro* incubations. In *A. lumbricoides*, urea is excreted both via the excretory pore and the intestine, whilst ammonia excretion is primarily via the intestine.

In *Nematodirus* sp. and in *F. hepatica*, anaerobic conditions cause a decrease in urea production. The presence of glucose in the incubation medium of *F. hepatica* suppresses ammonia excretion but does not affect urea production[70].

3.6.3. Uric Acid Production

Small quantities of uric acid are excreted by some cestodes and trematodes (but not *F. hepatica*). With the exception of *Nematodirus* sp., where uric acid constitutes some 3% of the total excreted nitrogen, parasitic nematodes do not excrete detectable quantities of uric acid. The uric acid excreted by parasites probably comes from the breakdown of purines, and the low levels of uric acid production reflect either the complete catabolism of purines to urea or ammonia in most helminths or else is due to the efficiency of their purine salvage pathways (Section 4.6.1). Uric acid excretion tends to be highest in tissue-feeding helminths, presumably because of the high nucleic acid content of their diet.

3.6.4. Amine Production

The larvae of the cestode *T. taeniaeformis* and of the nematodes *A. lumbricoides, N. brasiliensis* and *T. spiralis* excrete a wide range of amines. Amine excretion has also been found in adult *T. spiralis* and in some plant parasitic nematodes, but not in free-living nematodes. In larval *T. spiralis*, amines may constitute as much as 7% of the total nitrogen excreted and may include methyl-, ethyl-, propyl-, butyl-, amyl- and heptylamine, ethylenediamine, cadaverine, ethanolamine and 1-amino-2-propanol. Some of these amines can arise from the decarboxylation of the appropriate amino acids, glycine, alanine, lysine and threonine, giving rise to methylamine, ethylamine, cadaverine and 1-amino-2-propanol, respectively. The direct decarboxylation of serine to ethanolamine has never been reported in animal tissues. So, the synthesis of ethanolamine and of propylamine, butylamine, amylamine, heptylamine and of ethylenediamine must involve specialised, and as yet unknown, pathways. One possible source of amines might be the reduction of azo or nitro compounds.

The excretion of amines is extremely unusual in animals and amines are, of course, very toxic. A possible function of amine production in helminths may be to neutralise the acidic excretory products. In vertebrates, amines are detoxified via monoamine oxidase or by conjugation with a glycone.

Two compounds related to amines, creatinine and betaine, have been found in *Echinococcus* cysts.

3.6.5. Excretion of Amino Acids and Peptides

Many helminths have been reported to excrete substantial amounts of nitrogen in the form of amino acids, peptides or proteins. Amino nitrogen constitutes 35% of the nitrogenous end-products of *Nematodirus* sp. and 28% of the total in *H. diminuta*.

The excretion of amino nitrogen either as amino acids or peptides is fairly common in invertebrates (constituting usually about 10% of the total excretory nitrogen), and comparable rates of amino nitrogen excretion are found, for example, in Echinoderms (24% of the total). The origin of the excretory amino nitrogen in helminths (and invertebrates generally) is not clear. The excretion of amino acids does, of course, provide a way of detoxifying ammonia in animals that do not make urea or uric acid. The synthesis of end-products like urea and uric acid also requires metabolic energy. Some amino acids, such as alanine and proline, may be metabolic end-products. In *H. diminuta*, alanine constitutes 38% of the total amino acids in protonephridial fluid, and alanine and proline are the major amino acids in the protonephridial fluid of *F. gigantica*. Other amino acids may originate from the excretion of excess dietary amino acids. In insects, the excretion of excess dietary amino acids has been well established.

The amino nitrogen produced by helminths could also arise from the partial products of digestion (from faeces or vomit) or from the activity of extracorporeal enzymes. Alternatively, amino nitrogen could be leaking out of the moribund helminth and not be a normal excretory product.

In many invertebrates and possibly helminths as well, amino acids are involved in the regulation of intracellular osmotic pressure. Disruption of the osmotic balance when helminths are removed from their hosts and incubated *in vitro* could well result in amino acid leakage.

The significance of amino nitrogen production by helminths is thus uncertain. In trematodes and cestodes, at least some of the amino acids are excreted via the protonephridial system and may represent 'true' excretory products. Much of the amino nitrogen produced by helminths probably comes from the partial products of digestion, and it is perhaps significant that peptide excretion occurs extensively in nematodes and trematodes, both of which possess an intestine, but not in cestodes, which have no intestine and do not produce digestive enzymes.

3.6.6. Rates of Nitrogenous Excretion in Parasitic Helminths

The rate of nitrogenous excretion in helminths often seems to be considerably higher than that of free-living invertebrates. Values for parasitic nematodes range from 9 to 300 mg N/100 g wet weight/24 h, for trematodes from 100 to 150 mg N/100 g wet weight/24 h and for cestodes from 40 to 200 mg N/100 g wet weight/24 h. Comparable figures for free-living invertebrates are, for crustaceans, 3–60 mg N/100 g fresh weight/24 h and, for annelids, 5–57 mg N/100 g fresh weight/24 h. However, the figures for helminths are generally extrapolated from short-term incubations and, in most of the studies, the animals are not feeding and are, therefore, not in nitrogen balance. So, it is not really possible to conclude that nitrogen catabolism, as judged by total nitrogen excretion, is, in fact, any higher in parasitic helminths than in free-living organisms.

3.7. SUMMARY AND CONCLUSIONS

The pathways of energy production in parasitic helminths are probably better known than any other aspect of parasite biochemistry. In the adult parasite, carbohydrate is the major, and in most cases probably the only, energy source. No adult parasitic helminth appears to be able to catabolise fatty acids by β-oxidation, and amino acid breakdown is relatively unimportant. Parasites are extremely sensitive to inhibitors of carbohydrate catabolism since they have no alternative energy source. Several anthelmintics are thought to work by inhibiting carbohydrate catabolism, and this is a fertile area for anthelmintic research.

Carbohydrate catabolism in parasitic helminths is essentially anaerobic and the pathways involved are all linear, leading to the production of a variety of organic end-products (mostly acids, but occasionally alcohols). In contrast, aerobic catabolic pathways, such as the tricarboxylic acid cycle or the β-oxidation sequence, are cyclic and result in complete degradation of substrate. In most parasitic helminths, the classical tricarboxylic acid cycle is not a significant route for carbohydrate catabolism.

The excretion of a range of organic acids by parasitic helminths can be correlated with the need to maintain a favourable redox balance within the tissues. By coupling the reoxidation of NADH to the reduction of different organic substrates, a variety of end-products can be produced, and this allows the parasite a degree of flexibility in balancing its redox couples.

Helminths that live in sites such as the gut or urinary system are in environments with low O_2 tensions (Section 1.1.1) and it is not surprising that their energy metabolism is largely anaerobic. However, many helminths, for example *S. mansoni* and larval *T. spiralis*, occupy unambiguously aerobic sites in the body, such as the bloodstream or muscles, and yet their metabolism is still essentially anaerobic. It has been suggested that, in the case of larval *T. spiralis*, the anaerobic metabolism may be a preparation for the adult stage which lives in the intestine. When *T. spiralis* larvae are eaten by their next host, they moult and become adult within 36 h. The trematode *S. mansoni* may have arisen from forms which were once gut parasites and, therefore, originally anaerobic. Many parasitic helminths fix carbon dioxide during carbohydrate breakdown, and it is possible that these pathways have evolved not in response to the low environmental pO_2 but as a result of the high pCO_2 found in animal tissues (Sections 1.1.2 and 5.2.2).

An alternative idea is that the loss of the tricarboxylic acid cycle in parasitic helminths is a form of biochemical economy. Heterotrophs are faced with two problems, to obtain their energy source (food) and to catabolise the food source in order to release the energy. In free-living animals, obtaining the food source may be the limiting factor and so there is a need to release the maximum amount of energy from the food obtained. Parasites, on the other hand, have an abundant supply of food and so the need to extract the maximum amount of energy from the food molecule is not so great. For parasites, it may be energetically more profitable to use abbreviated metabolic pathways, rather than maintain the complex enzyme systems of the tricarboxylic acid cycle and β-oxidation sequence. A concept that can be applied to the metabolic systems of parasites is that of the energy utilisation ratio[64]. For a series of reactions, such as glycolysis,

$$\text{energy utilisation ratio} = \frac{\Delta F - \Delta H}{\Delta F}$$

where ΔF is the free-energy change for overall catabolism and ΔH is the energy not available for coupling. As the number of steps in the pathway increases, the smaller the ratio will tend to become. Parasites with their simplified metabolic systems could be said to have elected for an increase in the energy utilisation ratio.

Despite the essentially anaerobic nature of carbohydrate catabolism in helminths, all of them appear to use oxygen when it is available. Many helminths have now been shown to possess cytochrome chains and are capable of oxidative phosphorylation. The cytochrome chains of the large intestinal helminths such as *A. lumbricoides, F. hepatica* and *M. expansa* are, however, unusual in that they have multiple terminal oxidases. The relative importance of oxidative processes in the energy metabolism of helminths is difficult to assess and is probably different in different species. The persistence of anaerobic metabolism in helminths, even when oxygen is available, may be due to the inability of oxidative phosphorylation to supply all of the energy requirements of the parasite; or it may be the result of peculiarities in the control mechanisms of helminth pathways.

In contrast to the adult parasite, the free-living and intermediate stages of parasites are usually aerobic, with a functional tricarboxylic acid cycle and β-oxidation sequence and mammalian-type cytochrome chains, So, although the adult parasite may lack a β-oxidation sequence or complete tricarboxylic acid cycle, it none the less still possesses the information necessary to synthesise these pathways since they are present in the free-living stages of the life-cycle.

3.8. GENERAL READING

Barrett, J. (1976). 'Energy metabolism in nematodes.' In *The Organization of Nematodes*. Ed. N. A. Croll, pp. 11–70. New York; Academic Press

Barrett, J. (1977). 'Energy metabolism and infection in helminths'. *Symp. Br. Soc. Parasitol.*, **15**, 121–44

Van den Bossche, H. (1976). *Biochemistry of Parasites and Host–Parasite Relationships*. Amsterdam; North-Holland

von Brand, T. (1973). *Biochemistry of Parasites*, 2nd edn. New York; Academic Press

Bryant, C. (1975). 'Carbon dioxide utilization and the regulation of respiratory metabolic pathways in parasitic helminths.' *Adv. Parasitol.*, **13**, 35–69 ·

Bryant, C. (1978). 'The regulation of respiratory metabolism in parasitic helminths.' *Adv. Parasitol.*, **16**, 311–31

Coles, G. C. (1973). 'The metabolism of Schistosomes: A review.' *Int. J. Biochem.*, **4**, 319–37

Coles, G. C. (1975). 'Fluke biochemistry—*Fasciola* and *Schistosoma*.' *Helminthol. Abstr.*, **A44**, 147–62

Wright, D. J. and Newall, D. R. (1976). 'Nitrogen excretion, osmotic and ionic regulation in nematodes.' In *The Organization of Nematodes*. Ed. N. A. Croll, pp. 163–210. New York; Academic Press

3.9. REFERENCES

1. Lapp, D. F. and Mason, S. L. (1978). *J. Parasitol.*, **64**, 645–50
2. Rew, R. S. and Saz, H. J. (1974). *J. Cell Biol.*, **63**, 125–35
3. Köhler, P. and Saz, H. J. (1976). *J. Biol. Chem.*, **251**, 2217–25
4. Köhler, P. (1977). *Int. J. Biochem.*, **8**, 141–7
5. Barrett, J. (1973). *Int. J. Parasitol.*, **3**, 393–400
6. Harpur, R. P. and Leigh-Browne, G. (1971). *Exptl Parasitol.*, **29**, 208–14
7. De Mata, S. Z., Saz, H. J. and Pasto, D. J. (1977). *J. Biol. Chem.*, **252**, 4215–44
8. Barrett, J. and Beis, I. (1973). *Compar. Biochem. Physiol.*, **44A**, 331–40
9. Prichard, R. K. (1978). *Parasitology*, **76**, 277–88
10. Schaefer, F. W., Saz, H. J., Weinstein, P. P. and Dunbar, G. A. (1977). *J. Parasitol.*, **63**, 687–9

11. Barrett, J., Coles, G. C. and Simpkin, K. G. (1978). *Int. J. Parasitol.*, **8**, 117–23
12. Köhler, P., Bryant, C. and Behm, C. A. (1978). *Int. J. Parasitol.*, **8**, 399–404
13. Tkachuck, R. D., Saz, H. J., Weinstein, P. P., Finnegan, K. and Mueller, J. F. (1977). *J. Parasitol.*, **63**, 769–74
14. Ward, P. F. V. and Huskisson, N. S. (1978). *Parasitology*, **77**, 255–71
15. Fioravanti, C. F. and Saz, H. J. (1976). *Arch. Biochem. Biophys.*, **175**, 21–30
16. Fioravanti, C. F. and Saz, H. J. (1978). *J. Exptl Zool.*, **206**, 167–78
17. Umezurike, G. M. and Anya, A. O. (1978). *Compar. Biochem. Physiol.*, **59B**, 147–51
18. Barrett, J. (1975). *J. Parasitol.*, **61**, 545–6
19. Barrett, J. (1978). *Parasitology*, **76**, 269–75
20. Rew, R. S. and Saz, H. J. (1977). *J. Parasitol.*, **63**, 123–9
21. Barrett, J. (1978). *Z. Parasitenkunde*, **155**, 223–7
22. Körting, W. and Barrett, J. (1977). *Int. J. Parasitol.*, **7**, 411–7
23. Bryant, C. and Behm, C. A. (1976). In *Biochemistry of Parasites and Host-Parasite Relationships*. Ed. H. Van den Bossche, pp. 89–94. Amsterdam; North-Holland
24. Ackman, R. G. and Gjelstad, R. T. (1975). *Anal. Biochem.*, **67**, 684–7
25. Coles, G. C. and Simpkin, K. G. (1977). *Int. J. Parasitol.*, **7**, 127–8
26. Ryboš, M., Leštan, P. and Dubinský, P. (1974). *Biológica Bratislava*, **B29**, 129–32
27. Komuniecki, R. W. and Roberts, L. S. (1977). *Compar. Biochem. Physiol.*, **58B**, 35–8
28. Goil, M. M. and Harpur, R. P. (1978). *Parasitology*, **77**, 97–102
29. Goil, M. M. and Harpur, R. P. (1978). *Z. Parasitenkunde*, **57**, 117–20
30. Barrett, J. and Beis, I. (1973). *Compar. Biochem. Physiol.*, **44B**, 751–61
31. Saxon, D. J. and Dunagan, T. T. (1975). *Compar. Biochem. Physiol.*, **50B**, 299–303
32. Saxon, D. J. and Dunagan, T. T. (1976). *Compar. Biochem. Physiol.*, **55B**, 377–80
33. Cheah, K. S. (1975). *Compar. Biochem. Physiol.*, **51B**, 41–5
34. Cheah, K. S. (1975). *Biochim. Biophys. Acta*, **387**, 107–14
35. Cheah, K. S. and Prichard, R. K. (1975). *Int. J. Parasitol.*, **5**, 183–6
36. Gerwel, C., Michejda, J. and Boczoń, K. (1975). *Wiadomśki Parazytologiczne*, **21**, 669–77
37. Threadgold, L. T. and Arme, C. (1974). *Exptl Parasitol.*, **35**, 475–91
38. Seed, J. L., Boff, M. and Bennett, J. L. (1978). *J. Parasitol.*, **64**, 283–9
39. Ramalingam, K. (1970). *Experientia*, **26**, 828
40. Paul, J. M. and Barrett, J. (1980). *Int. J. Parasitol.*, in press
41. Robinson, J. M. and Bogitsh, B. J. (1978). *Exptl Parasitol.*, **45**, 169–74
42. Harpur, R. P. and Jackson, D. M. (1976). *Compar. Biochem. Physiol.*, **54B**, 455–60
43. Von Kruger, W. M. A., Gazzinelli, G., Figueiredo, E. A. and Pellegrino, J. (1978). *Compar. Biochem. Physiol.*, **60B**, 41–6
44. Harpur, R. P. (1974). *Compar. Biochem. Physiol.*, **48A**, 133–43

45. Barrett, J. and Körting, W. (1977). *Int. J. Parasitol.*, **7**, 419–22
46. Barrett, J. and Körting, W. (1976). *Int. J. Parasitol.*, **6**, 155–7
47. Körting, W. and Barrett, J. (1979). *Z. Parasitenkunde*, **57**, 243–6
48. Oudejans, R. C. H. M. and Van Der Horst, D. J. (1974). *Compar. Biochem. Physiol.*, **47B**, 139–47
49. Fried, B. and Shapiro, I. L. (1975). *J. Parasitol.*, **61**, 906–9
50. Fried, B. and Appel, A. J. (1977). *J. Parasitol.*, **63**, 447
51. Fried, B. and Butler, M. S. (1977). *J. Parasitol.*, **63**, 831–4
52. Butler, M. S. and Fried, B. (1977). *J. Parasitol.*, **63**, 1041–5
53. Popiel, I. and James, B. L. (1976). *Z. Parasitenkunde*, **51**, 71–7
54. Mustafa, T., Komuniecki, R. and Mettrick, D. F. (1978). *Compar. Biochem. Physiol.*, **61B**, 219–22
55. Bishop, S. H. (1975). *J. Parasitol.*, **61**, 79–88
56. Ertel, J. and Isseroff, H. (1974). *J. Parasitol.*, **60**, 574–7
57. Isseroff, H. and Ertel, J. C. (1976). *Int. J. Parasitol.*, **6**, 183–8
58. Isseroff, H., Sawma, J. T. and Reino, D. (1977). *Science*, **198**, 1157–9
59. Brown, J. N. and Smith, T. M. (1973). *Compar. Biochem. Physiol.*, **45B**, 487–9
60. Cornish, R. A. and Bryant, C. (1975). *Int. J. Parasitol.*, **5**, 355–62
61. Nations, C., Hicks, T. C. and Ubelaker, J. C. (1973). *J. Parasitol.*, **59**, 112–6
62. Sanchez Moreno, M. and Barrett, J. (1979). *Parasitology*, **78**, 1–5
63. Kurelec, B. (1972). *Compar. Biochem. Physiol.*, **43B**, 769–80
64. Read, C. P. (1961). In *Comparative Physiology of Carbohydrate Metabolism in Heterothermic Animals*, pp. 3–34. Seattle; University of Washington Press
65. Berl, S. and Bueding, E. (1961). *J. Biol. Chem.*, **191**, 401–18
66. van Vugt, F., van der Meer, P. and van den Berg, S. G. (1979). *Int. J. Biochem.*, **10**, 11–8
67. Boczoń, K. and Michejda, J. W. (1978). *Int. J. Parasitol.*, **8**, 507–13
68. Bollerup, G. and Burr, A. H. (1979). *Can. J. Zool.*, **57**, 1057–69
69. Sawma, J. T., Isseroff, H. and Reino, D. (1978). *Compar. Biochem. Physiol.*, **61A**, 239–43
70. Moss, G. D. (1970). *Parasitology*, **60**, 1–9

4 Nutrition and Biosynthesis

Parasites often grow extremely rapidly and can produce large numbers of eggs or larvae. A female A. *lumbricoides*, for example, lays 1.6×10^6 eggs per day and a developing tapeworm, *H. diminuta*, increases its weight 2×10^4 fold in 10 days. This gives some indication of the high synthetic rates of which parasites are capable. However, although synthetic pathways are well developed quantitatively in helminths, the range of compounds that they synthesise is relatively limited.

4.1. DIGESTION AND ABSORPTION OF NUTRIENTS

Like all heterotrophs, parasites require a supply of low molecular weight nutrients. Trematodes and most nematodes have a digestive system and produce a range of digestive enzymes. Other helminths, such as cestodes, acanthocephalans, nematomorphs and some nematodes, have no functional gut, they produce no digestive enzymes of their own and have to rely entirely on the host to provide them with low molecular weight compounds.

4.1.1. Digestive Enzymes

The comparative biochemistry of digestive enzymes is a very much neglected subject. Most parasites are too small to allow direct sampling of digestive enzymes from their gut lumen and so, often, whole animal extracts have had to be used. However, in whole homogenates, enzymes may be derived not only from the gut lumen, but also from the tissues. Tissue digestive enzymes are involved with the final intracellular digestion of nutrients and with the turnover of cellular constituents.

Many parasites discharge digestive enzymes into the environment either during extracorporeal digestion or to assist penetration into and migration through host tissues. Larval parasites also produce a variety of hatching and exsheathing enzymes. The action of penetration enzymes or of hatching and exsheathing enzymes may lead to the release of potentially useful nutrients and these enzymes will be considered in Section 4.1.2.

Proteolytic Enzymes

The breakdown of proteins requires the action of both endopeptidases and exopeptidases. The endopeptidases break peptide bonds in the middle of the peptide chain, whilst the exopeptidases split off single amino acids from the ends of the chain. Carboxypeptidases cleave amino acids from the C terminal (carboxyl) end of the protein, and the aminopeptidases split off amino acids from the N terminal (amino) end. The combined action of these enzymes gives a mixture of free amino acids and di- and tripeptides. The di- and tripeptides are finally split by di- and tripeptidases; in the mammal, the di- and tripeptidases are located in the brush borders of the mucosal cells.

In general, the proteolytic enzymes of helminths have not been characterised. Proteolytic activity has been demonstrated in oesophageal extracts of *A. caninum* and *A. lumbricoides* and may play a role in extracorporeal digestion. In *T. vulpis*, protease activity is concentrated at the anterior end and again may be involved in extracorporeal digestion. Proteases have been demonstrated in extracts of *Haplometra cylindracea, Haematoloechus medioplexus, F. hepatica* and the cercariae of *S. mansoni*, but whether these are gut or tissue enzymes was not shown. Similarly, trypsin and chymotrypsin activity have been found in extracts of *S. mansoni*, but their location is not known. Histochemically, proteases have been located in the digestive caecae of the trematodes *F. hepatica, L. constantiae* and *Philophthalmus burrili*[1]. Definite intestinal proteases have been isolated from the nematodes *A. lumbricoides, Graphidium strigosum, Strongylus edentatus* and *Leidynema appendiculata*. Although these proteases have not been fully characterised, they appear to resemble mammalian trypsin in their general properties. True peptic proteases have not been found in helminths and acid proteases are not common in invertebrates (although they have been found, for example, in some molluscs). In vertebrates, proteases are secreted initially as inactive proenzymes, which are subsequently activated—trypsinogen, for example, is converted to trypsin. Similar inactive precursors have yet to be described in parasitic helminths. Although some of the helminth proteases, so far described, are undoubtedly tissue proteases, none have been shown to have the properties of mammalian cathepsins. Cathepsins are the proteases found in lysosomes and are only maximally active in the presence of sulphydryl reagents.

Peptidases show a range of specificities and there is no simple classification. Peptidases have been found in homogenates of trematodes (*F. hepatica, H. cylindracea, S. mansoni* eggs) and acanthocephalans (*Neoechinorhynchus* sp.), but have only been investigated to any significant extent in parasitic nematodes. Glycylglycine peptidase, glycylproline aminopeptidase and leucine aminopeptidase have been found in the intestine of *Leidynema appendiculata*, whilst four peptidases have been characterised from the intestine of *A. lumbricoides*, glycylglycine peptidase, alanylglycine peptidase, leucine aminopeptidase and a general tripeptidase. The leucine aminopeptidase of *A. lumbricoides* intestine is primarily insoluble and may be associated with the brush borders of the intestinal cells. In addition to the intestine, leucine aminopeptidase is found in the uterus, excretory canals and hypodermis of adult *A. lumbricoides*. Two separate leucine aminopeptidases occur in the uterus of *A. lumbricoides* and these uterine enzymes differ in several respects (pH optimum, metal ion activation, kinetic constants) from the intestinal enzyme. The cyst fluid of *E. granulosus* is said to contain a leucine aminopeptidase as well as proteases; the possible role of these enzymes in this parasite is obscure. Leucine aminopeptidase is involved in the hatching and exsheathing of several nematode larvae (Section 4.1.2) and is also said to be present in the tegument of the acanthocephalan *P. minutus* and in the tegument, but not the gut, of *Schistosoma rodhaini*.

An interesting substrate-specific protease occurs in the gut of *S. mansoni*. This enzyme (globinase) has an acid pH optimum (pH 3.9) and appears to be highly specific for haemoglobin and globin, and serum proteins are not attacked. This substrate-specific protease has aroused interest for two reasons. First, since the enzyme is highly specific for its substrate, it might prove possible to develop an anthelmintic which would specifically inhibit it. Secondly, significant amounts of this enzyme are released into the bloodstream by the parasite, so purified protease could form the basis of a sensitive skin test for schistosomiasis. The end-products of haemoglobin degradation by the schistosome protease are peptides, rather than amino acids. Complete degradation of globin would require the presence of a second protease. There is some evidence in schistosomes for a second protease but, alternatively, they could absorb peptides. Peptide absorption has, however, not been demonstrated in *S. mansoni*, although they have been shown to take up ^{14}C-leucine when fed labelled reticulocytes.

In *S. mansoni*, haemoglobin digestion is wholly extracellular, whilst in *F. hepatica* it is both extra- and intracellular. *F. hepatica* also has a protease capable of breaking down haemoglobin (pH optimum 3.6-4) and this is again excreted in large quantities. Haemoglobin digestion has been followed histochemically in a number of nematodes and trematodes, and, depending on the species, the main end-product can be haematin, haemosiderin or an unidentified iron compound.

Carbohydrate Breakdown

In the mammalian gut, starch and glycogen are rapidly broken down by α-amylase, releasing maltose, maltotriose and α-limit dextrins. The disaccharides, together with others in the diet, are hydrolysed to monosaccharides by disaccharidases located in the brush borders of the intestinal cells.

An α-amylase has been found in intestinal extracts of a number of nematodes (*A. lumbricoides, S. edentatus, L. appendiculata, G. strigosum*), in homogenates of larval *Anisakis* and *A. galli*, and also in the pseudocoelomic fluid of *A. lumbricoides* and *P. equorum*. Of the disaccharidases, a maltase has been found in intestinal extracts of *L. appendiculata* and four disaccharidases, maltase, invertase, trehalase and isomaltase (palatinase), have been located in the brush borders of *A. lumbricoides* intestinal cells. In *A. lumbricoides*, trehalase is found not only in the intestine, but in the muscles, ovary, oviduct and testis (Section 3.1.1). A number of disaccharidases have been identified in homogenates of larval and adult *T. spiralis*[2] (maltase, invertase, trehalase, lactase, isomaltase), *T. vulpis* (maltase, invertase, lactase), the acanthocephalan *M. hirudinaceus* (maltase, trehalase) and the cestode *Stilesia globipunctata* (trehalase)[3]. With homogenates it is not, of course, possible to say whether these disaccharidases are concerned with digestion or with some other metabolic function. Trehalase, in particular, is involved both in digestion and trehalose utilisation in the tissues (Section 3.1.1).

A number of glycosidases have been identified in homogenates of *T. vulpis* (β-glucuronidase, β-galactosidase) and *N. brasiliensis* (β-acetylaminodeoxyglucosidase, β-glucuronidase, β-galactosidase, α-mannosidase); β-glucuronidase has also been shown, histochemically, in various tissues and stages of schistosomes. The function of these glycosidases is not clear, but they could be involved in the breakdown of mucopolysaccharides.

Cellulases, chitinases and pectinases occur in plant parasitic nematodes.

Lipases and Esterases

Lipases, capable of hydrolysing esters of long chain fatty acids, occur in the intestine of several nematodes (*A. lumbricoides, L. appendiculata, S. edentatus*) and the oesophagus of *A. caninum*. However, few details of their properties are known. Tissue lipases, possibly involved in triacylglycerol mobilisation, have been reported from nematodes, trematodes, cestodes and acanthocephalans. The presence of lipases in cestodes (*H. diminuta*) has, however, been disputed by some workers[4]. Lysophospholipase and phospholipase A and C, but not D, have been demonstrated in *A. lumbricoides* (Section 4.3.5), and phospholipase activity has also been claimed in *H. diminuta*. Phospholipase A removes the fatty acids from phospholipids, phospholipase C hydrolyses the phosphoric acid/glycerol link, whilst phospholipase D removes the polar head group leaving a phosphatidic acid.

Related to lipases are the esterases, which hydrolyse esters of short chain fatty acids. The esterases are usually divided into non-specific esterases and choline esterases. Non-specific esterases can be further subdivided on the basis of substrate specificity and selective inhibition into carboxyl esterases (ali-esterase or B esterase), aryl esterases (C esterase) and acetyl esterase (A esterase). These esterases preferentially hydrolyse esters of straight chain acids, aromatic acids and acetic acid, respectively. Each of these groups of esters probably consists of several different enzymes with overlapping specificities.

Non-specific esterases have been described in various tissues of nematodes, trematodes, cestodes and acanthocephalans and have been extensively studied, histochemically. Esterases have also been separated electrophoretically in a number of species[5] and in *A. lumbricoides* different tissues, including pseudocoelomic fluid, have their own esterase isoenzyme pattern[6]. Unfortunately, despite the many studies on esterase distribution, the physiological role of non-specific esterases is unknown. The natural substrate for some of the esterases is possibly cholesterol esters, whereas others may normally hydrolyse amides (amidases). Several peptidases, including leucine aminopeptidase, also show esterase activity.

The choline esterases can also be divided into two types on the basis of substrate specificity and inhibition studies. Acetylcholine esterase preferentially hydrolyses acetylcholine and is inhibited by high substrate concentrations. Choline esterase (pseudocholine esterase), on the other hand, shows a higher activity with butylcholine than with acetylcholine, and is not inhibited by excess acetylcholine. In mammals, acetylcholine esterase is found in the nervous system, choline esterase in the plasma. Both acetylcholine esterase and choline esterase have been demonstrated in a variety of tissues from nematodes, trematodes and cestodes. Many, but by no means all, intestinal nematodes contain large amounts of acetylcholine esterase in their oesophageal and subventral glands. These nematodes appear to excrete large amounts of acetylcholine esterase *in vitro* (*T. colubriformis, T. axei, Trichostrongylus retortaeformis, O. radiatum, N. brasiliensis, N. battus, N. americanus*)[7]. As in the case of the specific protease from *S. mansoni*, the production of acetylcholine esterase by these nematodes is interesting for two reasons. First, since invertebrate (and helminth[8]) acetylcholine esterases are generally more sensitive to inhibition by organophosphates than the mammalian enzyme, this enzyme is a possible site for chemotherapy. Secondly, the secretion of large amounts of acetylcholine esterase by these nematodes leads to the production of specific antibodies by the host, and this could again be the basis of a sensitive skin test. The significance of acetylcholine esterase secretion by intestinal nematodes is not known. Acetylcholine esterase might reduce peristalsis of the host intestine, or it may reduce the host's immune response. In *N. brasiliensis* and *N. battus*, acetylcholine esterase production varies with the host's immune status. Alternatively, acetylcholine esterase, by reducing acetylcholine levels in the intestine, may stimulate glycogen breakdown and increase the free glucose levels. Acetylcholine is normally present in intestinal secretions and it may be involved in regulating uptake mechanisms.

Nucleic Acid Breakdown

Digestion of nucleic acids usually involves initial degradation to nucleotides via ribonuclease, deoxyribonuclease or a polynucleotidase. The nucleotides are then hydrolysed by nucleotidases and nucleosidases to pyrimidine or purine bases, pentose and phosphate. In the vertebrate intestine, the pentose sugar is usually rapidly rephosphorylated. Nucleic acid digestion has not been investigated at all in parasitic helminths and there is only one report of a ribonuclease and a deoxyribonuclease from homogenates of *T. muris*. A 5'-nucleotidase has been demonstrated histochemically in larval *Anisakis, F. gigantica, R. cesticillus, H. contortus, T. spiralis* and in the eggs of *S. mansoni*.

Phosphatases

The two most widely studied phosphatases in helminths are the non-specific acid and alkaline phosphatases[9,10]. These enzymes are widely distributed in the gut (including the brush border in *A. lumbricoides*), tegument and tissues of nematodes, trematodes, cestodes and acanthocephalans. Rather like esterases, the physiological role of acid and alkaline phosphatases is not clear. In helminths, as in mammals, acid phosphatase is usually associated with lysosomes, and alkaline phosphatase is often indicative of membrane transport mechanisms. Both acid and alkaline phosphatases act not only as phosphohydrolases but also as transphosphorylases, and it is the transphosphorylase activity of these enzymes which may be of more biological importance than the phosphatase activity.

Inorganic pyrophosphatase activity has been found in nematodes, trematodes and acanthocephalans. ATPase activity is also universally distributed in helminths and, again, probably represents a variety of enzymes.

Tegumental Enzymes

It is now well established in mammals that the brush borders of the mucosal cells contain di- and tripeptidases, disaccharidases and phosphohydrolases. The final hydrolysis of peptides and disaccharides takes place within the brush borders, and there may be a spatial relationship between the brush border enzymes and the amino acid and monosaccharide absorption sites. There is some evidence that, in the nematode intestine, peptidases, disaccharidases and phosphatases are located in the brush borders of the intestinal cells. Cestodes and acanthocephalans, on the other hand, do not secrete digestive enzymes of any sort. Nevertheless, within the teguments of these parasites are enzymes, some of which may have a digestive function.

In *H. diminuta*, there are surface phosphatases capable of hydrolysing exogenous sugar phosphates, nucleotides and artificial substrates. The phosphatases are thought to be in close proximity to the sugar and nucleoside uptake sites. The products of hydrolysis can, therefore, be rapidly absorbed by the tapeworm, rather than diffusing back into the surrounding medium. The phosphatase and uptake sites are not, however, functionally linked. There is some evidence that there may be up to three different nucleotide phosphohydrolases in the tegument of *H. diminuta*, all capable of hydrolysing external nucleotides.

A tegumental phosphohydrolase, which hydrolyses exogenous glucose-6-phosphate, has been found in the acanthocephalan *M. dubius*, and a tegumental phosphatase has also been found in *S. mansoni* (Section 4.1.10). Acid and alkaline phosphatases occur widely in the teguments of trematodes, cestodes and acanthocephalans. In adult cestodes and acanthocephalans, alkaline phosphatase is usually the most active, whilst acid phosphatases tend to predominate in the trematode tegument. In *F. hepatica*, acid and alkaline phosphatases are found both in the tegument and the glycocalyx. At one time it was thought that helminths possessed either acid or alkaline phosphatase activity, but it is now clear that both are usually present. The relative activities of acid and alkaline phosphatases in the teguments of cestodes change during development. The role of acid and alkaline phosphatases, if any, in digestion and absorption is uncertain.

The cestode *H. diminuta* also possesses what appears to be an intrinsic tegumental ribonuclease[140] and a monoacylglycerol hydrolase. There is, however, no evidence that these two enzymes are involved in the digestion and transport of nutrients.

Intact *H. diminuta* lacks any detectable aminopeptidase or dipeptidase activity. The acanthocephalan *M. dubius*, however, shows significant aminopeptidase activity and will hydrolyse leucine- and alanine-containing peptides present in the incubating medium. Again, the aminopeptidase activity and the leucine–alanine transport sites appear to be separate, but in close spatial proximity. Activated larvae of *M. dubius* (cystacanths) also possess a similar surface dipeptidase.

A leucine aminopeptidase has been described in the tegument of *S. rodhaini* and *P. minutus* and aminopeptidases have been described on the surface of trematode rediae. The latter are thought to be involved in extracorporeal digestion. Although intact adult cestodes show no protease or dipeptidase activity, homogenates of tapeworms (*T. saginata, T. pisiformis, D. caninum, D. latum, M. benedeni*) show considerable dipeptidase activity, as well as weak protease activity. These are probably involved in tissue protein turnover and not in absorption and digestion. The plerocercoids of *Spirometra erinacei* appear to have a protease associated with the tegument of the scolex and this may be related to tissue penetration[11].

The acanthocephalan *M. dubius* can metabolise maltose, and a few cestodes are also said to be able to metabolise exogenous disaccharides (*Cittotaenia* sp., maltose and sucrose; *Phyllobothrium foliatum*, maltose). However, whether this involves tegumental disaccharidases of intrinsic or host origin is not known.

Although cestodes and acanthocephalans do not secrete digestive enzymes, they do have, in their teguments, enzymes that can hydrolyse external substrates. Similar enzymes may also occur in the teguments of trematodes. Like the brush borders of mammalian mucosal cells, there may be a spatial relationship between the enzyme and the relevant uptake sites. Not all of the enzymes in the tegument are necessarily concerned with digestion or transport, and the non-absorptive cuticle of *A. lumbricoides*, for example, contains esterases, as well as a polyphenol oxidase.

Contact Digestion and Contact Inhibition

In the mammalian intestine, pancreatic enzymes become adsorbed onto the brush borders of the mucosal cells. This has the advantage that the products of digestion are released in close proximity to the membrane-bound di- and tripeptidases and disaccharidases and associated transport sites. It has also been claimed that, when α-amylase is adsorbed onto the mucosal surface, it is stabilised in a favourable configuration, so that its catalytic activity is enhanced. However, the presence, in mucosal cells, of intrinsic α-amylases makes claims for increased activity following adsorption open to doubt. At the moment, the relative importance of luminal and contact (or surface) digestion in the mammalian intestine is in dispute.

Several species of cestode have been shown to adsorb α-amylase *in vitro* (*H. diminuta, H. microstoma, M. expansa, L. intestinalis*), and adsorption appears to lead to an increase in amylolytic activity. Intact tapeworms show no intrinsic α-amylase activity, so intrinsic enzymes cannot be responsible for the increased activity. The activation of α-amylase by *H. diminuta* requires live worms, is reversible and activation is prevented by polycations. The inhibition of activation by polycations suggests that the enzyme becomes bound to the glycocalyx. However, there is no evidence that α-amylase is stabilised in some form of kinetically favourable configuration when bound to *H. diminuta*. Although the reversibility of α-amylase activation shows that diffusible activators are not involved, the cestode glycocalyx may constitute a micro-environment, different from that of the bulk phase. In particular, localised pH changes could account for the apparent activation.

The tapeworm *H. diminuta* also interacts, *in vitro*, with trypsin, α- and β-chymotrypsin and lipase. Both trypsin and α- and β-chymotrypsin are irreversibly inactivated by *H. diminuta*. These proteolytic enzymes do not appear to become bound to the parasite in the same way as α-amylase, and polyions have no effect. One possibility is that there is a proteolytic enzyme inhibitor present in the glycocalyx. Another cestode, *Proteocephalus longicollis*, has also been shown to inactivate trypsin. Protease inhibition might be important in protecting the worms against digestion, although it could possibly limit the worms' ability to obtain amino acids. Intact mammalian mucosa has also been shown to have the ability to inhibit trypsin and chymotrypsin, and similarly this may be a protective device.

Lipase is reversibly inhibited by *H. diminuta* and, again, polyions have no effect. The physiological significance of lipase inhibition is, however, obscure.

In contrast, the acanthocephalan *M. dubius* shows no contact acceleration or contact inhibition with α-amylase, trypsin, α- and β-chymotrypsin or lipase, although it has been shown *in vivo* that *M. dubius* does absorb onto its surface relatively large amounts of host α-amylase. The presence of increased α-amylase levels in the immediate vicinity of the parasite would mean that the products of starch and glycogen breakdown are readily available to the helminth. The end-products of amylase digestion are, however, di- and trisaccharides and not free glucose. So, although this could be of advantage to *M. dubius*, which can metabolise maltose, *H. diminuta* possesses no intrinsic disaccharidases and can metabolise only glucose and galactose.

In the case of *H. diminuta*, absorption of host α-amylase, if it occurs *in vivo*, would seem to be of no obvious use. Rats infected with *H. diminuta* show no detectable increase in amylolytic activity in their intestines[12].

4.1.2. Hatching, Exsheathing and Tissue-penetrating Enzymes

The tissue-penetrating stages of helminths may contain enzymes active against the acellular components of connective tissue[141], although many nematode larvae invade the epidermis of their hosts by purely mechanical means. The tissue-penetrating enzymes of helminths are usually said to be of the collagenase type, rather than hyaluronidases. Collagenases have, for example, been described from immature *F. hepatica*, *S. mansoni* eggs and the larvae of *S. ratti*, *S. simiae*, *A. caninum* and *Anisakis* sp. In schistosome eggs, the collagenase is said to pass out through the pores in the egg shell. The cercariae of *S. mansoni* have a protease complex which has elastolytic and keratolytic properties, but it is doubtful if there is any collagenase activity[13]. The cercariae also produce a peptidase, a lipase and possibly a hyaluronidase. The protease of *S. mansoni* cercariae is reversibly inhibited by calcium[14], and the high calcium levels in the preacetabular glands (Section 2.1) may serve to inactivate the enzyme prior to secretion. Schistosome cercarial proteases are also inhibited by the mammalian plasma protease inhibitor.

The excretory gland of the nematode *S. edentatus* contains a tryptic-type protease, leucine aminopeptidase and esterase activity and these may be concerned with tissue penetration. There have also been claims of hyaluronidase activity in *S. edentatus* and *Strongylus equinus*. However, no collagenase or hyaluronidase activity could be detected in the onchospheres of *H. diminuta* or the infective larvae of *N. brasiliensis*[15] despite earlier suggestions that they might be present[16]. The infective larvae of *N. brasiliensis* do produce a lipase and there is considerable esterase activity in the pharynx. There are also unconfirmed reports of hyaluronidase activity in the infective larvae of *Dictyocaulus filaria*, *A. caninum* and *Ancylostoma duodenale*.

Studies on hatching and exsheathing enzymes have been almost exclusively restricted to nematodes. The hatching fluid from *A. lumbricoides* eggs contains a whole variety of enzymes[17], a tryptic-type protease, an esterase, α- and β-glycosidases, leucine aminopeptidase and a chitinase. These enzymes presumably attack different components of the egg shell during hatching. The chitinase is interesting, as it is absent in unembryonated eggs, but can be demonstrated in embryonated eggs and in first- and second-stage larvae. The purified chitinase degrades chitin to *N*-acetylglucosamine. Most other chitinases only degrade chitin to di- and trisaccharides and require a second enzyme, chitobiase, for complete breakdown. No chitinase activity occurs in adult female *A. lumbricoides* or *A. galli*, but activity has been reported from sperm cells. The function of sperm chitinase is unclear, since neither the sperm nor the oocyte contain chitin. Hatching fluid from *H. contortus* eggs contains a lipase and an aminopeptidase, but no chitinase[18]; and chitin is said to be absent from *H. contortus* egg shells. The eggs of acanthocephalans, which hatch in the intestines of arthropods, may also produce a chitinase. This raises the interesting possibility that the chitinase may not only act on the chitin in the acanthocephalan egg shell, but might also aid penetration through the peritrophic membrane.

The exsheathing fluid of nematode larvae is also a complex mixture of enzymes. Third-stage larvae of *H. contortus* and *T. colubriformis* are protected by being retained within the shed cuticle of the second-stage larva. When stimulated, both species of nematode produce an exsheathing fluid, probably from the excretory gland, which attacks the second-stage sheath in a narrow region near the anterior end. This results, initially, in the formation of a hyaline ring around the sheath, and eventually the cap falls off and the infective larva emerges. The exsheathing fluids appear to be species-specific; that is, fluid from *H. contortus* larvae will attack isolated *H. contortus* sheaths, but not *T. colubriformis* sheaths and vice versa. Exsheathing fluid from both species contains leucine aminopeptidase activity, and a lipase has also been described in *H. contortus* fluid[18,19]. Initially, it was thought that leucine aminopeptidase was the sole enzyme responsible for exsheathing. However, it seems likely that leucine aminopeptidase is only one of the enzymes concerned[142]. It is an interesting problem why exsheathing fluid only attacks the sheath in such a highly restricted region. Presumably, the cuticle which forms the hyaline ring is different in some way from the rest of the cuticle. Leucine aminopeptidase is also involved in moulting in *P. decipiens* larvae. Here, the secretion of the enzyme is governed by a neurosecretory cycle during the moult.

Hatching enzymes have not been demonstrated in trematode eggs, although it is often assumed that the hatching of operculate trematode eggs involves enzymatic attack on the cement substance around the edge of the lid. There is, however, no clear evidence that such a cement substance actually exists. In *F. hepatica*, the opening of the operculum is purely mechanical, due to swelling of the viscous cushion (Section 2.2.3). The hatching mechanisms of non-operculate trematode eggs has not been studied. The excystment of metacercarial cysts may involve parasite enzymes, but again this has not been investigated.

4.1.3. Anticoagulants and Antienzymes

All bloodsucking parasites produce anticoagulants of some sort to prevent premature clotting of blood. Anticoagulants have been described from trematodes (*Pneumoneces* sp.) and nematodes (*A. caninum, Bunostomum trigonocephalum*). The anticoagulant from *A. caninum* has been named ancylostomatin and it is a polypeptide, molecular weight 20 000–50 000. Ancylostomatin prevents the conversion of prothrombin to thrombin probably by interfering with activated factor X. An anticoagulant has also been demonstrated in homogenates of *S. mansoni* and this inhibits the conversion of factor XI to XIa by factor XIIa[20].

Antienzymes, that is, compounds that inhibit the digestive enzymes of the host, have been found in several nematodes and cestodes, but not, as yet, in any trematodes or acanthocephalans. A variety of such inhibitors occur in *A. lumbricoides*, where a pepsin inhibitor, at least two trypsin inhibitors, two or three chymotrypsin inhibitors and three separate carboxypeptidase inhibitors have been identified[21]. These inhibitors are all peptides of low molecular weight (4650–12 400), and one of the trypsin inhibitors has been purified and its amino acid sequence determined. The protease inhibitors of *A. lumbricoides* are found, not only in the body wall, but also in the intestine, ovary, uterus and pseudocoelomic fluid.

The biological significance of these protease inhibitors is not clear. Intestinal helminths can withstand tryptic digestion as long as they are alive and intact, but are rapidly digested when dead or if their tegument is damaged. At the moment, however, there is no good evidence to suggest that antienzymes are involved in this resistance to digestion. No secretion of antienzymes has been detected in *A. lumbricoides* or in cestodes, although it has been suggested that antienzymes in the glycocalyx might be responsible for the phenomenon of contact inhibition in *H. diminuta* (Section 4.1.1). In the nematode *S. edentatus*, trypsin and chymotrypsin inhibitors are found in the excretory gland cell and these inhibitors are released into the incubation medium[22]. It is possible that this protects the nematode from digestion by host enzymes. Alternatively, the inhibitor may, like the protease inhibitor from the mammalian pancreas, prevent the proteases in the digestive gland from being active before they are secreted. The antienzymes found in the tissues of other helminths may similarly have a role in the regulation of intracellular proteases.

Resistance to Digestion

The mechanisms by which intestinal helminths resist digestion in the gut are not really known. Enzyme action may be prevented by contact inhibition or the presence, in the outer parts of the tegument, of antienzymes. The mucopolysaccharides of the glycocalyx cover the surface of the parasite and this could prevent access of trypsin. The surface proteins of helminths might be resistant to tryptic digestion and helminths, unlike dietary protein, are not being exposed to sequential peptic and tryptic digestion. Finally, in the same way as the intestinal lining is being continuously renewed, the helminth tegument may be constantly turning over.

4.1.4. Nature of the Absorptive Surface

Cestodes

The cestodes have no digestive tract of any sort and all materials must be absorbed through the body surface. The body wall of cestodes is a syncitial tegument and the surface is covered with micro-villi; morphologically, the body wall of a cestode can be compared with the mammalian intestinal cell. In *H. diminuta*, the micro-villi increase the surface area of the parasite approximately 2.6 times, which is rather small in comparison with the mammalian intestine where the micro-villi increase the surface area about 25 fold.

The cestode tegument is impermeable to peptides, proteins and macromolecules. The uptake of material by pinocytosis has not been demonstrated in adult cestodes, although pinocytotic-like vesicles are found in the tegument. Pinocytosis has, however, been described in the plerocercoid of *S. solidus*.

Acanthocephala

Like the cestodes, the acanthocephalans have no digestive tract and their teguments are modified for absorption. The tegument of acanthocephalans is again syncitial, but is morphologically very different from that of cestodes. The acanthocephalan tegument does not possess micro-villi, but instead is covered with crypts, which again may help to increase the absorptive surface.

Unlike cestodes, pinocytosis has been described in adult acanthocephalans (*M. dubius*) and takes place via the surface pits. Associated with these pits are lysosomes and acid phosphatase activity[23].

The proboscis of acanthocephalans lies buried in the host's mucosa and it has been suggested that the proboscis may be a specialised region for absorption. A similar 'placental' function has been claimed for the penetrative scoleces of cestodes, but experimental evidence is lacking.

Trematodes

There are two potential absorptive sites in trematodes, the gut epithelium and the external tegument. As in the cestodes and acanthocephalans, the trematode tegument is syncitial and apparently modified for absorption. There are no micro-villi or crypts in the trematode tegument, but there may be irregular pits. In Stregeid trematodes, there is a specialised region of the tegument called the 'holdfast' which may play a major role in extracorporeal digestion and absorption. Histochemically, the holdfast has been shown to possess a variety of hydrolytic enzymes (esterase, aminopeptidase, alkaline phosphatase).

All of the studies, so far, on the uptake mechanisms of trematodes have dealt just with transport across the external tegument. The relative importance of the tegument and the gut in uptake has been little studied. In order to investigate tegumental uptake, the mouth of the trematode is ligatured and this can cause considerable damage to the surrounding tegument. This may result in leakage, from the tegument, of low molecular weight compounds and this should be borne in mind when interpreting the results of ligature experiments.

Pinocytosis has been described in the tegument of trematodes, but it is said not to occur in the caecae. The cells lining the digestive caecae have cytoplasmic processes which may be free or form loops, and presumably increase the absorptive area. Trematode gut cells go through cycles of secretory and absorptive activity, and digestion is probably both extra- and intracellular.

Nematodes

Typically, nematodes have a digestive tract, and have, therefore, two potential absorptive surfaces. However, in most nematodes, the cuticle (which is composed of modified keratinised cells) is permeable only to water and certain lipid-soluble anthelmintics. Transcuticular uptake of glucose and alanine has been demonstrated in *A. galli* and *A. lumbricoides*, but the rates are too low to be of any physiological significance.

Transcuticular uptake does take place in certain insect parasitic nematodes such as *Bradynema* sp. and larval *Mermis nigrescens*. In *Sphaerularia bombi*, nutrients are taken up from the insect haemocoel via an everted uterine membrane. There is also some evidence for transcuticular uptake in the adult filarial worms *B. pahangi* (glucose, leucine and adenine) and *D. immitis* (glucose)[143]. In the Trichuroidea, the trichurid and capillarid nematodes have a cuticular structure known as the bacillary band associated with the stichosome. The function of the bacillary band is not known, but it has been suggested that it may be involved in absorption and extracorporeal digestion.

The intestine of nematodes consists of a single layer of columnar cells on a basement membrane. The luminal surface of the intestinal cells is covered with micro-villi and, in *A. lumbricoides*, the micro-villi increase the surface area of the intestine 75-90 times. Covering the micro-villi is a glycocalyx. In *A. lumbricoides*, the anterior part of the intestine is mainly secretory, the posterior part mainly absorptive. Both apocrine and merocrine secretions have been described in the intestinal cells.

Nematodes do not have a continuous muscle sheet around the intestine and the pseudocoelomic fluid is in direct contact with the basement membrane. The nematode intestine is, therefore, an ideal cell monolayer with which to study transport mechanisms, the only diffusion barrier being the basement membrane. In *A. lumbricoides*, the basement membrane is composed of collagen-type polypeptides (Section 2.5.1).

4.1.5. Absorption Mechanisms

Tissues take up solutes by four different mechanisms, passive diffusion, mediated transport, pinocytosis and mass flow (solvent drag).

Passive Diffusion (Non-mediated Transport)

This is the movement of substances across the cell membrane by mechanisms that follow the laws of diffusion. Empirically, diffusion is described by the Fick equation:

$$\frac{dm}{dt} = -DA \frac{dc}{dx}$$

where dm/dt is the flow rate, A is the area, dc/dx is the concentration gradient and D is the diffusion coefficient. For diffusion, the rate of uptake is linear with concentration (*Figure 4.1*).

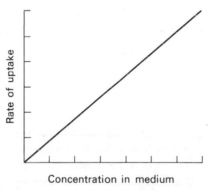

Figure 4.1 Passive diffusion

Passive diffusion is too slow for the uptake of most water- and lipid-soluble compounds by cells. However, there is usually a diffusion component involved in the uptake of nutrients and corrections must be made for it.

Mediated Transport

The transport of most solutes across cell membranes involves a carrier system and is called mediated transport. The carrier systems are proteins, but it is not known whether they go back and forth across the membranes like shuttles or whether, as is more likely, they permanently span the membrane. The carriers show specificity towards the compound or group of compounds that they transport. Mediated transport systems can be inhibited competitively by substances structurally related to the substrate and non-competitively by reagents which are capable of blocking or altering specific functional groups of proteins (such as dinitrofluorobenzene which blocks $-NH_2$ groups and p-hydroxymercuribenzoate which blocks $-SH$ groups). The temperature coefficient for mediated transport systems is similar to that for chemical reactions ($Q_{10} \approx 3$).

In mediated transport, there are a finite number of carrier sites and the system has a limited capacity. That is, it can be saturated and uptake is not linear with

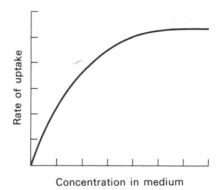

Figure 4.2 Mediated transport.

concentration as in passive diffusion (*Figure 4.2*). A double reciprocal plot of uptake (*R*) against concentration (*S*) gives a straight line, showing that mediated transport follows Michaelis–Menten kinetics:

$$R = \frac{[\text{S}] \, V_\text{m}}{K_\text{t} + [\text{S}]}$$

The maximum rate of absorption (V_m) is equivalent to the V_max of an enzyme and K_t (transport constant) is equivalent to K_m. So, K_t is a measure of the affinity of the carrier system for its substrate, and is the substrate concentration that gives the half-maximal rate of uptake. If several compounds are transported by the same carrier, they will compete for the carrier site and so act as competitive inhibitors for each others' transport. Inhibitor constants (K_i) can be calculated for the reversible inhibitors of mediated transport systems in the same way as inhibitor constants of enzymes. The K_i of a transport mechanism is the dissociation constant of the inhibitor–carrier complex, in the same way as the K_i for an enzyme is the dissociation constant for the inhibitor–enzyme complex.

Mediated transport of solutes may also be linked with a coflux or counterflux of ions.

Although carrier mechanisms show many of the kinetic properties of enzymes, they are not usually considered to be enzymes because their 'product' is the unaltered substrate in a different location.

Mediated systems transport compounds across membranes in both directions, so, for a mediated system, the unidirectional flux of a substrate is always greater than the net transport. A simple model of mediated transport is shown in *Figure 4.3*. In the model, there are saturatable carrier sites, analogous to the active sites of an enzyme, which have alternate access to one side of the membrane and then the other. The carrier can cross the membrane in two states, free or bound to substrate.

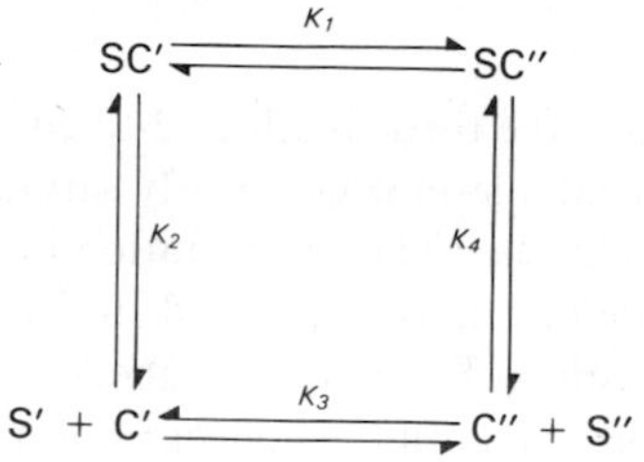

$$SC' \underset{}{\overset{K_1}{\rightleftharpoons}} SC''$$

$$K_2 \qquad\qquad K_4$$

$$S' + C' \underset{}{\overset{K_3}{\rightleftharpoons}} C'' + S''$$

$$K_1 = \frac{[SC'']}{[SC']} \qquad K_2 = \frac{[SC']}{[S'][C']}$$

$$K_3 = \frac{[C'']}{[C']} \qquad K_4 = \frac{[SC'']}{[C''][S'']}$$

Figure 4.3 Model of mediated transport. The inside and outside of the membrane are denoted by a single prime (') and by double primes ("), respectively. C is the carrier, S is the substrate; K_1 and K_3 are distribution constants, and K_2 and K_4 are dissociation constants for the carrier-substrate complex.

The affinity of a carrier for its substrate may be different on the two sides of the membrane.

This simple carrier model can be used to explain a number of phenomena related to mediated transport, namely, exchange diffusion, counterflow and accelerative exchange diffusion.

Exchange Diffusion

If a tissue is allowed to take up labelled substrate until a steady state is reached, and it is then placed in unlabelled substrate (at the same concentration), a 1:1 exchange occurs between the labelled substrate in the tissue and the unlabelled substrate in the medium. This 1:1 exchange occurs without any net transport and is called exchange diffusion or mediated efflux. It can be explained by the model in *Figure 4.3* operating at equilibrium. If the passage of the unloaded carrier (C) across the membrane was relatively slow, compared with the loaded carrier (SC), the model for exchange diffusion reduces to *Figure 4.4*.

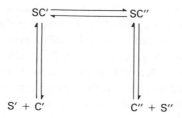

Figure 4.4 Model of exchange diffusion—symbols are as in *Figure 4.3*.

Counterflow

To demonstrate counterflow, the tissue is allowed to equilibrate with a labelled, non-metabolisable substrate at a level which nearly saturates the carrier. When an accumulation ratio of unity is reached (concentration of labelled substrate is the same in the tissue and in the medium), unlabelled substrate or a related substrate is added to the incubation medium. Efflux of the labelled substrate, against its concentration gradient, then occurs, until the concentration of labelled substrate is the same inside and outside (*Figure 4.5*). The explanation for counterflow is that, after the addition of the unlabelled substrate, competition for the carrier site by external substrates is not balanced by competition on the inside; therefore, labelled substrate comes out faster than it goes in. Counterflow experiments show how, if two substrates share a common carrier, a maintained gradient of one may force the translocation of the other.

The experimental demonstration of counterflow and exchange diffusion is very strong evidence for a mediated transport system.

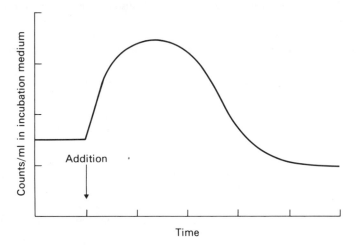

Figure 4.5 Counterflow—unlabelled substrate is added to the medium at the arrow.

Accelerative Exchange Diffusion

This is another transport phenomenon involving an exchange between external and internal substrate which can be explained by the model in *Figure 4.3*. With the substrate concentrations below saturation level, the influx rate of substrate may depend on its internal concentration, $[S'']$. A decrease in $[S'']$, although it leads to an increase in the transmembrane concentration gradient for S, results in a decreased influx. This can be explained by assuming that the binding of the substrate to the carrier (K_2 and K_4) is rapid compared with reorientation of the carrier, and that the passage of the unloaded carrier across the membrane (C) is relatively slow compared to the loaded carrier (as in *Figure 4.4*). Reducing S'' will decrease the level of

CS″, so the return of the carrier (to be unloaded outside) will be reduced. If S″ is decreased, carrier availability on the outer surface will decrease, so the influx of substrate will be reduced.

Mediated transport can be divided into active and passive.

Active Mediated Transport

This is what is usually meant by active transport. In addition to the three basic characteristics of mediated transport, namely, saturation kinetics, specificity and inhibition, active mediated transport shows three other features:

(i)   transport takes place against a concentration gradient,
(ii) it requires metabolic energy, and
(iii) it is unidirectional or vectorial.

The energy for active mediated transport can be provided in a number of ways. Transport may be coupled directly to ATP hydrolysis, or it can involve phosphorylation either of the carrier protein or, in the case of bacterial group translocation, of the substrate. Alternatively, the energy for active transport can be provided by an ionic gradient, which is itself maintained by an active mechanism or, as in mitochondria, it can be driven by respiration, the translocation of electrons generating the membrane potential. The simple model of mediated transport (*Figure 4.3*) can easily be extended to include active mediated transport (*Figure 4.6*).

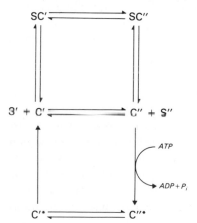

Figure 4.6 Model of active mediated transport—symbols are as in *Figure 4.3*. C* is activated carrier.

Passive Mediated Transport

In contrast to active mediated transport, passive mediated transport only occurs with the diffusion gradient, does not require metabolic energy and is not vectorial, taking place in both directions across the membrane. The advantage of passive mediated transport is that diffusion equilibrium is reached much more quickly than it would be by diffusion alone.

Pinocytosis

This is a method of taking up large colloidal particles, although small solute molecules may be taken up at the same time. Pinocytosis has been described in the tegument of larval cestodes, trematodes and acanthocephalans, but is not a significant route of entry for low molecular weight compounds.

Mass Flow

Solute molecules can also be transported passively when there is a large solvent flow through a membrane. This type of transport is characteristic of rather permeable membranes and occurs, for example, in the vertebrate kidney.

Summary

There are, therefore, a number of methods whereby substrates can be transported across membranes, and compounds may be transported by more than one method. This can make experimental identification of uptake mechanisms difficult and the absorption mechanisms may change under different conditions. Uptake via a mediated system which is not appreciably saturated with substrate under the experimental conditions will appear to be passive diffusion. As substrate concentrations increase, the diffusion component of transport increases. Active mediated transport mechanisms may, under conditions of energy shortage, function as passive mediated mechanisms. This last point may be particularly important in parasites, where uptake experiments are often conducted under what, to the parasite, are very unphysiological conditions.

4.1.6. Uptake in Helminths

Substrates are transported by the absorptive layer from the external medium to the underlying tissues. Absorptive layers are, therefore, asymmetric, having both input and output faces. The mechanisms by which substrates are taken up from the outside by the absorptive layer may well be different from the mechanisms by which substrates leave the layer for the underlying tissues. There is good evidence, for example, that amino acid uptake in the mammalian intestine involves active transport into the mucosal cells, but passive mediated transport from the cells into the submucosa. Helminth studies have concentrated on the uptake of substrates by absorptive layers, and the problems of transport from the tegument to the tissues have not been considered.

    Covering any absorptive surface is a stationary layer of fluid, which does not mix with the bulk phase. Substrates can only cross the stationary or unstirred layer by diffusion, and the stationary layer presents a considerable amount of diffusion resistance. The stationary layer is usually several orders of magnitude thicker than the cell membrane. In *H. diminuta*, the stationary layer has been estimated at between 10 and 400 μm thick, depending on the conditions[24]. Since substrates have to diffuse across the stationary layer, the actual concentration of substrate at the membrane surface may be considerably less than the concentration of substrate in the bulk phase. The presence of the unstirred layer affects the determination of uptake kinetics, leading to an overestimation of K_t and V_m and to an underestimation of the passive permeability coefficient. Failure to take into account the presence of an unstirred layer has meant that the majority of the published kinetic constants for helminth uptake mechanisms must be treated cautiously. In a recent study on *H. diminuta*, where the presence of the stationary layer was taken into account, K_t for glucose uptake was found to be 0.1 mM[25]. Previous estimates of K_t for glucose uptake in *H. diminuta* had given a value an order of magnitude larger, around 1 mM.

The thickness of the unstirred layer depends on the physical conditions. In the rat intestine, it has been estimated that the presence of the unstirred layer effectively reduces the absorptive area of the mucosa to the tips of the micro-villi. In the rat intestine, an anatomical absorptive area of 1200 cm^2/100 mg is reduced to an effective absorptive area of 9.5 cm^2/100 mg. With *H. diminuta*, the same calculations give an anatomical surface area of 101 cm^2/100 mg and an effective absorptive area of 39 cm^2/100 mg. On a weight-for-weight basis, *H. diminuta* may have a higher effective absorptive area than the rat intestine[25].

The cell surface of the absorptive layer is also covered by a cell coat or glycocalyx. The glycocalyx is a complex mixture of polysaccharides, glycoproteins and glycolipids and it is an integral part of the cell membrane. Together, the cell membrane and glycocalyx form what has been described as the 'greater membrane'. At physiological pH, the glycocalyx acts as a polyanion and, under experimental conditions, colloids and polycations are strongly bound to it. During uptake, substrates have to traverse the glycocalyx and in some, or perhaps most, cases they may interact with it.

A study of transport kinetics thus requires a consideration of the substrate distribution in several separate compartments. External to the absorptive surface there are at least three compartments; the bulk phase, the stationary layer and the glycocalyx. Within the absorptive tissue itself, there are again at least two compartments to consider; the intracellular water and the extracellular water. In practice, separate determination of substrate levels in the intra- and extracellular water is not normally possible. So, for most uptake experiments, it has to be assumed that the concentration of solute is the same in both of these two tissue compartments. However, this may not necessarily always be the case and solute could accumulate intracellularly during transport. Moreover, it has to be assumed, in uptake studies, that the solute is in free solution in the tissue and is not being bound intracellularly. Osmotic volume changes during uptake experiments can also lead to errors. In *H. diminuta*, attempts have been made to estimate the size of the different fluid compartments and to evaluate the errors[26,27]. The transport of substrates from the external medium, across the absorptive layer and into the underlying tissues is thus a complex, multi-step process.

In helminths, most of the work on uptake has been done on cestodes and, in particular, on the rat cestode *H. diminuta*. Parasites such as cestodes (and acanthocephalans) have no gut and live in the lumen of their host's intestine. These parasites produce no extracellular digestive enzymes and their uptake mechanisms must compete directly with those of the host's intestine for available nutrients. In the mammalian mucosa, compounds may be transported by an intercellular trans-epithelial route. That is, the compounds do not actually enter the cytoplasm of the mucosal cells, but pass between them. Cestodes, trematodes and acanthocephalans all have syncitial teguments and an intercellular transport route is not possible.

4.1.7. Carbohydrate Uptake

Carbohydrate absorption has been most extensively studied in tapeworms. In the mammalian intestine, the di- and trisaccharides are finally hydrolysed by enzymes located in the brush borders of the mucosal cells. The di- and trisaccharidases are spatially, and possibly functionally, linked with the monosaccharide transport sites and so the products of digestion are rapidly absorbed. Nevertheless, significant amounts of monosaccharide occur free in the lumen. In the rat, this varies from 10 to 50 mM glucose after a meal, to 1 mM during fasting. The free glucose comes partly from di- and trisaccharidases present in the lumen and partly from back-diffusion from the membrane-bound enzymes. Intestinal secretions contain only small amounts of hydrolytic enzymes, but sloughed-off mucosal cells and, to a lesser extent, bacteria contribute to the luminal di- and trisaccharidase activity. Gut parasites compete with the intestinal uptake mechanisms only for the luminal mono-saccharides; most of the monosaccharides released by the brush border enzymes never become free in the gut. The amount of glucose that diffuses back into the intestine can be as little as 5% of the total available[28]. The glycocalyx may be one of the factors that limits back-diffusion. However, parasitised guts often show defective absorptive processes, and this may increase the availability of free glucose in the lumen.

Cestodes

The carbohydrate uptake mechanisms seem to be fairly similar in all of the cestodes so far studied (*H. diminuta, H. microstoma, C. verticillatum, T. crassiceps* larvae, *T. taeniaeformis* adults and larvae). In all cases, glucose and galactose are taken up by active mediated transport and the major features of active mediated transport have been demonstrated. Uptake follows Michaelis–Menten kinetics, occurs against a concentration gradient, requires metabolic energy, is specific for D-hexose and can be competitively inhibited by glucose analogues and non-competitively inhibit-ed by protein precipitants. In *H. diminuta*, glucose uptake shows two distinct pH optima (pH 7.5 and 8.5) and has a Q_{10} greater than 2.4. Exchange diffusion and accelerative exchange diffusion, phenomena indicative of mediated transport (Section 4.1.5), have been demonstrated in *C. verticillatum*. Exchange diffusion has also been shown in *T. taeniaeformis*.

Since glucose and galactose are readily metabolised by tissues, non-metabolisable glucose analogues such as 2-deoxyglucose and 3-O-methylglucose have been extensively used to characterise hexose transport systems. Differences have been reported in the interaction of these analogues with uptake systems from different species of tapeworm. These discrepancies may reflect differences in uptake mechanisms between species, but are more likely to be due to experimental differences and to the use of analogues of variable purity. In general, α- and β-methylglucoside, 1-deoxyglucose and 6-deoxyglucose inhibit glucose transport in tapeworms, whilst 2-deoxyglucose, 3-O-methylglucose, glucosamine and N-acetylglucosamine are without effect. In *H. diminuta*, D-allose is also said to be inhibitory.

In all cestodes studied, glucose and galactose are transported via a common carrier system which is sodium-dependent and potassium- and phloridzin-sensitive. In *H. diminuta* and in *C. verticillatum*, the coupling coefficient for glucose transport, i.e. [sodium influx] / [glucose influx] = 2, and is independent of the sodium concentration[29,30]. In the mammalian intestine, the coupling coefficient is unity, but again is independent of sodium concentration. Several workers have reported a small glucose uptake rate in *H. diminuta* in sodium-free media. However, *H. diminuta* can secrete sodium ions in sodium-free media (Section 4.1.12) and there may be significant amounts of sodium in the glycocalyx[31].

Not all workers have been able to demonstrate potassium inhibition of glucose uptake in *H. diminuta*[31], but it has been reported by Starling[32] and has been clearly shown in *T. crassiceps*. In the mammalian mucosal cell, when sodium ions enter, electroneutrality is achieved by the passive entry of chloride ions. Glucose transport in *H. diminuta* is chloride-dependent[29], with an apparent coupling coefficient [Cl⁻ influx] / [glucose influx] = 2. However, Uglem[31] has suggested that the co-transport of sodium and glucose into the tegument of *H. diminuta* is coupled with sodium efflux, and it is this that maintains the electroneutrality.

The uptake of glucose by mammalian mucosal cells is similarly sodium-dependent, and glucose and sodium are transported by a common carrier through the apical plasma membrane. Sodium is pumped out of the mucosal cell by a sodium 'pump' located in the basal and lateral membranes. The sodium 'pump' uses metabolic energy to create an electrochemical gradient, which in turn drives the carrier system. Glucose leaves the mucosal cell, through the basal membrane, by passive mediated transport. The two components involved in glucose transport by mammalian mucosal cells, the apical carrier and the basal sodium 'pump', can be differentiated by specific inhibitors. Phloridzin blocks the coupled sodium/glucose uptake when applied to the apical (mucosal) surface of the intestinal epithelium, but not when applied to the basal (serosal) side. It is thought that phloridzin competes with glucose for the carrier site. Ouabain, on the other hand, specifically inhibits membrane sodium/potassium ATPases and inhibits glucose uptake when applied to the basal side, but not on the apical side. Mucosal cells are thus biochemically, as well as structurally, polarised. The tapeworm tegument shows a similar functional polarisation for sodium-coupled transport[33]. In both *H. diminuta* and *H. microstoma*, ouabain inhibits glucose and galactose uptake when applied to the tissue side of the tegument, but not when applied to the brush border side. The sodium gradient hypothesis of hexose transport is not, however, universally accepted, and some workers think that the role of sodium is in intracellular energy production.

The cysticercoids of *H. diminuta* take up glucose and galactose by an active mediated transport system, similar to that of the adult. There is some evidence that in the cysticercoid there may be two transport systems present, both transporting glucose and galactose. In adult *H. diminuta*, K_t of the hexose transport system changes as the worm matures. This could be explained by changes in the relative proportions of two transport systems, one with a high K_t, the other with a low K_t. However, there is no evidence, at the moment, for two separate transport sites in adult *H. diminuta*[34]. Two transport systems for hexoses, with similar specificities but different K_t values, have also been proposed in the mammalian intestine.

Glucose uptake *in vivo* by *H. diminuta* has been resolved into two components, active mediated transport and mass flow[35]. The passive diffusion component of glucose entry into *H. diminuta* is negligible. Under experimental conditions, mass flow may account for as much as 30% of the total glucose uptake. This figure is very similar to that found for the mammalian intestine, where mass flow accounts for about 25% of glucose transport and the diffusion component is again negligible. In the intestine, mass flow is thought to occur via the tight junctions between the mucosal cells. The site of mass flow in the syncitial cestode tegument is not known.

In contrast to glucose and galactose, fructose enters cestodes by passive diffusion. Adult *H. diminuta* are virtually impermeable to fructose, and *C. verticillatum* and *T. taeniaeformis* only sparingly so. The larvae of *T. crassiceps*, however, are fairly readily permeable to fructose, and the uptake of glucose and galactose by this parasite also shows a large diffusional component.

The hexose uptake mechanisms of cestodes thus show similarities with those of the mammalian intestine. In both cases, glucose and galactose share a common carrier which is sodium-dependent and is inhibited by phloridzin and potassium, the latter acting as a competitive inhibitor for sodium. The mucosal cell and the cestode tegument are both functionally polarised with an apical hexose transporter and a basal sodium pump. In mammals, as well as glucose and galactose, some twelve different glucose analogues are actively transported. In cestodes, only glucose and galactose have been shown to be accumulated against a concentration gradient. Glucose analogues, such as α- and β-methylglucoside and 1- and 6-deoxyglucose, competitively inhibit glucose uptake but, except for β-methylglucoside, there is no information as to whether these analogues are actually transported. The uptake of β-methylglucoside by *H. diminuta* has been demonstrated and shows the same characteristics as glucose transport[36].

There are also differences between the hexose transport systems in cestodes and the mammalian intestine. The coupling coefficient between sodium and glucose is 1 in the mammalian system and 2 in cestodes, whilst the analogue 3-*O*-methylglucose is actively transported in the mammalian intestine, but does not seem to interact with the tapeworm system. Fructose is not metabolised by cestodes and enters only by passive diffusion. The mammalian gut actively transports fructose by a specific fructose carrier. D-xylose is also taken up to a limited extent, by active transport, in the intestine, but its uptake by cestodes does not seem to have been studied.

Glycerol uptake by *H. diminuta* contains a passive diffusion component and a passive mediated transport component. Mediated uptake involves two separate uptake sites which are distinct from the hexose porter. One of the glycerol transport systems is sodium-sensitive, the other sodium insensitive. The uptake of glycerol by *T. taeniaeformis* also involves a passive diffusion component and a passive mediated transport component distinct from the hexose site. The significance of the two glycerol transport systems in *H. diminuta* remains unknown. Dual glycerol uptake sites exist in trypanosomes, and glycerol uptake in the mammalian intestine also involves both passive diffusion and mediated transport.

Acanthocephalans

In many ways, the acanthocephalans are very similar to tapeworms. The adults live in the lumen of the gut, they produce no extracellular digestive enzymes and they absorb low molecular weight nutrients through the general body surface, which in both groups is a syncitium. It is, therefore, rather surprising to find that hexose uptake by *M. dubius* is very different from that of cestodes[32,37,38]. In *M. dubius*, hexose uptake is via a passive mediated mechanism, which is neither phloridzin- nor sodium-sensitive. There are two separate uptake sites, which have been designated the glucose site and the fructose site, respectively. The glucose site transports, in order of decreasing affinity, glucose, 2-deoxyglucose, mannose, *N*-acetylglucosamine, 3-*O*-methylglucose, fructose and galactose. The fructose site, on the other hand, transports, in order of decreasing affinity, fructose, galactose, *N*-acetylglucosamine, 3-*O*-methylglucose, glucose and 2-deoxyglucose. It is possible that the fructose site is a secondary site for hexoses and may, for example, be primarily a pentose uptake site. The hexose uptake system of *M. dubius* thus transports a variety of sugars (2-deoxyglucose, 3-*O*-methylglucose, mannose, fructose, *N*-acetylglucosamine) which do not interact with cestode transport systems. The rapid conversion of glucose to trehalose by acanthocephalans may maintain a favourable glucose gradient into the worm. The trehalose can then act as a glycosyl shuttle between the tegument and the free glucose pools[38]. Glucose uptake by another acanthocephalan, *P. minutus*, is also via a mediated system, but has not been studied in detail.

Trematodes

The tegumental transport of hexoses by trematodes has been investigated in at least three species, *F. hepatica, F. gigantica* and *S. mansoni*. In *F. hepatica*, hexose uptake is by passive mediated transport and is sodium- and phloridzin-insensitive. Like *M. dubius*, there are probably two separate hexose transport sites in *F. hepatica*. One site, the glucose site, transports glucose, galactose, 3-*O*-methylglucose, glucosamine and mannose; the other site, the fructose site, transports fructose and probably ribose. Glucose, galactose and 3-*O*-methylglucose may bind non-productively to the fructose site, inhibiting fructose uptake, but are not themselves transported. Xylose enters *F. hepatica* by passive diffusion only.

In *F. gigantica*, glucose uptake is primarily via the tegument[39], and the same is probably true for *F. hepatica* and *S. mansoni*. Glucose uptake in *F. gigantica* is via mediated transport and is said to be phloridzin-sensitive. Glucose uptake by the cestodarians *Gyrocotyle fimbriata* and *Gyrocotyle parvispinosa* is also said to be phloridzin-sensitive[40]. These two cestodarians are reported to be able to absorb glucose, galactose, α-methylglucoside and, at a slower rate, xylose, lactose, mannose and inulin. The mechanisms have not, however, been investigated.

Hexose uptake by *S. mansoni* has been the subject of conflicting reports. Initially, glucose, galactose, fructose, glucosamine, ribose and 3-O-methylglucose were reported to cross the tegument by passive mediated transport, but there was also a large diffusion component. Other workers found that glucose, β-methylglucoside and fructose entered by diffusion alone.

Glucose is rapidly metabolised by *S. mansoni* and it is difficult to demonstrate accumulation against a concentration gradient. However, 2-deoxyglucose and glucose appear to share the same carrier in *S. mansoni,* so the non-metabolisable 2-deoxyglucose can be used to study the process. The uptake of 2-deoxyglucose appears to be by active mediated transport and is phloridzin- and sodium-sensitive. Coupled sodium and 2-deoxyglucose uptake has been demonstrated and the coupling coefficient is 1. Glucose would also, presumably, be accumulated by a similar active mechanism if it were not so rapidly metabolised.

The miracidia of *S. mansoni* take up glucose, but the mechanism is not known. Active mediated glucose uptake has, however, been shown in the sporocysts of *M. similis*. Glucose, galactose and fructose are reported to enter via a single site which also interacts with α-methylglucoside, fucose, mannose and 3-O-methylglucose.

Nematodes

The only detailed studies on hexose uptake by nematodes is on the uptake of sugars by the intestine of *A. lumbricoides*. In this nematode, glucose is taken up from the gut by active mediated transport and is sodium- and phloridzin-sensitive. Fructose, 3-O-methylglucose and possibly xylose are also taken up by active transport. The conversion of glucose to trehalose in *A. lumbricoides* may, as suggested in Acanthocephala, maintain a favourable glucose gradient. Trehalose, however, cannot act as the energy source for active transport of hexoses across the intestine[41].

In contrast to all the other helminth systems studied, the gut of *A. lumbricoides* appears to be virtually impermeable to galactose. Correlated with this is the fact that no lactase has been found in the brush border disaccharidases of *A. lumbricoides*. Mediated glucose transport has also been described across the cuticle of larval *M. nigrescens*.

Summary

There would seem to be considerable variation in the hexose transport mechanisms of helminths. Active mediated hexose transport occurs in cestodes, nematodes and the sporocysts of *M. similis*, there are conflicting reports in *S. mansoni* and there is no active transport in *M. dubius* or *F. hepatica*. There is only one hexose transport site in cestodes and *M. similis*, but two in *M. dubius*, *F. hepatica* and possibly *S. mansoni* as well. Of the glucose analogues, 2-deoxyglucose is transported by *M. dubius* and *S. mansoni*, but not by cestodes (or by the mammalian mucosa). In mammals, a free hydroxyl group at the C_2 position is essential for transport. 3-*O*-methylglucose is not transported by cestodes, but is by *A. lumbricoides, F. hepatica* and possibly *S. mansoni*. These variations may represent fundamental differences in uptake mechanisms between species or they may be due to experimental differences. Many of the buffers used in *in vitro* incubations, especially 'tris', may interact with uptake systems. Active mediated transport is a labile process and, as discussed earlier, under adverse conditions, an active mediated transport system may function as a passive mediated system. Similarly, a mediated system which is not appreciably saturated with substrate will appear to be passive diffusion.

4.1.8. Amino Acid Uptake

Amino acid uptake has again been most extensively studied in tapeworms. Dietary proteins are digested in the intestine to a mixture of amino acids (10–25%) and peptides (75–90%). The peptides are finally hydrolysed to amino acids by di- and tripeptidases located in the brush borders of the mucosal cells. As in carbohydrate breakdown, the peptidases and the transport sites are in close proximity, but some amino acids diffuse back into the lumen. The amino acid composition of the intestinal lumen seems to be under a certain degree of homeostatic control. (*Table 4.1* gives a classification of amino acids according to their side chains.) It has been found that, although the concentration of free amino acids in the intestine varies with the feeding cycle, the molar ratios of the different amino acids stays relatively constant. The reason for this is twofold. First, the contribution of dietary protein to the luminal free amino acid pool is relatively small and is largely swamped by endogenous protein. The endogenous protein comes, in part, from the pancreatic and intestinal secretions (200 g of protein per day in man) and, in part, from the turnover of the intestinal epithelium. In man, the mucosal epithelium grows at the

Table 4.1 Classification of amino acids according to the nature of their side chains

---

1. NEUTRAL
(*a*) Aliphatic:
     Alanine, glycine, *isoleucine, leucine*, serine, *threonine, valine*
(*b*) Aromatic:
     Phenylalanine, tryptophan, tyrosine
(*c*) Sulphur-containing:
     Cysteine, cystine, *methionine*
(*d*) Imino group*:
     Betaine†, hydroxyproline, proline, sarcosine†

2. ACIDIC
     Aspartic acid, glutamic acid

3. BASIC
     Arginine, citrulline†, *histidine*, hydroxylysine, *lysine*, ornithine†

Essential amino acids (man) are in italics.
*The imino group are not true amino acids, since the amino group is not free.
†Not true constituents of proteins.

rate of about 1% per hour (90 g protein per day). Secondly, there is a bidirectional flux (exchange diffusion) of amino acids across the mucosa, between the intestinal tissue and the lumen. (The existence of this amino acid flux has not, however, been confirmed in some recent studies.) Amino acids derived from endogenous protein and from the mucosa effectively buffer any amino acid change due to exogenous protein in the diet. The actual molar ratios of amino acids in the intestine may differ in different hosts and could be a factor involved in host recognition and host specificity.

The presence of parasites in the intestine can lead to changes in the luminal free amino acid pool. This is due both to uptake of amino acids by the parasite and to disruption of the host's uptake mechanisms.

This concept of amino acid homeostasis in the intestine may, in fact, be an over-simplification. If the intestinal amino acid pool is treated as a single unit, the molar ratios of the amino acids appear similar before and after a protein meal. However, there may be considerable regional differences in both the concentration and in the molar ratios of amino acids, and these reflect the changing physiological functions of the different regions of the intestine during digestion. The amino acid ratios in the lumen of the posterior part of the small intestine seem to be rather more stable than in the anterior part.

Cestodes

The earliest studies demonstrating mediated uptake in helminths were on amino acid absorption by *H. diminuta*. Accumulation of amino acids by *H. diminuta* probably involves active mediated transport, and most of the features of mediated transport have been demonstrated. Uptake obeys Michaelis–Menten kinetics, is stereo-specific (for the α-amino group), can be inhibited both competitively and non-competi-tively, shows a distinct pH optimum and has a large temperature coefficient. In addition, both exchange diffusion and counterflow have been demonstrated. Accumulation against a concentration gradient has only been shown for methionine, proline, histidine, cycloleucine and 2-aminoisobutyrate. Attempts to demonstrate accumulation against a concentration gradient for the other amino acids have not apparently been made. Strictly, only five amino acids have been shown to be transported by an active process, although the other amino acids are probably transported actively as well. To what extent diffusion is involved in amino acid uptake by *H. diminuta* is unclear. The uptake of proline and histidine involves a significant diffusional component, but whether other amino acids are also absorbed in part by diffusion is not known. In *H. diminuta*, low external concentrations of ATP stimulate amino acid uptake (methionine, leucine), and high concentrations inhibit uptake[147].

The uptake of amino acids by cestodes is not affected by hexoses or peptides. In the mammalian gut, monosaccharides decrease amino acid uptake. This is probably due to competition for the limited energy available, rather than to the presence of a multifunctional carrier. Also in the mammalian gut, peptides inhibit amino acid uptake and there may be specific peptide uptake sites. There is, however, no evidence as yet that cestodes can take up peptides. The larval stages (cysticerci) of some

Table 4.2 Amino acid porters of *H. diminuta*

			Carrier			
	Dicarb-oxylic	Glycine	Serine	Leucine	Phenyl-alanine	Basic
High affinity	Aspartate, glutamate, methionine	Glycine, methionine	Serine, threonine, alanine, methio-nine, valine, proline	Leucine, isoleucine, methionine, (cyclo-leucine)	Phenyl-alanine tyrosine, histidine, methionine	Arginine, lysine, histidine
Low affinity	Serine, alanine, glycine	Serine, threonine, alanine	Glycine	Glycine, serine, threonine, alanine, valine	Leucine, isoleucine	

cestodes (*T. taeniaeformis, T. crassiceps, E. granulosus*) may be capable of absorbing proteins[42] and host protein can be detected in cyst fluid.

There are at least six separate amino acid uptake sites in *H. diminuta*, although there is a certain degree of overlap in their specificities; this is summarised in *Table 4.2*. There is a basic amino acid site, which also transports histidine, a dicarboxylic amino acid system with a low affinity for certain neutral amino acids and at least four neutral amino acid transport systems. Not all of the amino acids that interact with a particular site are necessarily transported. It is quite probable that amino acids bind reversibly to some of the sites without being translocated (non-productive binding). Thus K_t of an amino acid (its transport constant) may be different from K_i (its inhibitor constant).

Experiments with single substrates and single inhibitors are useful in determining the specificity of particular amino acid transport sites. However, they do not show how the system will function in a complex environment, where there may be several potential inhibitors. All of the amino acids transported by any one site will act as competitive inhibitors for one another. In order to get a balanced amino acid uptake from a mixture, the molar ratios must remain constant. This feature of amino acid uptake, of course, makes the concept of intestinal amino acid homeostasis such an attractive hypothesis.

The uptake of a single amino acid from a complex mixture of interacting amino acids can be described by an equation, derived from classical Michaelis–Menten kinetics:

$$v = \frac{V_m}{K_t/[S] + 1 + K_t[S_1]/^1K_i[S] + K_t[S_2]/^2K_i[S] + \ldots + K_t[S_n]/^nK_i[S]}$$

where v is the velocity of the inhibited uptake, V_m is the maximum velocity of uninhibited uptake, K_t is the transport constant for the amino acid whose uptake is being studied, ^1K_i, ^2K_i, etc. are the inhibitor constants for the interacting amino acids, [S] is the concentration of the amino acid being studied, and [S_1], [S_2], etc. are the concentrations of the interacting amino acids. Experimentally, this equation describes quite accurately the uptake of methionine by *H. diminuta* and *H. citelli*, from complex amino acid mixtures.

Exchange diffusion of amino acids between the tissue amino acid pool of *H. diminuta* and the surrounding medium has been demonstrated both *in vitro* and *in vivo*. Because of this coupled flux, the free amino acid pool in the tapeworm is in dynamic equilibrium with the amino acid pool of the intestinal lumen, which in turn is in equilibrium with the blood. Equilibrium does not mean that the amino acid concentrations are necessarily the same in the different pools, or even that they are simply related. A specific concentration and ratio of amino acids in the gut lumen leads to a specific, but not necessarily the same, concentration and ratio of amino acids in the cestodes' free amino acid pool. The non-metabolisable amino acid, cycloleucine, rapidly reaches a steady state in the tissues of *H. diminuta*, the intestinal lumen and the rat blood plasma. A similar equilibrium has been demonstrated using serine. Not all of the amino acids in the tissues are freely exchangeable and, in both *H. diminuta* and *T. crassiceps* larvae, there is evidence that proline is compartmentalised and only part is available for exchange.

Imbalance in the intestinal amino acid pool will rapidly be reflected in an imbalance in the tapeworms' free amino acid pool. This has been demonstrated experimentally, by feeding rats infected with *H. diminuta* large doses of amino acids or amino acid mixtures. The addition of amino acid supplements to the diets of infected rats also impairs the growth of *H. diminuta*. Presumably the imbalance in the worms' amino acid pool caused by these supplements leads to an impairment of protein synthesis. However, no such impairment of protein synthesis can be shown in short-term experiments[43]. There is also a positive rank correlation between the amino acids in the intestinal lumen and those in the worm pool, although the total size of the worm free amino acid pool is, of course, much smaller.

From the point of view of amino acid fluxes, a tapeworm bears the same sort of relationship with the blood plasma amino acid pool of the host, as does one of the host's own organs, such as the liver or kidney. A change in the amino acid pool of one component will affect all of the others, since they are all part of a dynamic equilibrium.

The kinetics of amino acid uptake by *H. diminuta* vary with age and with the host species from which they came. The basis for these changes in amino acid transport systems during maturation or growth in different hosts is unknown. It does, however, emphasise the necessity of using standardised techniques (Section 1.3).

The cysticercoids of *H. diminuta* absorb amino acids by active mediated transport, but the uptake sites have not been characterised.

Amino acid uptake has been studied in two other tapeworm species, *C. verticillatum* and *T. crassiceps* larvae. In *C. verticillatum*, amino acids are taken up by active mediated transport and there are at least two transport systems, one for basic amino acids and one for neutral amino acids. Other amino acid uptake sites may exist, but more data will be required before they can be characterised. The natural host of *C. verticillatum* is the dogfish, and the tissues of the dogfish contain around 300 mM urea. Approximately 4% of the dry weight of *C. verticillatum* is urea and it is an important constituent in maintaining osmotic balance. Urea uptake by *C. verticillatum* is, however, entirely by passive diffusion. Interestingly, urea is toxic to cestodes of birds and mammals.

The uptake of amino acids by *T. crassiceps* larvae is also probably by active mediated transport. At least four uptake sites have been identified, one for the basic amino acids, one for the acidic amino acids and two for the neutral amino acids. Of the two neutral amino acid sites, one has a high affinity for aliphatic amino acids, and the other has a high affinity for aromatic amino acids. Amino acid uptake by *T. crassiceps* larvae has an appreciable diffusion component, and proline and gluta-mate may be taken up solely by diffusion. Hexose uptake by this cysticercus also showed a large diffusion component (Section 4.1.7).

Compared with the generalised mammalian system, the amino acid uptake mechanisms of cestodes appear to be unique in two respects. First, the cestode system shows virtually equal affinity for D- and L-amino acids and, secondly, amino acid uptake does not appear to be coupled to ion transport. In mammals, amino acid uptake mechanisms characteristically have a high affinity for L-amino acids and only a low affinity for the D-isomer. Uptake in mammals is also usually coupled to the movement of sodium and/or an anion such as chloride. However, some amino acids (glycine, lysine or proline) can be taken up in mammals by a sodium-independent pathway. In tapeworms, there is no evidence that either anions or cations are necessary for amino acid influx or accumulation. The possible role of the γ-glutamyl cycle in amino acid transport is dealt with in Section 4.4.2.

Cestode and mammalian amino acid uptake systems are similar in that they both involve multiple uptake sites with overlapping affinities. The mammalian intestine and *H. diminuta* have a basic amino acid site, an acidic amino acid site and multiple sites for the neutral amino acids. In the rat intestine, there are at least three neutral amino acid uptake sites, one for low molecular weight neutral amino acids, one for high molecular weight neutral amino acids and a separate site for proline. In *H. diminuta*, four neutral amino acid sites have been characterised, and these sites show general similarities with those of the mammalian gut but differ in detail (*Table 4.2*). The neutral amino acid uptake sites of *H. diminuta* also show some general similarities with the systems characterised in Ehrlich ascite tumour cells. Here, there are three neutral amino acid uptake sites, an A site (alanine preferring), an L site (leucine preferring) and an ASC site (alanine, serine, cysteine). In addition, ascite cells may have a separate glycine site.

Acanthocephalans

Compared with cestodes, amino acid uptake mechanisms have not been well characterised in other helminths. The acanthocephalans *M. dubius* and *M. hirudin-aceus* absorb amino acids by a mediated system, although there is a significant diffusion component at high substrate concentrations. Methionine and leucine have been shown to be absorbed against a concentration gradient, but whether other amino acids are also taken up by active mediated transport has not been determined. As in cestodes, amino acid uptake by acanthocephalans is not sodium-sensitive. The different amino acid uptake sites have not been characterised in acanthocephalans, but the uptake of methionine from amino acid mixtures by *M. dubius* can be predicted from the derived Michaelis–Menten equation. There has only been one, unsuccessful, attempt to demonstrate exchange diffusion of amino acids in *M. dubius.*

Trematodes

Only very limited data are available for amino acid uptake by trematodes. In both *Fasciola hepatica* and *Fascioloides magna*, amino acid uptake takes place primarily via the tegument, ligation of the gut having no effect on absorption rates. In both species, amino acid uptake appears to be by passive diffusion. This is, of course, in marked contrast to the situation in cestodes and acanthocephalans. However, the efflux of cycloleucine from preloaded *F. hepatica* shows a distinct biphasic curve. This could be taken as indicative of some form of mediated process, but could equally well be due to compartmentation of the amino acid after absorption (Section 2.4.1).

In *S. mansoni*, amino acid absorption is again primarily via the tegument. Amino acids are taken up by a mixture of mediated transport and diffusion[44]. A number of amino acids (alanine, aspartate, glutamate, cycloleucine, leucine, methionine, phenylalanine, valine) can be accumulated against a concentration gradient and, in some cases (alanine, arginine, aspartate, cycloleucine, valine), uptake appears to be sodium-sensitive. This sodium dependency is different from all other helminths so far studied. The amino acid uptake sites in *S. mansoni* have not been well character-ised, but there are at least three separate sites, and possibly as many as five[45].

There have been a few studies on amino acid accumulation by larval trematodes. The schistosomulae of *S. mansoni* take up methionine via a mediated system, but the sporocysts of *Microphallus pygmaeus* and *Cercaria emasculans* take up amino acids by passive diffusion only.

The monogenean *Diclidophora merlangi*, which is a gill parasite, can absorb both amino acids (alanine, leucine) and glucose from sea water, via the tegument[46]. The amino acid uptake is mediated. Detectable levels of amino acids occur in natural sea water (0.1–4 μM) and many invertebrates appear to be able to absorb amino acids from sea water through their general body surface. The tegumental porter systems of parasitic trematodes and cestodes may represent an elaboration of mechanisms present in free-living marine platyhelminths.

Nematodes

In the nematodes, amino acid uptake has been looked at in the gut, muscles and reproductive tissue of *A. lumbricoides* and in larval *M. nigrescens*. In the gut of *A. lumbricoides*, amino acid uptake is a mediated process, but whether it can take place against a concentration gradient and whether it is ion-sensitive is not known.

The uptake by reproductive and muscle tissue of the non-metabolisable amino acid, cycloleucine, has shown that this compound enters reproductive tissue by active transport and muscle tissue by passive diffusion. Amino acids are, of course, not an energy source for *A. lumbricoides* muscles (Section 3.1.2).

Larval *M. nigrescens* take up amino acids through the cuticle by a mediated process[47]. These larvae also accumulate glucose via a transcuticular mediated process and this is probably related to their site of parasitism, the insect haemocoel.

4.1.9. Lipid Uptake

Like amino acids, the lipid composition of the intestinal lumen may stay relatively constant, although there is considerably less evidence for the homeostatic regulation of luminal lipids than for luminal amino acids. Nevertheless, intestinal secretions, and particularly bile, contain considerable amounts of lipid and these may serve to buffer the effects of dietary lipids.

In the mammalian intestine, the hydrolytic products of triacylglycerol digestion, i.e. monoacylglycerols, fatty acids and glycerol, form mixed micelles with the bile salts. These micelles disrupt at the mucosal surface, the fatty acids and monoacyl-glycerols entering by diffusion, the bile salts remaining in the lumen. Some bile salts enter the mucosal cells by diffusion, and active absorption of bile salts takes place in the ileum. The tapeworms, *H. diminuta* and *H. microstoma*, have no mechanism for the active uptake or excretion of bile salts and appear relatively impermeable to them[48]. Bile salts do, however, bind to the tegument of tapeworms and this influences the rate of uptake of glucose and possibly of amino acids as well. Bile salts, adsorbed onto the tegument may also play a role in the uptake of long chain fatty acids by tapeworms. Different bile salts can have different effects, and commercial bile salt preparations are often extremely impure.

The mammalian intestine can transport citrate, 2-oxoglutarate, succinate and pyruvate, but they are largely metabolised on uptake. In mammals, ammonium ions may assist the uptake of short chain acids.

Cestodes

Adult *H. diminuta* and cysticercoids absorb short chain fatty acids (acetate, propionate, butyrate) by a mixture of diffusion and mediated transport. Undissociated acids may be taken up by diffusion and dissociated acids by mediated transport. The larvae of *T. crassiceps* also have an acetate uptake site.

Long chain fatty acids are again taken up in *H. diminuta* by a mixture of diffusion and mediated transport. In the tapeworm, the absorbed acids are rapidly synthesised into triacylglycerols. There is some evidence that mediated long chain fatty acid transport in *H. diminuta* shows allosteric activation, similar to that proposed for purine and pyrimidine transport (Section 4.1.10). Palmitate uptake, for example, is stimulated in the presence of oleate, linoleate and linolenate. This is in contrast to the mammalian intestine where fatty acids are thought to enter by diffusion alone and no transport mechanisms have been found. The cysticercoids of *H. diminuta* also take up long chain fatty acids, but the mechanism has not been studied[49].

Monoacylglycerols are rapidly taken up by *H. diminuta* from micellar solution, but they appear to be rapidly hydrolysed in the tegument. In the mammalian mucosa, absorbed monoacylglycerols are not hydrolysed, but are reacylated to give diacylglycerols and triacylglycerols, thus conserving energy (Section 4.3.2). *H. diminuta* rapidly takes up lysolecithins from micelles and these are again probably hydrolysed like the monoacylglycerols.

Cholesterol is absorbed by *H. diminuta* from micellar solution, but nothing is known of the mechanism. Cholesterol is also taken up by *E. granulosus* cysts. In the mammalian intestine, sterol uptake usually involves prior esterification.

Acanthocephalans

It has been claimed that the proboscis is a specialised region for lipid uptake, but there is no evidence for this. In *Acanthocephalus ranae*, triacylglycerol may be taken up through the general body wall, apparently without prior hydrolysis[50]. The mechanism is not known but could possibly be pinocytosis.

Trematodes

Virtually nothing is known about lipid absorption in trematodes. The only reports have been from *F. hepatica*, where short chain acids (acetate, propionate, butyrate) are taken up by a mixture of diffusion and mediated transport.

Nematodes

The uptake of plalmitic acid has been studied in *A. lumbricoides* gut preparations. The movement of palmitate into the mucosal cells of *A. lumbricoides* appears to be passive, but transport from the cells into the pseudocoelom requires energy. The gut cells of *A. lumbricoides*, like mammalian mucosal cells, thus show functional polarisation. The kinetics of the transport mechanisms for fatty acids at the two surfaces in *A. lumbricoides* gut has, unfortunately, not been investigated.

Gut preparations of *A. lumbricoides* take up cholesterol and β-sitosterol by a passive process, but monoacylglycerols do not appear to be absorbed without prior hydrolysis. The encysted muscle larvae of *T. spiralis* also take up cholesterol.

4.1.10. Purine, Pyrimidine and Nucleoside Transport

Nucleic acids are broken down in the intestine by nucleases, nucleotidases and nucleosidases to give nucleotides, nucleosides and, finally, pyrimidine and purine bases (*Table 4.3*), although some workers claim that nucleotides are not a product of intestinal digestion.

Cestodes

The tapeworm *H. diminuta* absorbs purines and pyrimidines by a combination of passive diffusion and mediated transport. The pyrimidine–purine transport mech-

Table 4.3 Biochemically important nucleosides and nucleotides

	Base	Nucleoside (base + sugar*)	Nucleotide (base + sugar* + phosphate)
Pyrimidine	Cytosine	Cytidine	Cytidylic acid (CMP)
	Thymine	Thymidine	Thymidine monophosphate
	Uracil	Uridine	Uridylic acid (UMP)
Purine	Adenine	Adenosine	Adenylic acid (AMP)
	Guanine	Guanosine	Guanylic acid (GMP)
	Hypoxanthine	Inosine	Inosinic acid (IMP)

*The sugar is ribose, the corresponding deoxyribose analogues are involved in DNA synthesis.

anism is the most complex of the transport systems so far characterised in *H. diminuta*. It involves at least three carriers, two of which have multiple substrate sites. However, it is not known if pyrimidine and purine transport is sodium-sensitive in *H. diminuta* (or in any other helminth).

The uptake of uracil by *H. diminuta* is stimulated at high substrate concentrations, and by related pyrimidines such as thymine, 5-bromouracil and 5-aminouracil. The rate of uptake by *H. diminuta* of 5-bromouracil, thymine and adenine, as a function of concentration, shows sigmoid kinetics. These observations can be accounted for by assuming that two binding sites are involved in the uptake of these compounds. One site is a transport site, the other is an activator site, and there is some form of allosteric interaction between them. As a result of extensive inhibitor studies, Pappas *et al.*[51] have suggested a model for the uptake of pyrimidines and purines in *H. diminuta* (*Table 4.4*). In this model, there are three separate carriers. A thymine–uracil carrier transports thymine, uracil and uracil analogues (5-bromouracil and probably 5-aminouracil). These compounds are all taken up via an allosteric mechanism and the carrier has an activator site for these compounds as well as a transport site.

Table 4.4 Pyrimidine and purine porters of *H. diminuta*

Thymine–uracil carrier		Hypoxanthine carrier I		Hypoxanthine carrier II
Transport site	Activator site	Transport site	Activator site	
Thymine	Thymine	Adenine	Adenine	Hypoxanthine
Uracil	Uracil	Guanine		Purine?
5-Bromouracil	5-Bromouracil	Hypoxanthine		(Adenine)
5-Aminouracil	5-Aminouracil	6-Methyluracil?		
		Uracil?		
(Adenine)		5-Bromouracil?		
(Hypoxanthine)				
(6-Methyluracil?)				
(Purine?)				

Compounds in parentheses bind non-productively (i.e. they are not transported).

Table 4.5 Interactions of purine and pyrimidine uptake in *H. diminuta*

Substrate being absorbed	'Effector'							
	Thymine	Uracil	5-Bromo-uracil	5-Amino-uracil	6-Methyl-uracil	Hypoxan-thine	Adenine	Purine
Thymine	±	±	±	+	−	−	−	−
Uracil	±	±	±	+	−	−	−	−
5-Bromo-uracil	+	0	+	+	−	−	−	−
Hypoxan-thine	0	−	−	0	−	−	−	−
Adenine	0	−	−	0	−	−	±	0
Guanine	0	−	−	0	−	−	−	0

The entries are as follows: +, uptake stimulated; −, uptake inhibited; ±, uptake inhibited or stimulated depending on the effector/substrate ratio; 0, no effect.

Thymine has a much higher affinity than uracil for both the transport site and the activator site. Adenine and hypoxanthine bind non-productively to the thymine–uracil carrier, that is, they inhibit the uptake of thymine and uracil but are not themselves transported. Purine and 6-methyluracil also bind to this site, probably non-productively. The pyrimidine, 6-methyluracil, acts like a purine at the thymine–uracil locus. The nature of the groups at carbons 5 and 6 in the uracil ring may be important in determining binding with the purine and pyrimidine carriers.

There are two distinct hypoxanthine carriers. Carrier I transports hypoxanthine, guanine and adenine, the latter by an allosteric mechanism. Uracil, 5-bromouracil and 6-methyluracil also bind to this site and may be transported. Hypoxanthine carrier II transports hypoxanthine and binds adenine non-productively. Purine also binds to this site, but it is not known if it is transported.

This model represents the simplest scheme that will adequately explain the interactions reported in the uptake of purines and pyrimidines in *H. diminuta* (*Table 4.5*). It is, of course, possible that the carrier mechanisms are, in fact, more complex. 5-Bromouracil interacts differently at the thymine–uracil locus than do thymine and uracil. Low concentrations of thymine, 5-bromouracil or 5-aminouracil did not inhibit the uptake of 5-bromouracil, as is the case with thymine and uracil. 5-Bromouracil uptake is, however, stimulated at high effector concentrations. Uracil, in contrast, does not affect the uptake of 5-bromouracil. It may be necessary to postulate a separate 5-bromouracil site to explain these differences, or they could be due to the relatively low affinity of the pyrimidine analogues for the different binding sites.

There seems to be no transport mechanism for cytosine in *H. diminuta* and it enters by passive diffusion.

Purines and pyrimidines are taken up by mammalian cells via an active mediated process. Uptake is sodium-sensitive, but it has not been established how many carriers are involved. In mammalian cells, there is cross-reactivity between the purine and pyrimidine porters, and there is evidence for at least two purine carriers. So there are similarities between the mammalian and tapeworm purine and pyrimidine transport systems. However, nothing comparable to the allosteric activation of the thymine–uracil carrier and of adenine uptake in *H. diminuta* has been reported in mammals. Stimulation of uracil uptake by thymine also occurs in *H. citelli*, but not apparently in *H. microstoma.*

Nucleoside transport in Hymenolepid tapeworms (*H. diminuta, H. citelli, H. microstoma*) is again mediated, it is sodium-dependent[52] and involves at least two carriers. One carrier has a high specificity for purine nucleosides, the other for pyrimidine nucleosides[53]. The uptake of uridine by *H. diminuta* shows a diurnal rhythm[54]. Transport via the purine nucleoside carrier in *H. diminuta* is stimulated by hypoxanthine, and transport via the pyrimidine nucleoside carrier is stimulated by thymine. Stimulation by free bases of the nucleoside carrier systems in the other two species of tapeworms could not, however, be demonstrated. Thymine is also said to stimulate pyrimidine nucleoside transport in the protozoan *Trypanosoma lewisi.*

In *H. diminuta*, the pyrimidine nucleosides are transported much faster than the free bases. Nucleotide phosphohydrolases are present in the tegument of *H. diminuta* and may be in close proximity to the nucleoside carriers (Section 4.1.1).

In mammalian cells, nucleoside transport is also mediated, but involves a single common carrier rather than multiple carriers as in tapeworms.

Trematodes

The only data on purine and pyrimidine uptake in trematodes are for *S. mansoni.* Pyrimidines appear to be taken up solely by diffusion, although there may be a mediated system for cytosine. Purine bases and nucleosides are transported by a mixture of diffusion and mediated transport. As a result of reciprocal inhibitor studies, five carriers have been proposed to account for purine and nucleoside uptake in *S. mansoni (Table 4.6)*[55]. This model is, however, probably incomplete, and guanosine and thymidine may also be taken up by mediated transport. The tegument of *S. mansoni* contains a phosphohydrolase capable of hydrolysing external nucleotides and, like *H. diminuta*, the phosphohydrolase may be in close proximity to the nucleoside carriers. The sporocysts of *S. mansoni* can take up thymidine and the adults of *Megalodiscus temperatus* take up thymidine and adenosine, but the mechanisms are not known.

Table 4.6 Purine and nucleoside porters in *Schistosoma mansoni*

Carrier	Substrates
I	Guanine, hypoxanthine, (adenine, adenosine, purine)
II	Adenine, adenosine
III	Adenine, (purine)
IV	Adenosine, uridine
V	Adenosine

Compounds in parentheses are bound non-productively (i.e. they inhibit uptake, but are not themselves transported).

Nematodes

There is no information on purine or pyrimidine transport in nematodes. Thymidine is said not to be taken up by *B. pahangi* or *D. immitis.*

4.1.11. Vitamins and Related Compounds

The only detailed kinetic data on vitamin uptake by helminths are for the absorption of water-soluble vitamins by *H. diminuta*. Thiamine (B_1) and riboflavin (B_2) are taken up by a mixture of mediated transport and diffusion, whilst pyridoxine (B_6) and nicotinamide (B_3) enter by diffusion alone. The absence of a mediated transport system for pyridoxine is interesting, since *H. diminuta* has a specific requirement for pyridoxine (Section 4.7). In the mammalian intestine, there is a specific absorption site for thiamine, whilst pyridoxine enters by diffusion as in the tapeworm. In the intestine, it has been suggested that there is an exocrino-enteric circulation of B group vitamins. B group vitamins would, therefore, be available to intestinal parasites even when they were absent from the host's diet. The presence of such a circulation of B group vitamins is not, however, certain.

Vitamin B_{12} (cobalamin) is often accumulated in large amounts by certain parasites, in particular pseudophyllidean cestodes (Section 2.7.1). The tapeworm *D. latum* has such a high affinity for B_{12} that it causes B_{12} deficiency (pernicious anaemia) in its host. The uptake of B_{12} by *D. latum* and the larvae of *S. mansonoides* (spargana) seems to involve a mediated process[56]. In contrast, cyclophyllidean cestodes (*H. diminuta, T. saginata, T. taeniaeformis*) do not absorb B_{12} to any significant extent. The uptake of B_{12} has also been demonstrated in the plerocercoids of *L. intestinalis* and in *F. gigantica*. In nematodes, B_{12} often accumulates in the pseudocoelomocytes. In *A. lumbricoides*, B_{12} uptake is via the intestine. In the mammalian intestine, the uptake of B_{12} requires initial binding to a glycoprotein, called intrinsic factor, and, once in the tissues, B_{12} is transported bound to carrier proteins (transcobalamin I and II). Uptake of B_{12} by *S. mansonoides* larvae (which is a tissue parasite) and *A. lumbricoides* does not seem to require initial binding to intrinsic factor or a carrier protein, and both parasites can take up the free vitamin. It is said that *D. latum* can split B_{12} from intrinsic factor, *A. lumbricoides* cannot split B_{12} from intrinsic factor and it is doubtful if *S. mansonoides* larvae can split B_{12} from its carrier protein. Presumably, there must be enough free B_{12} in the tissues for *S. mansonoides* larvae. A mucoprotein that binds B_{12} has been tentatively identified from the gut of *A. lumbricoides* and, following uptake, B_{12} becomes bound to protein, both in *A. lumbricoides* and *S. mansonoides.*

An interesting compound that is taken up by some helminths is serotonin (5-hydroxytryptamine). Both *S. mansoni* and larval *M. corti* take up serotonin by a mediated process which involves two carriers, one with a high affinity for substrate and one with a low affinity[57,58].

4.1.12. Ion and Water Transport

The transport of electrolytes and water in helminths has not been as extensively studied as the transport of non-electrolytes.

Cestodes

Sodium uptake by tapeworms is closely linked with hexose transport (Section 4.1.7). Bicarbonate absorption in *H. diminuta* is via a hydrogen ion secretory mechanism (*Figure 4.7*)[59]. Hydrogen ion secretion in *H. diminuta* is also partially coupled with sodium absorption. Whether this is partial direct coupling or the result of indirect coupling is not known. Coupled hydrogen ion secretion and sodium absorption is usual in tissues. However, *H. diminuta* is unusual in that it is largely dependent on external carbon dioxide as the source of tissue protons for the hydrogen ion pump[60].

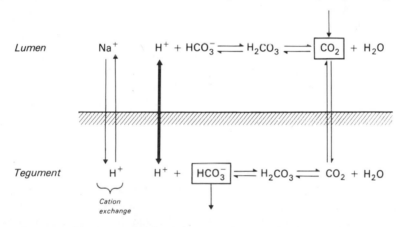

Figure 4.7 Bicarbonate uptake via hydrogen ion secretion in *H. diminuta*.

Chloride uptake by *H. diminuta* passively follows sodium uptake, although bicarbonate was the major anion accompanying sodium uptake during *in vivo* studies. In sodium-free media, there is a net secretion of sodium chloride. Chloride is also secreted in chloride-free media by *H. diminuta*.

The electrolyte transport systems of *H. diminuta* are thus very similar to those of other transport epithelia. The size of the active sodium transport pool in the tegument of *H. diminuta* is comparable to that of toad urinary bladder epithelia and the steps involved in sodium transport are the same in the two tissues[61].

Water uptake in *H. diminuta* is coupled to solute transport, although ion uptake can occur in the absence of water uptake. The fluid accumulated by *H. diminuta* is hypertonic with respect to the surrounding medium. In vertebrate tissues, the intercellular spaces are thought to be involved in maintaining the standing osmotic gradients required for solute-linked water transport. The syncitial tegument of cestodes does not have intercellular channels, so an alternative scheme will have to be proposed to account for active water movement through this tissue. The absence of cell junctions in the tegument of cestodes may help restrict water and ion exchange with the underlying tissues and make it a more efficient osmoregulatory surface[60].

A high environmental carbon dioxide level, with consequent acidification of the tissues, is a problem faced by intestinal helminths. The ability of *H. diminuta* to secrete hydrogen ions may be a factor in regulating internal pH.

Hydatid cysts (*E. granulosus*) have a low permeability to sodium and chloride ions but a high permeability to water. The permeability to water is said to be increased by mammalian ADH[62].

Trematodes

There is some ultrastructural evidence that *F. hepatica* may have similar ion and water transport mechanisms to *H. diminuta*.

Acanthocephalans

The only work on acanthocephalans is on *M. dubius*, which appears to be able to accumulate both sodium and potassium ions from the external medium by an active process. The sodium and potassium pumps of *M. dubius* are not coupled, and water uptake appears to follow solute transport. This rather unusual system would repay re-investigation.

Nematodes

The active uptake or elimination of ions has not been demonstrated in nematodes, although regulation of body fluid ions certainly takes place and *A. lumbricoides*, for example, can regulate its internal K^+, Mg^{2+}, Ca^{2+} and Cl^-. A number of nematodes show volume regulation in hypotonic media, and the gut, excretory system and specialised hypodermal gland cells have all been suggested as sites of urine production.

Intestinal sac preparations from *A. lumbricoides* can transport water from the luminal to the pseudocoelomic side. Water uptake is isosmotic and coupled to solute uptake, but in *A. lumbricoides* preparations, glucose rather than sodium appears to be the major osmotic effector. During fluid transport, the intercellular spaces in the gut preparations swell[63]. So in *A. lumbricoides* gut, as in mammalian preparations, the intercellular spaces appear to be involved in establishing and maintaining the local osmotic gradients required for water movement.

An electrical potential of 15–30 mV develops across isolated *A. lumbricoides* gut ribbons, the lumen positive with respect to the pseudocoelom. Flux studies indicate that both Na^+ and Cl^- contribute to the observed potential.

4.1.13. Significance of Uptake Mechanisms

Much work has been done on uptake mechanisms in helminths and a considerable volume of data has been accumulated. Unfortunately, as is often the case in parasite biochemistry, relatively few species of helminth have been studied. The most investigated species is undoubtedly the rat tapeworm *H. diminuta*. This cestode has a whole series of different carrier systems for hexoses, amino acids, purines, pyrimidines, nucleosides, fatty acids, water-soluble vitamins and ions. Some of the porter systems, such as the purine and pyrimidine carriers, are extremely complex. In this and probably other parasites, there seems to have been a diversification of absorption mechanisms rather than a simplification. The high specificity of the hexose transport mechanisms in *H. diminuta* also contrasts with the low specificity of its hexokinase (Section 3.1.10).

The uptake mechanisms of trematodes, acanthocephalans and nematodes have not been so well characterised as those of cestodes, but the evidence suggests a similar variety of transport systems. The apparent absence of any mediated system for amino acid transport in *F. hepatica* may well be due to experimental difficulties.

On a unit weight basis, the uptake of nutrients by *H. diminuta* is equal to, or in some cases greater than, that of the rat intestine. No conclusions can be drawn from a comparison of the relative affinities (K_t) of the tapeworm and intestinal transport mechanisms since almost none of the relevant data have taken into account the presence of the stationary layer (Section 4.1.6). However, it does appear that the tapeworm porters may have a higher affinity for substrate than the intestinal carriers.

The uptake mechanisms of a tissue reflect its metabolic needs. This is well shown in *A. lumbricoides* where the reproductive tissue, which has a high rate of protein synthesis, transports amino acids actively, whilst in muscle tissue, which does not catabolise amino acids, entry is by passive diffusion. In broad terms, the uptake mechanisms of intestinal helminths are similar to the transport mechanisms of the intestinal mucosa, although there are considerable differences in detail, amino acid transport in cestodes, for example, being sodium-insensitive, whereas in the mucosa it is sodium-dependent. The significance of these differences is not clear. The absorptive teguments of cestodes, trematodes and acanthocephalans are of different embryological origin from the mammalian mucosa and this may be relevant. Little or nothing is known of transport mechanisms in non-parasitic invertebrates, so whether or not these transport mechanisms are unique to parasitic helminths or are standard in invertebrates is unknown. Some of the apparent differences between the uptake systems of helminths and those of mammals may also be due to experimental differences, and certain systems such as fatty acid transport and pyrimidine and purine transport have been studied in much more detail in helminths than in mammals.

However, both mammalian and helminth transport systems have carriers with broad and often overlapping specificities. This may have two advantages. First, it prevents flooding of the internal pool by a single compound. As all of the compounds transported by a single carrier are competitive inhibitors of one another, the uptake of any one is modulated by the relative concentrations of all of the rest. Secondly, by having carriers with wide specificities, the total number of carriers required is reduced.

Uptake mechanisms are generally constitutive in metazoa and inducible in microorganisms. It is not known if parasitic helminths can alter either the numbers or relative proportions of the different uptake sites under different conditions. Nor, in fact, are there any data on the number of uptake sites per unit area in helminths, although this information is available for mammalian tissues. The fact that the kinetic parameters of uptake mechanisms change in *H. diminuta* with age and with host species suggests that some alterations in the transport systems are possible. These changes, however, need not necessarily involve alterations in the number or type of transport sites, but could reflect differences in the properties of the stationary layer or changes in surface morphology.

Mediated transport mechanisms transport compounds across membranes in both directions, giving rise to the phenomena of exchange diffusion and counterflow. The result of this mediated bidirectional flux is that, in a parasite such as *H. diminuta*, the internal substrate pools are in equilibrium with the intestinal substrate pools, which in turn are in equilibrium with the host's tissue. So, with respect to low molecular weight substrates, the parasite and the host are in a state of dynamic equilibrium.

4.2. BIOSYNTHESIS OF CARBOHYDRATES

Quantitatively, the synthesis of carbohydrates is probably the most prominent anabolic process in parasites. Playing a central role in carbohydrate synthesis is glucose-6-phosphate. Gluconeogenic substrates are converted first to glucose-6-phosphate, which is the starting point for monosaccharide, disaccharide and polysaccharide synthesis.

4.2.1. Synthesis from Non-hexose Precursors

In parasitic helminths, dietary hexoses are the main substrate for glyconeogenesis. However, helminths, like other organisms, are able to synthesise hexoses from non-sugar precursors. In helminths, glucose-6-phosphate is broken down by glycolysis as far as phosphoenolpyruvate and in many species to pyruvate. The reversal of glycolysis can be used to synthesise glucose-6-phosphate from pyruvate or phosphoenolpyruvate. However, two of the steps in glycolysis, phosphofructokinase and pyruvate kinase, are thermodynamically unfavourable for glucose-6-phosphate synthesis and under physiological conditions they are essentially irreversible.

The phosphofructokinase step can be reversed by another enzyme, fructose-1,6-bisphosphatase. This enzyme is widely distributed in helminths (Section 5.1.3) and together with phosphofructokinase may form a substrate cycle between fructose-6-phosphate and fructose-1,6-bisphosphate:

$$\text{fructose-6-phosphate} \underset{\text{FBPase}}{\overset{\text{PFK}}{\rightleftarrows}} \text{fructose-1,6-bisphosphate}$$

Two other enzymes that can form a substrate cycle are hexokinase and glucose-6-phosphatase:

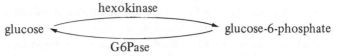

glucose $\rightleftharpoons$ glucose-6-phosphate (with hexokinase above and G6Pase below)

Glucose-6-phosphatase occurs in helminths and is necessary for the formation of free glucose from gluconeogenesis or from glycogen. The significance of substrate cycles is not altogether clear; they may increase the sensitivity of the pathways to modulation (Section 5.1.3) or they might be involved in heat production or the removal of excess ATP.

The other irreversible enzyme in glycolysis is pyruvate kinase. In mammals, the pyruvate kinase step is bypassed during gluconeogenesis by a sequence involving pyruvate carboxylase and phosphoenolpyruvate carboxykinase. In the mammalian mitochondrion, pyruvate is carboxylated by pyruvate carboxylase to give oxaloacetate:

$$\text{pyruvate} + CO_2 + ATP \rightleftharpoons \text{oxaloacetate} + ADP + P_i$$

The oxaloacetate is reduced to malate which then leaves the mitochondrion for the cytoplasm where it is reoxidised back to oxaloacetate. The oxaloacetate is then converted via phosphoenolpyruvate carboxykinase to phosphoenolpyruvate. In mammals, this sequence of reactions brings about the effective reversal of the pyruvate kinase step:

$$\text{pyruvate} + GTP + ATP \rightarrow \text{phosphoenolpyruvate} + GDP + ADP + P_i$$
$$\text{(sum)}$$

This permits gluconeogenesis from lactate (via pyruvate) and from tricarboxylic acid cycle intermediates (via oxaloacetate).

In parasites, like *A. lumbricoides* and *F. hepatica*, which fix carbon dioxide, phosphoenolpyruvate carboxykinase is a key enzyme in catabolism (Section 3.1.4). Phosphoenolpyruvate carboxykinase is also found in helminths such as *S. mansoni* and *L. carinii*, which are essentially homolactic fermenters, and is probably universally distributed in helminths. In contrast, the importance of pyruvate carboxylase in helminths is uncertain. It has been reported in *M. expansa* and *E. granulosus*, but could not be detected in *A. lumbricoides* or the plerocercoids of *S. solidus*. An alternative to pyruvate carboxylase in helminths, for the carboxylation of pyruvate, could be the malic enzyme. The malic enzyme is again widely distributed in helminths, but in both helminths and mammals it normally functions in the direction of malate decarboxylation:

$$\text{malate} + NAD(P)^+ \rightleftharpoons \text{pyruvate} + CO_2 + NAD(P)H + H^+$$

The malic enzyme has a relatively low affinity for carbon dioxide, so pyruvate carboxylation is limited. However, in gut helminths, with their high ambient carbon dioxide levels, the carboxylation of pyruvate via the malic enzyme remains a possibility. Malate could then be converted to glucose as outlined above.

Parasitic helminths thus have all the enzyme systems necessary to carry out glyconeogenesis from glycolytic or tricarboxylic acid cycle intermediates. Substrates like the glucogenic amino acids, which can be catabolised to glycolytic or tricarboxy-lic acid cycle intermediates (Section 3.4), should also be glycogenic. In addition, some helminths, such as *A. lumbricoides, F. hepatica* and *S. mansonoides*, can convert succinate to propionate (Section 3.1.4). This pathway is reversible, so in these helminths propionate is also a potential glyconeogenic substrate. However, despite the presence of all of the relevant enzymes, there have been few demonstrations of glyconeogenesis from substrates, other than hexoses, in parasitic helminths. The conversion of propionate to glycogen has been shown in fourth-stage *Cooperia punctata* larvae[64], pyruvate and glutamate have been reported as glyconeogenic in *H. diminuta* and glycerol is glyconeogenic in larval *T. taeniaeformis*. In *H. diminuta*, glutamate is presumably converted to 2-oxoglutarate by glutamate dehydrogenase and hence via the tricarboxylic acid cycle to oxaloacetate. The pathway of pyruvate metabolism is not known, it could involve carboxylation via the malic enzyme or there may be a pyruvate carboxylase present. In *T. taeniaeformis* there is an active glycerol kinase (Section 3.2.4), so glycerol could be converted to glycerol-3-phos-phate and enter glycolysis via dihydroxyacetone phosphate. Finally, acetate has been reported as being glyconeogenic in *E. granulosus* scoleces, but the possible pathway is again not known.

Glyoxylate Cycle

In contrast to the other glycolytic and tricarboxylic acid cycle intermediates, there is no net conversion of acetyl-CoA into glycogen in most animal tissues. This is because the conversion of acetyl-CoA to oxaloacetate, via the tricarboxylic acid cycle, involves two decarboxylation steps (isocitrate dehydrogenase and 2-oxoglutar-ate decarboxylase). By the time oxaloacetate has been formed from citrate, two carbon dioxide molecules have been lost and there is no net synthesis. However, a net synthesis of glycogen from acetyl-CoA can be achieved via the glyoxylate cycle (*Figure 4.8*). This effectively 'short circuits' the tricarboxylic acid cycle by bypass-ing the two decarboxylation steps. The glyoxylate cycle involves two extra enzymes, isocitrate lyase and malate synthase. Isocitrate lyase cleaves isocitrate to succinate and glyoxylate, whilst malate synthase condenses a second acetyl-CoA with glyoxy-late to give malate.

The glyoxylate cycle occurs in micro-organisms and in germinating seeds, but until recently it was not thought to occur in animals. During the first 10 days of development of *A. lumbricoides* eggs, glycogen and trehalose are extensively catabolised. However, from the tenth day of development until the egg becomes infective (21 days at 30 °C) the carbohydrate reserves are resynthesised (*Figure 3.13*). The resynthesis of trehalose slightly precedes the resynthesis of the glycogen. Careful carbon balance studies showed that the carbohydrate was resynthesised at the expense of the triacylglycerol fatty acids. In *A. lumbricoides* eggs, some 12% of the triacylglycerol fatty acids are short chain volatile fatty acids (2-methylbutyrate and 2-methylvalerate). These volatile fatty acids are potentially glyconeogenic in that they can be degraded to propionate. However, the volatile fatty acids could only account for a small proportion of the resynthesised carbohydrate and the

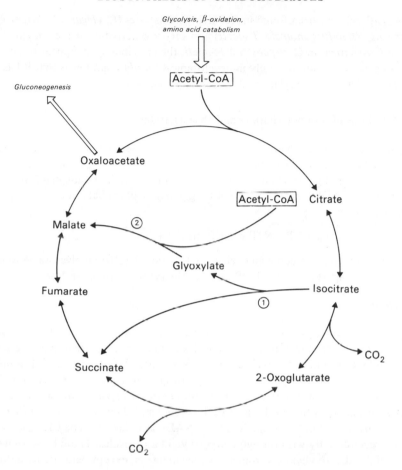

Figure 4.8 The glyoxylate cycle: 1, isocitrate lyase; 2, malate synthase.

volatile acids have mostly been catabolised before resynthesis begins. So, the majority of the resynthesised carbohydrate is derived from long chain fatty acids and developing *A. lumbricoides* eggs have a functional glyoxylate cycle. There is an active β-oxidation sequence and tricarboxylic acid cycle in *A. lumbricoides* eggs (Sections 3.1.13 and 3.3.4) and the two enzymes of the glyoxylate cycle, isocitrate lyase and malate synthase, are also present. The activities of the glyoxylate cycle enzymes in developing eggs peak at a time which corresponds to the peak resynthesis of carbohydrate from lipid. Most of the resynthesised glycogen appears in the muscles as β-glycogen[65]. There is no evidence for glyoxysomes in *A. lumbricoides* larvae and the glyoxylate cycle enzymes appear to be mitochondrial[66]. This means that isocitrate dehydrogenase and isocitrate lyase are competing for the same substrate within the mitochondrion. How this possible branch point might be controlled is not known.

The glyoxylate cycle is not present in adult *A. lumbricoides*. Isocitrate lyase and malate synthase have been found in free-living nematodes (*C. elegans, C. briggsae, P. redivivus, Rhabditis anomala, T. aceti*) and very low activities of the enzymes occur in *F. hepatica*. In *C. elegans* and *T. aceti*, the enzymes again appear to be mitochondrial. However, it is only in developing *A. lumbricoides* eggs that it has been shown that the glyoxylate cycle is actually functional.

4.2.2. Synthesis of Monosaccharides and Disaccharides

The ability of helminths to interconvert glucose, fructose, mannose and galactose has already been discussed (Section 3.1.10). Syntheses involving sugars usually require an energised glycosyl unit in the form of a nucleoside diphosphate sugar. The synthesis of NDP-sugars is catalysed by glycosyl-1-phosphate nucleotidyl trans-phosphorylase:

$$\text{sugar-1-P} + \text{NTP} \rightleftharpoons \text{NDP-sugar} + \text{PP}_i$$

The interconversion of glucose and galactose (Section 3.1.10) involves nucleoside diphosphate sugars (in this case UDP) as does the synthesis of ascarylose.

Ascarylose

Ascarylose (3,6-dideoxy-L-arabinohexose) is an unusual sugar isolated from ascaro-sides. Ascarosides are the non-polar glycosides found in the egg shells and ovaries of ascarid and oxyurid nematodes (Section 2.3.5). Ovarian homogenates of *A. lumbri-coides* can synthesise ascarylose from glucose or glucose-1-phosphate, probably by a pathway similar to that found in the bacterium *Pasteurella pseudotuberculosis*. Initially, this involves the synthesis of CDP-glucose and then conversion to CDP-ascarylose by a reaction requiring NAD and NADP as cofactors. The CDP-ascarylose can then react directly with the aglycones to yield ascarosides. There have been no reports of 3,6-dideoxyhexoses from any other metazoa, except parasitic nematodes.

Glucosamine

Nematodes and acanthocephalans both have chitin in their egg shells and so can presumably synthesise glucosamine.

In insects and micro-organisms, glucosamine is synthesised from fructose-6-phosphate and does not involve an NDP-sugar:

$$\text{fructose-6-P} + \text{glutamine} \rightarrow \text{glucosamine-6-P} + \text{glutamate}$$

The pathway of glucosamine synthesis in helminths has not been investigated.

Trehalose

Nematodes and acanthocephalans often contain relatively large amounts of trehalose (Section 2.2.1). Trehalose synthesis has been investigated in *A. lumbricoides, M. dubius* and *M. hirudinaceus*. In these helminths, the pathway of trehalose synthesis seems to be the same as in insects and in yeast:

glucose-6-P + UDP-glucose $\rightleftharpoons$ trehalose-6-P + UDP (*trehalose synthase*)

trehalose-6-P + H_2O $\rightleftharpoons$ trehalose + P_i (*trehalose-6-phosphatase*)

Some bacteria use GDP-glucose rather than UDP-glucose in trehalose synthesis. In *A. lumbricoides*, ovarian tissue has the highest trehalose synthase activity and there is only low activity in the muscles and intestine. In *M. dubius*, trehalose synthesis appears to be restricted to the body wall. Like glycogen synthase (Section 4.2.3), trehalose synthase is probably under allosteric control.

Sugar Alcohols

Sorbitol can be synthesised by *A. lumbricoides* and larval *P. decipiens* (Section 3.1.10) and there is indirect evidence that *H. diminuta* can synthesise inositol from glucose. The free-living nematode *T. aceti* can synthesise ribitol.

4.2.3. Synthesis of Polysaccharides

Glycogen

The major energy reserve in parasitic helminths is glycogen, and exogenous hexoses are rapidly synthesised into glycogen in most, if not all, species. In *H. diminuta*, glycogen can be synthesised from glucose at the rate of 1 g/100 g wet weight/h. There are, however, differences in the ability of helminths to utilise exogenous hexoses, other than glucose, for glycogen synthesis. The nematode *A. lumbricoides* can synthesis glycogen from glucose, fructose, sorbose, maltose and sucrose. *L carinii* can also synthesise glycogen from exogenous glucose and mannose, but not from fructose or galactose. Galactose is glyconeogenic in *F. hepatica* and *T. taeniae-formis*. However, in the trematode *Megalodiscus temperatus*, glucose is incorporated into glycogen, but galactose is primarily incorporated into mucopolysaccharides. Finally, the acanthocephalan *M. dubius* can synthesise glycogen from glucose, fructose, mannose and maltose.

Despite the importance of glycogen synthesis in helminths, the mechanism of glycogen synthesis has only been investigated in any detail in *H. diminuta*[67,68]. In *H. diminuta*, glycogen synthesis follows the same steps as in mammalian tissue, starting with glycose-6-phosphate:

glucose-6-P $\rightleftharpoons$ glucose-1-P   (*phosphoglucomutase*)

glucose-1-P + UTP $\rightleftharpoons$ UDP-glucose + PP_i (*glucose-1-P uridylyl transferase*)

UDP-glucose + (glucose)$_n$ $\rightarrow$ (glucose)$_{n+1}$ + UDP (*glycogen synthase*)
                glycogen

Glycogen synthase requires a primer chain of at least four α 1–4 glucose units. Only α 1–4 links are made by glycogen synthase, α 1–6 links require the presence of a second enzyme, α 1–4 glucan branching enzyme (Q enzyme). This enzyme is presumably present in helminths and has been demonstrated histochemically in *H.*

diminuta[149]. In mammals, ADP-glucose is only about 50% as active as UDP-glucose in glycogen synthesis, although ADP-glucose may be the preferred donor in some micro-organisms. Whether ADP-glucose can act as a donor in helminth systems has not been investigated.

In mammals, glycogen synthase is under both allosteric and covalent modulation (*Figure 4.9*). I (glucose-6-phosphate independent) and D (glucose-6-phosphate dependent) forms of glycogen synthase have been demonstrated in *H. diminuta*, but details of the interconversion and control of the two forms have not been worked out.

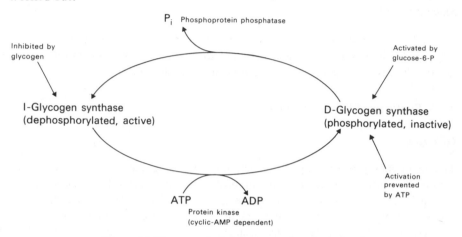

Figure 4.9 The control of glycogen synthase in mammals.

In some helminths, glyconeogenesis from glucose is stimulated by carbon dioxide. This is the case in *H. diminuta, H. citelli* and several other cestodes, as well as in the trematode *Cryptocotyle lingua*. Presumably, this reflects the role of carbon dioxide in energy production in these helminths. However, not all helminths require carbon dioxide for glyconeogenesis; *T. taeniaeformis* shows only slight stimulation by carbon dioxide, whilst *M. dubius* shows none at all. Carbon dioxide may even inhibit glycogen synthesis in the rediae of *Parorchis acanthus* and *C. lingua*.

Complex Polysaccharides

Helminths are capable of synthesising complex polysaccharides such as chitin and glycoproteins, but little is known of the pathways involved. Labelled galactose has been shown to be incorporated into tegumental glycoproteins in cestodes (*H. diminuta, T. crassiceps* larvae) and trematodes (*F. hepatica, M. temperatus*)[69,70]. Labelled sulphate has also been shown to be incorporated into the tegument of *F. hepatica*.

Glycosyl transferase, the enzyme responsible for building the carbohydrate side chain of glycoproteins, has been demonstrated in the tegument of *S. mansoni*[71]. This enzyme requires, as a cofactor, the phosphate ester of a long chain isoprenoid alcohol (dolichol phosphate). This phosphorylisoprenol acts as a carrier for the glycosyl unit:

phosphorylisoprenol + GDP-mannose $\rightleftharpoons$ mannosylphosphorylisoprenol + GDP

The glycosyl unit is then added to the oligosaccharide side chain of a glycoprotein:

mannosylphosphorylisoprenol + oligosaccharide
$\rightarrow$ phosphorylisoprenol + lengthened oligosaccharide

The blood fluke, *S. mansoni* can incorporate host blood group substances into its tegument and thereby avoid the host's immune response. The presence of glycosyl transferases and phosphorylisoprenols in the tegument has led to the speculation that these enzymes may be responsible for the incorporation of host antigen by transferring the carbohydrate side chains from host glycolipid or glycoprotein to parasite glycoproteins.

4.3. BIOSYNTHESIS OF LIPIDS

Lipid synthesis is an important process in most organisms and the same is true for helminths. Although the parasitic stages of helminths do not use lipid as an energy reserve (Section 3.1), they nevertheless synthesise triacylglycerols and there is, of course, a constant turnover of structural lipids. In addition, certain lipid derivatives are metabolically active (prenoids, steroids, prostaglandins).

Virtually all the work on lipid synthesis in parasitic helminths has involved isotope studies and the enzymes themselves have not been investigated.

4.3.1. Fatty Acid Synthesis

The synthesis of volatile fatty acids, as end-products of carbohydrate breakdown by helminths, has been discussed in Section 3.1.3. Parasitic helminths appear to have a much-reduced ability to synthesise long chain fatty acids *de novo*. In mammals, saturated long chain fatty acids (acids with no double bonds) are synthesised by a cytoplasmic fatty acid synthetase complex. The saturated fatty acids are formed by the sequential addition of malonyl-CoA to an acetyl-CoA (for even-numbered acids) or a propionyl-CoA (for odd-numbered acids) primer. The major steps of the malonyl-CoA pathway are summarised in *Table 4.7*. In fatty acid synthesis, the acyl intermediates are not CoA esters, but acyl carrier proteins (ACP).

In most organisms, the fatty acid synthetase cycle stops at palmitate (C_{16}), this acid then being the precursor for both saturated and unsaturated long chain acids. In the mammal, there are two systems for fatty acid elongation, one microsomal, the other mitochondrial. The microsomal system requires malonyl-CoA, but unlike the fatty acid synthetase complex uses CoA as the acyl carrier and not ACP. The mitochondrial system catalyses the sequential addition of acetyl-CoA to the fatty acid, using steps that are the reversal of β-oxidation, but involving different enzymes (Section 3.3.2).

In vertebrates, monoenoic acids (one double bond) are synthesised from saturated

Table 4.7 Malonyl-CoA pathway of fatty acid synthesis

Malonyl-CoA is synthesised from acetyl-CoA:

    (i)   acetyl-CoA + HCO_3^- + H^+ + ATP $\rightleftharpoons$ malonyl-CoA + ADP + P_i

Malonyl-CoA is added sequentially to an acetyl- (or propionyl-) CoA primer. The acyl carrier is not CoA but an acyl carrier protein (ACP):

    (ii)   acetyl-CoA + ACP $\rightleftharpoons$ acetyl-ACP + CoA

The acetyl group is then transferred to one of the synthase enzymes of the complex:

    (iii)   acetyl-ACP + synthase $\rightleftharpoons$ acetyl-synthase + ACP

Malonyl-CoA is first activated:

    (iv)   malonyl-CoA + ACP $\rightleftharpoons$ malonyl-ACP + CoA

Condensation reaction:

    (v)   malonyl-ACP + acetyl synthase $\rightarrow$ acetoacyl-ACP + synthase + CO_2

First reduction step:

    (vi)   acetoacyl-ACP + NADPH + H^+ $\rightleftharpoons$ D-β-hydroxybutyryl-ACP + $NADP^+$

Followed by dehydration:

    (vii) D-β-hydroxybutyryl-ACP $\rightleftharpoons$ crotonyl-ACP + H_2O

Finally, second reduction:

    (viii) crotonyl-ACP + NADPH + H^+ $\rightleftharpoons$ butyryl-ACP + $NADP^+$

The butyryl group is then transferred from the ACP to the synthetase (iii) and the cycle repeats, stopping when palmitate (C_{16}) is reached.

fatty acids by a specific mono-oxygenase. This system requires NADPH, is microsomal and involves cytochrome b_5:

$$palmitoyl\text{-}CoA + NADPH + H^+ + O_2 \rightarrow palmitoleyl\text{-}CoA + NADP^+ + H_2O$$

The polyenoic acids of mammals belong to four series and are synthesised from the precursor acids (palmitoleic, $C_{16:1}$; oleic, $C_{18:1}$; linoleic, $C_{18:2}$; linolenic $C_{18:3}$) by further desaturation and chain lengthening. Man can synthesise palmitoleic and oleic, but linoleic and linolenic are essential fatty acids. Linoleic and/or linolenic are also essential fatty acids for most insects.

Cestodes and Trematodes

In contrast to vertebrates, none of the parasitic platyhelminths so far studied (*F. hepatica, S. mansoni, H. diminuta*, larval and adult *S. mansonoides*) can synthesise long chain fatty acids *de novo*. Nor can these helminths desaturate preformed long chain fatty acids. Fatty acid synthesis in the parasitic platyhelminths is restricted to chain lengthening by the sequential addition of acetyl-CoA. The cestode *H. diminuta*, for example, can convert palmitate (C_{16}) and stearate (C_{18}) into saturated fatty acids with up to 26 carbons, and *F. hepatica* can synthesise $C_{20:1}$ and $C_{20:2}$ from $C_{18:1}$ and $C_{18:2}$. The mechanism for chain lengthening in these parasites is not known, but it may be similar to the mammalian mitochondrial elongation system (Section 3.3.2). In *S. mansoni*, there seems to be a preference for elongation of the linoleic series of acids[72].

The first enzyme in the malonyl-CoA pathway of fatty acid synthesis, acyl-CoA carboxylase (*Table 4.7* (i)), has, however, been isolated from *S. mansonoides*[73]. This enzyme is capable of carboxylating acetyl, propionyl and butyryl-CoA. Whether it is involved in fatty acid synthesis or whether it is concerned primarily with propionate production (Section 3.1.4) is not certain.

The inability to synthesise long chain fatty acids or to desaturate preformed fatty acids is not restricted to parasitic platyhelminths. The free-living turbellarian *Dugesia dorocephala* can also neither synthesise nor desaturate long chain fatty acids[74]. So it may be a feature of the phylum as a whole and not a parasitic adaptation. A wide variety of mono- and polyunsaturated fatty acids have been identified in the lipids of trematodes and cestodes, and presumably they have an absolute requirement for a corresponding wide range of essential fatty acids. Free-living platyhelminths may similarly need a large number of essential fatty acids. In this context, it is interesting that one of the products which acoel turbellarians get from their algal symbionts are polyunsaturated fatty acids.

Nematodes

The only information on fatty acid synthesis in nematodes is from *A. lumbricoides*. Like parasitic platyhelminths, *A. lumbricoides* can lengthen fatty acids by sequential addition of acetyl-CoA. There is also some evidence that *A. lumbricoides* may be able to synthesise long chain fatty acids by the mevalonate pathway. However, even if this is confirmed, the rate of *de novo* synthesis is very low. Whether parasitic nematodes can desaturate preformed fatty acids is not clear. Free-living nematodes can synthesise polyunsaturated fatty acids and there are claims that *A. lumbricoides* can convert linoleic ($C_{18:2}$) into $C_{20:4}$ (possibly arachidonic) via $C_{18:3}$. The free-living nematodes would appear to be unique in that free-living protozoa are the only other animals that can synthesise polyunsaturated fatty acids *de novo*. Acetyl-CoA carboxylase has been purified from the free-living nematode *T. aceti*[144].

Acanthocephalans

Nothing is known about fatty acid synthesis in acanthocephalans.

General

Parasitic platyhelminths and possibly other groups of parasitic helminths are unable to synthesise long chain fatty acids *de novo*, nor can they desaturate saturated fatty acids. Helminths can, however, lengthen preformed fatty acids by the sequential addition of acetyl-CoA. The inability of helminths to synthesise or to desaturate fatty acids may explain, at least in part, why the fatty acid composition of helminths often resembles, very closely, that of their hosts (Section 2.3.1). Although helminths have only a limited ability to synthesise fatty acids, they can make their own complex neutral lipids and phospholipids from simple precursors. Helminths may also be able to control, to a certain extent, the fatty acid composition of their lipids. They can do this by regulating the uptake of the different fatty acids from their environment and by preferential acylation of free fatty acids in their own free fatty acid pool.

There is no information on fatty acid synthesis in larval helminths. So it is not known if the synthetic pathways absent in the parasitic adult are present or not in the free-living stages. In the platyhelminths, the lack of *de novo* fatty acid synthesis and the inability to desaturate fatty acids may be a peculiarity of the phylum as a whole. However, this is based on studies on only one free-living planarian. The desaturation of fatty acids requires molecular oxygen and many parasites live in oxygen-poor environments. Bacteria can, however, synthesise monoenoic acids anaerobically by dehydration of intermediate length acyl fatty acids (polyenoic acids are not found in bacteria). The eukaryotic fatty acid desaturase system involves the microsomal cytochromes. Microsomal cytochromes have not been identified in helminths (Section 4.8) and parasitic helminths seem to be deficient in microsomal enzyme systems generally. The fatty acid chain lengthening system in helminths also resembles the mammalian mitochondrial system rather than the microsomal one.

The limited ability of helminths to synthesise and desaturate fatty acids presents problems with regards to environmental temperature change. When the ambient temperature increases, free-living animals synthesise more saturated fatty acids and thus raise the melting point of their lipids. If the ambient temperature falls, free-living animals lower the melting point of their lipids by increasing the proportion of unsaturated fatty acids. One of the responses of free-living animals to low temperature is an increase in the activity of the fatty acid desaturase system. During their life-cycle, parasitic helminths, particularly those parasitic in endotherms, are faced with large temperature changes (Section 5.2.3). Helminths are, however, unable to synthesise saturated fatty acids *de novo* or to desaturate preformed fatty acids. Helminths, and eukaryotes in general, are also unable to reduce unsaturated fatty acids to saturated ones. The only mechanisms available to parasitic helminths for modifying the melting point of their lipids is simple chain lengthening (which raises the melting point of the fatty acid) and altering the gross lipid composition of their membranes. Changing the relative proportions of the different phospholipid and steroid classes in the membrane would modulate the melting point. This, however, raises another problem and that is that helminths are also unable to synthesise sterols *de novo*.

4.3.2. Triacylglycerol Synthesis

Helminths rapidly incorporate exogenous labelled fatty acids into their triacylglycerols. In vertebrates, the main route for triacylglycerol synthesis is the phosphatidic acid/diacylglycerol pathway, summarised in *Figure 4.10*. The glycerol-3-phosphate for triacylglycerol synthesis can come from dihydroxyacetone phosphate via glycerol-3-phosphate dehydrogenase:

dihydroxyacetone phosphate + NADH + H⁺ ⇌ glycerol-3-phosphate + NAD⁺

or from free glycerol via glycerol kinase:

glycerol + ATP ⇌ glycerol-3-phosphate + ADP

Both glycerol-3-phosphate dehydrogenase and glycerol kinase occur in helminths.

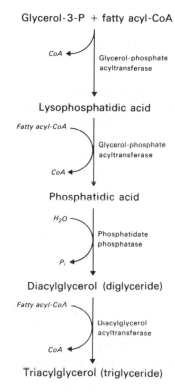

Figure 4.10 Triacylglycerol synthesis.

An alternative source of lysophosphatidic acid for the phosphatidic acid/diacyl-glycerol pathway is direct acylation of dihydroxyacetone phosphate, followed by reduction:

dihydroxyacetone phosphate + fatty acyl-CoA →
                              fatty acyldihydroxyacetone phosphate + CoA

fatty acyldihydroxyacetone phosphate + NADPH + H⁺ ⇌
                              lysophosphatidic acid + NADP⁺

However, it is not known if helminths can use this pathway for lysophosphatidic acid synthesis.

In the mammalian intestine, there is a different pathway for triacylglycerol synthesis, involving direct acylation of absorbed monoacylglycerols:

monoacylglycerol + fatty acyl-CoA $\rightleftharpoons$ diacylglycerol + CoA

diacylglycerol + fatty acyl-CoA $\rightleftharpoons$ triacylglycerol + CoA

In nature, most triacylglycerols are mixed, having two or more different acids esterified. It is not known how the identity and position of the different acids in triacylglycerols are specified.

Cestodes

In *H. diminuta*, fatty acids are much more rapidly incorporated into triacylglycerols than into phospholipids. Isotope studies indicate that triacylglycerols are synthesised via the phosphatidic acid/diacylglycerol pathway rather than via the monoacylglycerol route. The triacylglycerols of *H. diminuta* show a high degree of specificity and, of the fatty acids esterified at the C_2 position, 96% are unsaturated.

Lysolecithin (monoacylglycerol-3-phosphorylcholine), which occurs in high levels in intestinal contents, is rapidly absorbed and metabolised by *H. diminuta*. It has been postulated that *H. diminuta* (and other intestinal helminths) may be able to hydrolyse lysolecithin to lysophosphatidic acid, which can then be converted to triacylglycerol.

The dogfish tapeworm *C. verticillatum* has been shown rapidly to incorporate labelled docosohexaenoic acid ($C_{22:6\omega3}$) into mono-, di- and triacylglycerols and diacylglyceryl ethers. Docosohexaenoic acid is the predominant fatty acid found in dogfish (Section 2.3.1).

Nematodes

Triacylglycerol synthesis in *A. lumbricoides* is primarily via the phosphatidic acid/diacylglycerol pathway and the enzymes have all been demonstrated (glycerol kinase, glycerol-phosphate acyltransferase, phosphatidate phosphatase, diacylglycerol acyltransferase)[75]. There is some evidence that triacylglycerols are also synthesised by the monoacylglycerol pathway.

In *A. lumbricoides*, and a number of related nematodes, there are some unusual triacylglycerols which have volatile fatty acids (2-methylvalerate, 2-methylbutyrate, *n*-valerate) esterified at one of the three positions (Section 2.3.2). The volatile acids are produced by the muscles in *A. lumbricoides* and then pass to the ovaries for incorporation into triacylglycerols.

Trematodes and Acanthocephalans

Nothing is known about mechanisms of triacylglycerol synthesis in these groups.

4.3.3. Steroid Synthesis

All parasitic helminths so far investigated appear unable to synthesise steroids *de novo*. However, many helminths do synthesise isoprenoids of one sort or another.

In vertebrates, all the carbon atoms of cholesterol are derived from acetate, and

Table 4.8 Steoid synthesis

(i) *Formation of mevalonic acid*

acetyl-CoA + acetoacyl-CoA $\rightarrow$ hydroxymethylglutaryl-CoA + CoA

hydroxymethylglutaryl-CoA + 2NADPH + 2H$^+$ $\rightarrow$ mevalonic acid + CoA + 2NADP$^+$

(ii) *Conversion of mevalonate to squalene*

mevalonic acid + ATP $\rightarrow$ 5-phosphomevalonic acid + ADP

5-phosphomevalonic acid + ATP $\rightarrow$ 5-pyrophosphomevalonic acid + ADP

5-pyrophosphomevalonic acid + ATP $\rightarrow$

3-isopentenylpyrophosphoric acid + ADP + P$_i$ + CO$_2$

3-isopentenylpyrophosphoric acid $\rightleftharpoons$ 3-dimethylallylpyrophosphoric acid

3-isopentenylpyrophosphoric acid + 3-dimethylallylpyrophosphoric acid $\rightarrow$

geranyl pyrophosphate + PP$_i$

geranyl pyrophosphate + 3-isopentenyl pyrophosphate $\rightarrow$

farnesyl pyrophosphate + PP$_1$

(farnesyl pyrophosphate + H$_2$O $\rightarrow$ farnesol + 2P$_i$)

2 farnesyl pyrophosphate $\rightarrow$ presqualene pyrophosphate + PP$_i$

presqualene pyrophosphate + NADPH + H$^+$ $\rightarrow$ squalene + NADP$^+$ + PP$_i$

(iii) *Cyclisation of squalene*

squalene + O$_2$ + AH$_2$ $\rightarrow$ squalene-2,3-epoxide + H$_2$O + A

squalene-2,3-epoxide $\xrightarrow{\text{cyclises}}$ lanosterol

---

steroid synthesis can be divided into three phases: (1) the synthesis of mevalonate, which is the basic building block for the synthesis of isoprenoids; (2) the conversion of mevalonate to the long chain hydrocarbon, squalene; and (3) the cyclisation of squalene to give lanosterol, which is a precursor of cholesterol. These steps are summarised in *Table 4.8*.

Cestodes

The rat tapeworm *H. diminuta* cannot synthesise sterols from acetate or mevalonate. It does, however, synthesise farnesol. Farnesol, which is an intermediate in steroid synthesis (*Table 4.8*), is a sesquiterpenoid (three isoprenoid units). Initially, it was thought that *H. diminuta* produced the 2-*cis*,6-*trans*-isomer of farnesol, but it has now been shown that it synthesises only 2-*trans*,6-*trans*-farnesol[76]. The absence of any other isomers of farnesol in *H. diminuta* suggests that there is no sesquiterpenoid isomerase in this helminth. The normal isomer of farnesol for steroid synthesis is 2-*trans*,6-*trans*-, so the failure of *H. diminuta* to synthesise squalene is not due to steric hindrance.

Steroid synthesis has also been shown to be absent in *E. granulosus* (protoscoleces), *E. multilocularis*, *T. hydatigena* (cysticerci) and *S. mansonoides* (adults and larvae). In *E. granulosus* and *T. hydatigena*, acetate is converted to hydroxymethylglutarate, mevalonate and a compound similar to 2-*cis*,6-*trans*-farnesol.

Trematodes

There is no *de novo* synthesis of steroids in *E. revolutum* or *S. mansoni*. Whether trematodes can synthesise farnesol or farnesol-like compounds is not known.

However, there has been an unconfirmed claim that the sporocysts of *M. similis* incorporate labelled acetate into cholesterol.

Homogenates of adult *S. mansoni* can convert a number of mammalian steroids (4-androstene-3,17-dione, cortisone, estrone, pregnenolone, testosterone, 17-α-hydroxypregnenolone, 17-α-hydroxyprogesterone, cholesterol) into a variety of related metabolites. There are no reports of steroid hormones in *S. mansoni*, but it is possible that they could metabolise host hormones in the same way[145].

Nematodes

There is no synthesis of cholesterol from acetate or mevalonate by *A. lumbricoides*. Nor can *A. lumbricoides* dealkylate plant steroids to give cholesterol, as happens in phytophagous insects. There is some circumstantial evidence that *A. lumbricoides* can reduce cholesterol to cholestanol. Farnesol has not been detected in *A. lumbricoides*, and instead mevalonate is incorporated into a polyprenol, similar to solanesol. Solanesol is an all *trans* nonaprenol (an alcohol composed of nine isoprenoid units). Isoprenol alcohols of this type function as cofactors in glycosyl transferase reactions (Section 4.2.3).

Steroid synthesis has not been investigated in any other species of parasitic nematode. However, sterols are required as a growth factor for *N. glaseri, Rhabditis maupasi*[148] and the free-living stages of *N. brasiliensis*. Squalene and lanosterol will support the minimal development of *N. brasiliensis* L$_3$ larvae, suggesting they may have a limited ability to carry out the last part of the cycle (*Table 4.8*). No steroid synthesis could be detected in the free-living nematodes *T. aceti, C. briggsae* or *P. redivivus*, although there are unconfirmed reports that *T. aceti* and *P. redivivus* might be able to dealkylate plant steroids[146]. Testosterone and oestradiol stimulate growth in the free-living nematode *Cephalobus*.

Acanthocephalans

Neither *M. dubius* nor *M. hirudinaceus* can synthesise cholesterol from mevalonate, nor can *M. hirudinaceus* dealkylate plant sterols to give cholesterol. There is no information on the possible synthesis of farnesol or other isoprenoids by acanthocephalans.

General

Parasitic helminths seem incapable of synthesising steroids *de novo*. The ability to synthesise steroids, however, shows no clear-cut phylogenetic pattern. Present evidence suggests that steroid synthesis is absent in coelenterates, arthropods, platyhelminths (free-living and parasitic), nematodes (free-living and parasitic), acanthocephalans, molluscs, echinoderms and terrestrial annelids. The lack of steroid synthesis in parasitic helminths may be a peculiarity of the phyla, rather than an adaptation to parasitism.

In steroid synthesis, the cyclisation of squalene, via squalene epoxide, to give lanosterol has an absolute requirement for molecular oxygen (bacteria have anaerobic methods of steroid synthesis). The conversion of squalene to squalene epoxide is catalysed by the microsomal enzyme squalene mono-oxygenase. Many parasites live in an oxygen-poor environment and microsomal enzyme systems are often deficient in parasitic helminths. However, the block to steroid synthesis in helminths seems to be in squalene formation, rather than its cyclisation. Squalene will support the minimal development of *N. brasiliensis* larvae, and the free-living nematode *P. redivivus* can convert squalene epoxide to lanosterol (but not cholesterol)[77], so the cyclase may be retained. In insects, the block in steroid synthesis also appears to be prior to squalene formation. There is some evidence in insects for multiple blocks in the steroid pathway, and the same may be true for helminths. In mammals, squalene formation is not a regulatory site and steroid synthesis is controlled at the level of hydroxymethylglutaryl-CoA dehydrogenase.

Several helminths produce farnesol or related isoprenoids. Farnesol or its derivatives could have a hormonal role in helminths, and it is also a precursor for other isoprenoids such as ubiquinone and polyprenols (isoprenoid alcohols such as solanesol and dolichols).

In vertebrates, steroids are degraded to bile acids, which are conjugated and excreted. Bile acids also play a role in digestion. Nothing is known of steroid breakdown in helminths, and bile acids have not been reported from invertebrates.

Sterol Esters

Helminths readily incorporate exogenous fatty acids into sterol esters. Two pathways of sterol ester synthesis are known from animals, direct acylation of cholesterol:

$$\text{cholesterol} + \text{fatty acyl-CoA} \rightarrow \text{cholesterol ester} + \text{CoA}$$

or a transferase reaction:

$$\text{phosphatidylcholine} + \text{cholesterol} \rightarrow \text{cholesterol ester} + \text{lysophosphatidylcholine}$$

The mechanism of sterol ester formation in helminths has, however, not been investigated, although esterases capable of hydrolysing sterol esters have been found in parasites (Section 4.1.1).

Physiological Role of Prenoids and Steroids

The discovery of farnesol and farnesol-like compounds in helminths has aroused a great deal of interest[78]. Farnesol and its analogues show juvenile hormone activity in insects, and it was thought that there might be a parallel between the hormonal systems of insects and those of parasitic helminths. This has stimulated research along two lines. First, to look for compounds with juvenile hormone or ecdysone-like properties in helminths and, secondly, to see if compounds such as farnesol, juvenile hormone or ecdysone had any physiological effect on helminths.

Substances with juvenile hormone and ecdysone activity have been isolated from *H. contortus* larvae and ecdysone-like compounds have been isolated from larval *T. spiralis* and from *A. avenae* and *P. redivivus*. However, no ecdysone binding protein could be detected in the free-living *P. redivivus*[79]. β-Ecdysone itself has been purified from *A. lumbricoides* extracts, but the levels are vanishingly small (less than one-tenth that in intermoult crayfish). Such low levels of β-ecdysone could very easily have been derived from plant material in the hosts' diet (Section 2.3.7).

Juvenile hormone and juvenile hormone mimics affect the *in vitro* development of larval *T. spiralis* and *P. decipiens* and inhibit the growth of the free-living nematodes *P. redivivus* and *C. briggsae*; although the polyribosome profile of *P. redivivus* was not altered by juvenile hormone[79]. Juvenile hormone and juvenile hormone analogues also inhibit the hatching of a number of nematode eggs[80] and induce moulting in larval *Phocanema decipiens*[150]. Moulting in *N. dubius* is stimulated by α-ecdysone and inhibited by juvenile hormone. Farnesol and its derivatives induce abnormal gonad development in the plant parasitic nematode *Heterodera schachtii*. The *in vitro* growth of *T. spiralis* larvae is similarly affected by ecdysone and by steroid- and farnesol-like extracts prepared from larval *T. spiralis*. A farnesol-like compound, isolated from *E. granulosus*, is said to stimulate the *in vitro* development of *H. diminuta*, whilst a steroid-like extract was inhibitory. Recent workers have, however, found that low levels of farnesol or farnesol derivatives (equivalent to the levels in helminth tissues), did not affect the *in vitro* development of *H. diminuta*, but higher levels were toxic[81]. High levels of farnesol were also toxic to the insect parasitic nematode *N. glaseri*.

Farnesol, farnesol derivatives and ecdysone have a variety of effects on parasitic and free-living helminths. However, these effects appear to be relatively non-specific and may be the result of toxicity. No steroid or other prenoid hormones have been unambiguously identified in helminths and there is no good evidence to suggest that farnesol, or its derivatives, have any regulatory role in metabolism or development.

4.3.4. Ascaroside Synthesis

Ascarosides are a unique class of unsaponifiable lipids found in the female reproductive system and egg shells of ascarid and oxyurid nematodes (Section 2.3.5). In the egg, free ascarosides form the ascaroside membrane which is responsible for the extreme impermeability of the eggs. Prior to egg shell formation, the ascarosides occur in the developing oocyte as esters (mostly with acetate).

The ascarosides are a series of related α-glycosides, formed from ascarylose (3,6-dideoxy-L-arabinohexose) and a variety of long chain secondary monols or diols. Their synthesis probably involves a reaction between the aglycone and 3,6-dideoxyhexose nucleoside phosphate (Section 4.2.2). The aglycones are synthesised by a condensation reaction between the carbonyl carbon of one long chain fatty acid with the 2-methylene carbon of a second long chain fatty acid, followed by the elimination of carbon dioxide. The reaction requires CoA, ATP and NADH or NADPH. This condensation–decarboxylation sequence resembles the malonyl-CoA pathway for fatty acid synthesis (*Table 4.7*). The mechanism for introducing the hydroxyl groups and the methyl side chains into the aglycones is not known.

When the ascaroside membrane is formed, there is a virtually complete conversion of the ascaroside esters to free ascarosides. The esterases responsible for this have not been identified[82]. It has been suggested that the acetate released by de-esterification may be utilised in the synthesis of the chitin layer of the egg shell.

The melting point of ascaroside esters is about 40 °C and they are fluid at the body temperature of the host. Free ascarosides have melting points in the range 70–80 °C and so produce a solid membrane.

The ascaroside membrane of *A. lumbricoides* eggs is extremely impermeable. However, the initial process in the hatching of *A. lumbricoides* eggs is the sudden onset of permeability in the hitherto impermeable membrane. During this permeability change, no chemical or conformational alterations can be detected in the ascaroside membrane[83]. The induction of permeability in the ascaroside layer may, therefore, involve either a very localised chemical or conformational change, not detected by gross analytical methods, or it may be the result of mechanical damage to the membrane by the activated larva.

4.3.5. Phospholipid and Sphingolipid Synthesis

Parasitic helminths all seem able to incorporate the label from $^{32}P_i$- or ^{14}C-labelled fatty acids and glucose into the main phospholipid fractions. The tapeworm *H. diminuta*, for example, incorporates the label into phosphatidylcholine, lysolecithin, phosphatidylethanolamine, phosphatidylinositol, phosphatidylserine, diphosphatidyl-glycerol (cardiolipin) and cerebrosides. Different phospholipid classes become labelled at different rates, presumably reflecting varying rates of phospholipid turnover.

Phosphatidic acid is the usual starting point for phospholipid synthesis, and cytidine nucleotides serve as carriers for either the 'head' of the alcohol moiety or for the phosphatidic acid. The pathways of phospholipid synthesis in parasitic helminths have been little studied.

Phosphatidylcholine

Phosphatidylcholine synthesis has been demonstrated in *H. diminuta, S. mansonoides, C. verticillatum, F. hepatica,* the sporocysts of *M. similis* and *A. lumbricoides.*

In *F. hepatica*, phosphatidylcholine is synthesised from CDP-choline and 1,2-diacylglycerol[84]. The probable pathway is the same as in vertebrates:

$$\text{choline} + \text{ATP} \rightarrow \text{phosphocholine} + \text{ADP} \quad (\textit{choline kinase})$$

$$\text{phosphocholine} + \text{CTP} \rightarrow \text{CDP-choline} + \text{PP}_i \quad (\textit{choline-phosphate cytidyl transferase})$$

$$\text{CDP-choline} + \text{diacylglycerol} \rightarrow \text{phosphatidylcholine} + \text{CMP} \ (\textit{choline transferase})$$

Choline kinase, choline-phosphate cytidyl transferase and choline phosphotransferase have also all been demonstrated in *A. lumbricoides*[75].

An alternative pathway for phosphatidylcholine synthesis in the mammalian liver is the *N*-methylation of phosphatidylethanolamine (salvage pathway). There is, however, so far no evidence for this system in helminths.

Phosphatidylserine

The biosynthesis of phosphatidylserine has again been demonstrated in a variety of parasites (*H. diminuta, S. mansonoides, C. verticillatum, F. hepatica,* sporocysts of

M. similis, A. lumbricoides). In mammals, phosphatidylserine is synthesised by base exchange:

phosphatidylethanolamine + serine $\rightleftharpoons$ phosphatidylserine + ethanolamine

However, in *H. diminuta*, phosphatidylserine synthesis appears to be via phosphatidic acid[85], a pathway more characteristic of bacteria:

$$\text{phosphatidic acid} + \text{CTP} \rightarrow \text{CDP-diacylglycerol} + \text{PP}_i$$

$$\text{CDP-diacylglycerol} + \text{serine} \rightarrow \text{phosphatidylserine} + \text{CMP}$$

Phosphatidylethanolamine

H. diminuta, S. mansonoides, C. verticillatum, F. hepatica, the sporocysts of *M. similis* and *A. lumbricoides* have all been shown to synthesise phosphatidylethanolamine. In mammals, there are two pathways for phosphatidylethanolamine synthesis, the decarboxylation of phosphatidylserine:

$$\text{phosphatidylserine} \rightarrow \text{phosphatidylethanolamine} + \text{CO}_2$$

and synthesis from ethanolamine via a pathway identical to phosphatidylcholine formation:

$$\text{ethanolamine} + \text{ATP} \rightarrow \text{phosphoethanolamine} + \text{ADP}$$

$$\text{phosphoethanolamine} + \text{CTP} \rightarrow \text{CDP-ethanolamine} + \text{PP}_i$$

$$\text{CDP-ethanolamine} + \text{diacylglycerol} \rightarrow \text{phosphatidylethanolamine} + \text{CMP}$$

In *H. diminuta,* ^{14}C-serine is readily incorporated into ethanolamine. The direct decarboxylation of serine to ethanolamine does not occur in eukaryotes, and synthesis is probably via phosphatidylserine. CDP-ethanolamine has been identified in extracts of *T. saginata*. So there is some evidence for both routes of phosphatidylethanolamine synthesis in helminths.

Phosphatidylinositol

Phosphatidylinositol synthesis has been shown in *H. diminuta, S. mansonoides, F. hepatica* and the sporocysts of *M. similis*. In *H. diminuta*, inositol is synthesised from glucose (Section 4.2.2) and phosphatidic acid appears to be the other precursor. This suggests that the pathway of phosphatidylinositol synthesis in *H. diminuta* is the same as in mammals:

$$\text{phosphatidic acid} + \text{CTP} \rightarrow \text{CDP-diacylglycerol} + \text{PP}_i$$

$$\text{CDP-diacylglycerol} + \text{inositol} \rightarrow \text{phosphatidylinositol} + \text{CMP}$$

Cardiolipin (Diphosphatidylglycerol)

Cardiolipin is the predominant phospholipid of the inner mitochondrial membrane, but for some obscure reason it appears to be absent from the eggs of *F. hepatica*

(Section 2.3.3). Cardiolipin synthesis has been demonstrated in *H. diminuta, S. mansonoides* and the sporocysts of *M. similis*. In vertebrates, cardiolipin is synthesised from CDP-diacylglycerol and glycerol-3-phosphate, but the pathway in helminths has not been studied.

Plasmalogens

Plasmalogens are often found in quite large amounts in helminths and are phospholipids with an α-β unsaturated ether link (Section 2.3.3).

The liver fluke, *F. hepatica*, readily incorporates $^{32}P_i$ into ethanolamine plasmalogen, but labelled glycerol is not incorporated[84]. This is in agreement with the proposed pathway of plasmalogen synthesis in animals, where glycerol is introduced into plasmalogens via dihydroxyacetone phosphate. The dihydroxyacetone phosphate is acetylated, and there is then an exchange reaction with a fatty alcohol to form the ether link, followed by reduction of the ketone group. In mammals, the α-β unsaturated bond is inserted by a microsomal mixed-function oxidase, similar to the microsomal fatty acid desaturases. Helminths, however, are unable to desaturate fatty acids (Section 4.3.1), so how the double bonds are introduced into plasmalogens (and diglyceryl ethers) in helminths is not known. Bacteria have anaerobic pathways for plasmalogen synthesis as they do for fatty acid desaturation (Section 4.3.1).

Sphingolipids

These are lipids containing the complex amino alcohol sphingosine (Section 2.3.4). Serine is readily incorporated into sphingosine by *H. diminuta*. The pathway has not been investigated, but is probably the same as in vertebrates:

$$\text{palmitoyl-CoA} + \text{serine} \rightarrow \text{3-dehydrosphinganine} + \text{CoA} + CO_2$$

$$\text{3-dehydrosphinganine} + \text{NADPH} + H^+ \rightleftharpoons \text{sphinganine} + \text{NADP}^+$$

$$\text{sphinganine} + \text{FAD} \rightleftharpoons \text{FADH} + \text{sphingosine}$$

The intermediate sphinganine has been isolated from larval *T. taeniaeformis*. Sphingosine is the starting point for sphingolipid synthesis (sphingomyelin, cerebrosides, gangliosides). Sphingomyelin synthesis has been demonstrated in the sporocysts of *M. similis* and in *A. lumbricoides*. Sphingomyelin seems to be absent from *F. hepatica* (Section 2.3.4).

Cerebrosides are composed of sphingosine, a fatty acid and a hexose (Section 2.3.4). Cerebroside synthesis has been shown in the sporocysts of *M. similis* and in *H. diminuta*, and, in the latter, the hexose appears to be glucose. There are two alternative pathways for cerebroside synthesis in animals; the pathway in helminths has not been studied.

General

Parasitic nematodes, trematodes and cestodes can synthesise their own complex phospholipids, and the pathways involved are similar to those found in mammals.

Nothing, however, is known about phospholipid synthesis in acanthocephalans.

The phospholipids of *A. lumbricoides* differ from the neutral lipids in that they contain no volatile fatty acid residues. This suggests that there is a high degree of specificity in the incorporation of fatty acids into lipids.

Helminths often contain quite large amounts of lysolecithin (monoacylglycerol-3-phosphorylcholine). Lysolecithin is present in large amounts in intestinal contents (Section 4.1.9), but is also rapidly synthesised *de novo* by helminths (*H. diminuta, F. hepatica, M. similis* sporocysts, *A. lumbricoides*). Lysolecithin acyltransferase and lysophospholipase have been detected in *A. lumbricoides*[75].

Lysolecithin is usually formed by the hydrolysis of phosphatidylcholine (by phospholipase A) and is not a precursor of phosphatidylcholine synthesis. It has been suggested in mammals that there is a microsomal lysolecithin acylation/de-acylation system. This would catalyse the independent metabolic turnover of the two fatty acid residues of phosphatidylcholine and could be related to the control of the stereospecificity of fatty acids in glycerolipids. The high levels of lysolecithin in helminths suggest that a similar cycle may be present.

4.4. BIOSYNTHESIS OF AMINO ACIDS AND THEIR DERIVATIVES

Animals differ greatly in their ability to synthesise amino acids. Man and the albino rat can synthesise ten out of the twenty common amino acids, the remaining ten (arginine, histidine, isoleucine, leucine, lysine, methionine, phenylalanine, threonine, tryptophan, valine) being essential amino acids for these species. If an amino acid is essential, it does not necessarily mean the animal cannot synthesise it, the animal may simply not be able to synthesise enough of the amino acid, particularly during periods of growth. This is thought to be the case with arginine and histidine in man.

In general, the non-essential amino acids have relatively short synthetic pathways (less than 5 steps), whilst the essential amino acids have long synthetic pathways (5–10 steps). A survey of the amino acid requirements of animals (birds, insects and protozoa) indicates that all of them require the ten essential amino acids and many need additional amino acids as well. The chick, for example, requires glycine and glutamate in addition to the ten essential amino acids and, in insects, alanine, serine, aspartate, glutamate, proline, tyrosine and glycine have all been shown to be essential in various species. The essential amino acids for parasitic helminths are not known, nor, in fact, is it known which are the essential amino acids in free-living platyhelminths. However, there have been a few studies on nematodes and *C. briggsae* (free-living), *N. glaseri* (insect parasitic), *R. maupasi* (parasitic)[148] and *Aphelenchoides rutgersi* (plant parasitic) have all been found to require tyrosine, in addition to the ten essential amino acids. It is probably safe to assume that parasitic helminths will require the ten essential amino acids for normal growth and possibly others as well.

4.4.1. Synthesis of Amino Acids

The different amino acids are synthesised by different multienzyme sequences and, as is usual in metabolism, the synthetic pathways are different from the degradative pathways. Some of the intermediates from amino acid synthesis, like the intermediates of amino acid breakdown, are important precursors for other reactions. Amino acid synthesis is usually under tight metabolic control. First, from feedback inhibition, usually by the last metabolite in the pathway and, secondly, through repression of the pathway by exogenous amino acids.

The major precursors for amino acid synthesis are summarised in *Table 4.9*. There is, however, very little information on the ability of parasitic helminths to synthesise and interconvert amino acids.

Table 4.9   Biosynthesis of amino acids

Amino acid	Main precursors
Alanine	Pyruvate
Arginine	Glutamate → ornithine + carbamoyl-P
Aspartate	Oxaloacetate
Asparagine	Aspartate + NII_3
Cysteine	Serine + methionine
Glutamate	2-Oxoglutarate
Glutamine	Glutamate + NH_3
Glycine	Serine
Histidine	ATP + NH_3 → imidazoleglycerol-P
Isoleucine	Threonine → 2-ketobutyrate
Leucine	Pyruvate → 2-ketoisovalerate + acetyl-CoA
Lysine	(i) 2-Aminoadipic acid
	(ii) Diaminopimelic acid
Methionine	Aspartate → homoserine → cystathionine
Phenylalanine	Glucose → shikimic acid → prephenic acid
Proline	(i) Glutamate
	(ii) Ornithine
Hydroxyproline	Proline
Serine	(i) 3-P-glycerate → 3-phosphohydroxypyruvate
	(ii) Glycine
Threonine	(i) Aspartate → homoserine
	(ii) Glycine + acetaldehyde
Tryptophan	Glucose → shikimic acid → anthranilic acid → indole-3-glycerol-P
Tyrosine	Phenylalanine
Valine	Pyruvate → ketoisovalerate

The essential amino acids (man) are in italics.

Glycine

Low rates of conversion of serine to glycine have been reported in *H. diminuta*:

serine + tetrahydrofolate $\rightleftharpoons$ glycine + N^5, N^{10}-methylenetetrahydrofolate

This reaction is reversible and so also provides a pathway for serine synthesis.

Alanine

Alanine can be formed from pyruvate by reductive amination or by transamination.

The reductive amination of pyruvate has been demonstrated in *H. diminuta* and *A. lumbricoides*:

$$\text{pyruvate} + \text{NH}_4^+ + \text{NADH} \rightleftharpoons \text{alanine} + \text{NAD}^+ + \text{H}_2\text{O}$$

Pyruvate linked transaminases are widely distributed in parasitic helminths (Section 3.4.1), so it seems fairly certain that helminths can synthesise alanine from pyruvate. However, transaminases are probably more important in amino acid catabolism than in amino acid synthesis.

Arginine

The synthesis of arginine starts with ornithine and carbamoyl phosphate and involves the enzymes of the urea cycle (Section 3.6.2). The apparent absence or very low activity of carbamoyl-phosphate synthetase and ornithine transcarbamoylase in helminths[86,87] makes it unlikely that parasitic helminths are able to synthesise arginine *de novo*. Creatine, a derivative of arginine, has been identified in *A. lumbricoides*.

Aspartate

The transamination of oxaloacetate yields aspartate. 2-Oxoglutarate : aspartate and pyruvate : aspartate transaminases have a ubiquitous distribution in helminths (Section 3.4.1), and helminths are probably all able to synthesise aspartate from oxaloacetate.

Glutamate

This is formed by the transamination of 2-oxoglutarate and, as discussed above, 2-oxoglutarate linked transaminases have been found in all helminths investigated.

Methionine

This essential amino acid is synthesised by a complex series of reactions, starting with aspartate and proceeding via homoserine and cystathionine. There is no evidence that any helminth can synthesise methionine, but cell-free extracts of *A. lumbricoides* can convert 2-hydroxy-4-methylthiobutyrate and 2-keto-4-methyl-thiobutyrate to methionine[88]. The probable pathway is:

2-hydroxy-4-methylthiobutyrate + NAD$^+$ $\rightleftharpoons$

　　　2-keto-4-methylthiobutyrate + NADH + H$^+$ (*2-hydroxy acid dehydrogenase*)

2-keto-4-methylthiobutyrate + glutamate $\rightleftharpoons$

　　　　　　　　　　　　methionine + 2-oxoglutarate (*transaminase*)

These two steps do not, however, form part of the normal pathway either for methionine synthesis or for methionine breakdown.

Proline

Proline can be formed from glutamate or ornithine via Δ^1-pyrroline-5'-carboxylic acid. The pathway from ornithine to proline is particularly active in *F. hepatica* (Section 3.4.2). In *F. hepatica*, glutamate does not appear to contribute to proline formation and ornithine comes from the cleavage of dietary arginine. The situation in other helminths has not been studied.

Hydroxyproline

Proline must first be incorporated into protocollagen before it can be converted into hydroxyproline. The proline residue is hydroxylated by proline-4-mono-oxygenase, an enzyme which requires as cofactor or cosubstrate ascorbate, 2-oxoglutarate, CoA, Fe^{2+} and oxygen:

proline residue + O_2 + 2-oxoglutarate + CoA →
$$4\text{-hydroxyproline residue} + \text{succinyl-CoA} + CO_2 + H_2O$$

Proline-4-mono-oxygenase has been found in the cuticle, muscles and developing eggs of *A. lumbricoides*[89]. The enzyme from the muscles is inhibited by oxygen above 5 vol. per cent, whereas the cuticle and egg enzymes, on the other hand, are stimulated by oxygen.

4.4.2. Amino Acid Derivatives

In addition to being the building blocks of proteins, amino acids, and in particular the aromatic ones, are important precursors for the synthesis of other amino acids and of several biologically important compounds. Chief among the amino acid derivatives are amines, peptides and porphyrins (*Table 4.10*).

Amines

Some nematode and cestode larvae excrete significant quantities of amines, many of which are probably formed by the decarboxylation of amino acids (Section 3.4.3). Several physiologically active amines such as dopamine, adrenalin, noradrenalin, histamine and serotonin have been found in helminths (*Table 4.11*). These amines may function as neurotransmitters or they may have a hormonal role in metabolic regulation (Section 5.1.7). In nematodes, the mid- and hind-guts receive no nervous innervation, and amines may serve to coordinate activity.

Histamine

Histidine is decarboxylated to histamine via histidine decarboxylase:

$$\text{histidine} \rightarrow \text{histamine} + CO_2$$

This enzyme has been demonstrated in *A. lumbricoides* and in the trematodes *F. hepatica* and *M. monodi*.

Table 4.10   Role of amino acids in biosynthesis

Amino acid	Other amino acids synthesised from it	Other metabolites, synthesised in whole or in part from it
Alanine	Valine, leucine	
Arginine	Glutamate, creatine	Urea, octopine, agmatine, spermine, spermidine
Aspartate	Isoleucine, threonine, methionine, β-alanine	Pyrimidines, purines
Cysteine	Cystine	Taurine, thioethanolamine, mercapturic acid
Glutamate	Proline, ornithine, arginine, 4-aminobutyrate	Glutathione
Glycine	Creatine	Porphyrins, purines, riboflavin, glycocholic acid, hippuric acid, glutathione
Histidine	Serine, glutamate	Histamine, purines, ergothionine, carnosine, anserine
Lysine	Glutamate	Cadaverine, anabasine, coniine
Methionine	Cysteine, isoleucine, creatine	Choline
Ornithine	Arginine	Ornithuric acid, putrescene, hyoscyamine
Proline	Hydroxyproline, glutamate	
Phenylalanine	Tyrosine	
Serine	Glycine, cysteine	Purines, ethanolamine, choline, sphingosine
Threonine	Serine, isoleucine, glycine	
Tyrosine		Adrenalin, noradrenalin, thyroxin, thyronine, tyramine, melanin
Tryptophan		Serotonin, tryptamine, nicotinic acid, quinolinic acid, kynurenic acid, indole, skatole, indoleacetic acid, ommochromes
Valine		Pantothenic acid

Serotonin

Serotonin (5-hydroxytryptamine) is synthesised from tryptophan in two steps. Tryptophan is first hydroxylated to 5-hydroxytryptophan which is then decarboxylated:

$$\text{tryptophan} \rightarrow \text{5-hydroxytryptophan} \rightarrow \text{5-hydroxytryptamine} + CO_2$$

Serotonin synthesis has been studied in *M. corti* and *S. mansoni*, both of which appear to lack the initial hydroxylating enzyme. These helminths are, therefore, unable to synthesise serotonin and have specialised transport mechanisms to enable them to take up serotonin from the host[57,58]. The liver fluke *F. hepatica* can synthesise serotonin from 5-hydroxytryptophan, but not from tryptophan itself, and so also probably lacks the hydroxylating enzyme[151].

Tryptamine, an amine which has been found in larval *P. decipiens*, is formed by the direct decarboxylation of tryptophan, but the pathway has not been studied.

Table 4.11 Physiologically active amines found in parasitic helminths

	Adren-alin	Norad-renalin	Dop-amine	Trypt-amine	Sero-tonin	Hist-amine
Nematodes						
Ascaris lumbricoides	+	+				+
Ascaridia galli					+	
Aspiculuris tetraptera					+	
Haemonchus contortus	+	+				
Litomosoides carinii						
(adults)		+			+	+
(filariae)		+	+		+	+
Porrocaecum decipiens		+	+	+		
Trematodes						
Dicrocoelium dendriticum					+	
Fasciola hepatica		+	+			
Paragonimus ohirai			+			
P. westermani			+			
Schistosoma haematobium					+	
S. japonicum		+	+		+	
S. mansoni		+	+		+	
Cestodes						
Dipylidium caninum					+	
Hymenolepis diminuta					+	
H. nana					+	
Mesocestoides corti					+	
Spirometra mansonoides					+	

Dopamine, Adrenalin, Noradrenalin

These three amines are all formed in a series of reactions starting from tyrosine (*Figure 4.11*). The enzymes involved have, however, not been investigated in helminths.

Choline

Choline is synthesised from serine and the methyl group of methionine. Although this synthesis occurs in animals, choline is none the less a growth factor for mammals, birds and insects. The major role of choline is as a constituent of phospholipids (Section 4.3.5) and in the neurotransmitter, acetylcholine. Acetylcholine appears to be one of the neurotransmitters in trematodes, cestodes and nematodes but it is not known if helminths can synthesise choline. Acetylcholine is synthesised by choline acetylase:

$$\text{choline} + \text{acetyl-CoA} \rightarrow \text{acetylcholine} + \text{CoA}$$

Choline acetylase has been found in *F. hepatica* and *S. mansoni*, and both acetylcholine and propionylcholine have been isolated from *A. lumbricoides*[152].

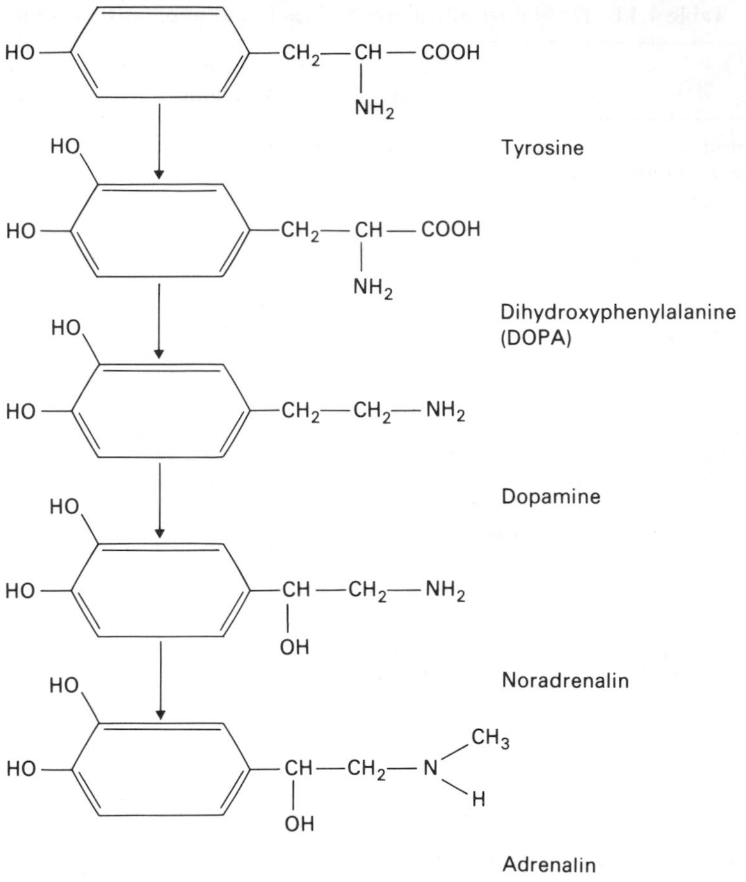

Figure 4.11 The formation of dopamine, adrenalin and noradrenalin.

Peptides

The most common of the physiological peptides is the tripeptide, glutathione (GSH). The occurrence and synthesis of glutathione in helminths has not been studied in detail. Glutathione has been detected in *M. benedeni, F. hepatica* and *A. lumbricoides*[90], and the demonstration of the glyoxalase reaction in *A. lumbricoides* muscle again indicates the presence of glutathione[91]. Glyoxalase catalyses the conversion of methylglyoxal to lactate and has an absolute requirement for glutathione:

methylglyoxal + GSH → S-lactoylglutathione → lactate + GSH

Glutathione is also a key intermediate in the γ-glutamyl cycle (*Figure 4.12*). It has been suggested that this cycle may be involved in the transport of amino acids across membranes, γ-glutamyl transpeptidase being a membrane-bound enzyme. Of the enzymes involved, three, γ-glutamyl transpeptidase, γ-glutamyl cyclotransferase and 5-oxoprolinase, have been demonstrated in *M. benedeni*, but these enzymes were not, however, present in *A. lumbricoides* or *F. hepatica*.

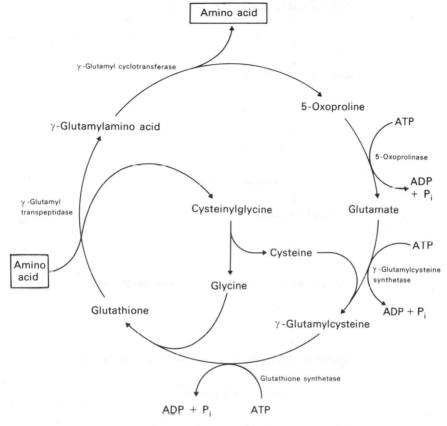

Figure 4.12 The γ-glutamyl cycle.

Porphyrins

The major precursor of porphyrins is glycine and the pathway is outlined in *Figure 4.13*. Porphyrinogens readily auto-oxidise to the corresponding porphyrins, a reaction catalysed by light. These oxidised porphyrins are not intermediates in the synthesis of protoporphyrin IX.

It seems doubtful if parasitic helminths can synthesise porphyrins from simple precursors. The trematodes *Fasciolopsis buski* and *Philophthalmus megalurus* incorporate neither δ-aminolevulinic acid nor ^{59}Fe into their haemoglobins. Haem has a growth stimulating effect on *H. microstoma* in culture. Haem porphyrins are also required for larval growth in *N. brasiliensis*[92], in *R. maupasi*[148] and in the free-living nematode *C. briggsae*. The sporocysts of *S. mansoni* may also take up haem.

Low levels of coproporphyrinogen oxidase, the enzyme that converts coproporphyrinogen III to protoporphyrinogen IX, have, however, been found in the tissues and eggs of *A. lumbricoides*[93]. Analysis of the perienteric fluid of *A. lumbricoides* has also shown the presence of protoporphyrin IX and small amounts of coproporphyrin III (presumably derived from coproporphyrinogen III). Uroporphyrin was not detected[94].

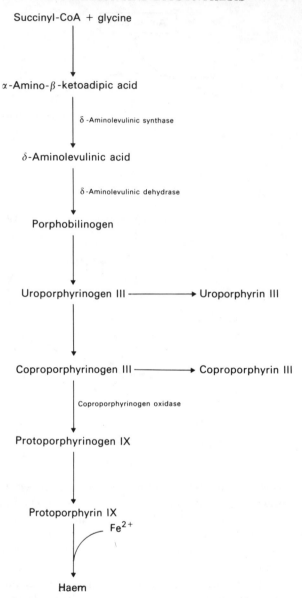

Figure 4.13 Porphyrin synthesis.

Nutritional experiments with *A. lumbricoides* have shown that this parasite rapidly synthesises haemoglobin, only if provided with a source of protoporphyrin IX. Earlier reports that *A. lumbricoides* might be able to synthesise haem from chlorophyll are probably not correct[95].

Adult *A. lumbricoides* use exogenous porphyrins for haem synthesis. So, although one of the enzymes and two of the intermediates of the porphyrin pathway have been found in *A. lumbricoides*, there is no evidence that this parasite synthesises porphyrins from simple precursors. A possible reason is that both δ-aminolevulinate synthetase (the rate-limiting enzyme in porphyrin synthesis) and δ-aminolevulinate dehydratase are strongly inhibited by haem. The synthetic pathway in *A. lumbricoides* could, therefore, be being repressed by exogenous haem.

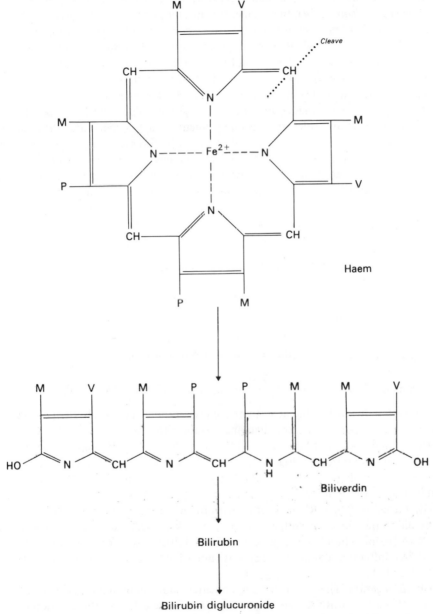

Figure 4.14 Formation of bile pigments. Side chains: M, methyl; V, vinyl; P, propionate.

Even though *A. lumbricoides* may not synthesise its own porphyrins, it can still carry out some porphyrin metabolism. Adult *A. lumbricoides* can incorporate iron into the porphyrin ring to synthesise haem, it can reduce ferrihaem to ferrohaem and can incorporate the haem nucleus into globin to give haemoglobin.

Nothing is known about the breakdown of haem in parasitic helminths. In mammals, the initial step in haem degradation involves opening of the porphyrin ring to give biliverdin (*Figure 4.14*). Bile pigments (bilirubin) have been identified in the intestine of *A. lumbricoides*, but whether these come from the degradation of parasite haemoglobin or whether they are derived from the host gut contents is not certain (see also Section 4.8). In addition to bilirubin, *A. lumbricoides* intestines also contain protoporphyrin IX and an unidentified metalloporphyrin[95]. The gut appears to be the site of haemoglobin production in this parasite.

It has been suggested that *A. lumbricoides* might be able to synthesise porphyrins from linear tetrapyrroles, such as bile pigments. The bile pigments in the gut of *A. lumbricoides* could then be intermediates in porphyrin synthesis. Exogenous haem would be broken down to a linear tetrapyrrole and new porphyrins synthesised by ring closure. However, there is no real evidence that this can occur in *A. lumbricoides* and such a pathway has never been described in any other organism.

4.5. BIOSYNTHESIS OF PROTEINS

Parasitic helminths are capable of rapid protein synthesis, and the incorporation of labelled amino acids into proteins has been demonstrated in a wide variety of nematodes, trematodes and cestodes.

The pathway of protein synthesis seems similar in all living systems and can be divided into four stages.

(i) *Activation* of amino acids by attachment to their corresponding *t*RNAs, a reaction catalysed by specific aminoacyl *t*RNA synthetases:

$$\text{amino acid} + t\text{RNA} + \text{ATP} \xrightarrow{\text{Mg}^{2+}} \text{aminoacyl } t\text{RNA} + \text{AMP} + \text{PP}_i$$

For each individual amino acid, there are one or more specific *t*RNA species (iso-accepting *t*RNAs). Why more than one specific *t*RNA should be necessary for each amino acid is not known, but different iso-accepting *t*RNAs occur in the cytoplasm and mitochondria. Aminoacyl *t*RNA synthetases are also present in multiple homologous forms (isoenzymes) and a given aminoacyl *t*RNA synthetase may not be equally active with all iso-accepting *t*RNAs.

(ii) *Initiation*. The *m*RNA, together with the initiating aminoacyl *t*RNA, becomes bound to the ribosome. In the cytoplasm of eukaryotes, the initiator is methionyl *t*RNA (in mitochondria and prokaryotes, the initiator is *N*-formylmethionyl *t*RNA). Initiation requires three specific initiating factors (proteins) as well as GTP and Mg^{2+}.

(iii) *Elongation*. This occurs by the sequential addition of aminoacyl *t*RNAs, as specified by the *m*RNA code. A peptidyl transferase catalyses the addition of each amino acid to the growing peptide chain. The process requires two specific elongation factors (proteins) as well as GTP. After each peptide bond is formed, the ribosome moves to the next position and this again requires GTP. Proteins are synthesised from the N (amino) terminal end.

(iv) *Termination*. Protein synthesis ends when the appropriate code is reached on the *m*RNA. The steps involved in the completion and detachment of the newly synthesised polypeptide chain are not fully understood and require at least three releasing factors (specific proteins).

Newly synthesised protein may require post-translational modification, such as the formation of sulphydryl cross-links and the removal of the initiator methionine residue. *In vivo* several ribosomes are often attached to each *m*RNA molecule, forming polyribosomes or polysomes.

4.5.1. General Protein Synthesis

In parasitic helminths, protein synthesis has only been investigated in any detail in cestodes. Cell-free systems capable of synthesising protein have been prepared from *E. granulosus* scoleces, larval *T. crassiceps* and adult *H. diminuta*[96,97]. These cestode systems seem basically similar to the scheme outlined above. Cestode protein syn-thesising systems involve polyribosomes, and stable polyribosomes have also been isolated from developing *A. lumbricoides* eggs. The cestode cell-free preparations often show a high degree of specificity for homologous *t*RNA. The actual rates of protein synthesis reported using helminth cell-free systems are comparable with other eukaryotic systems. Mitochondrial protein synthesis has not been studied in helminths.

Helminth *m*RNA has also been successfully translated in heterologous systems. The *m*RNA from larval *T. crassiceps* has been translated in a cell-free system derived from rabbit reticulocytes[98] whilst *A. lumbricoides* egg shell protein *m*RNA and specific collagen *m*RNA from the free-living nematode *Panagrellus silusiae* have been translated in cell-free wheatgerm systems[99]. Translation of purified hel-minth *m*RNA in heterologous systems may offer a method of preparing pure antigenic polypeptides for immunological studies.

Protein synthesis in gut ribbons of *A. lumbricoides* can, apparently, take place anaerobically[100].

Protein synthesis in cestodes is very similar to the scheme described for mammals and micro-organisms, and the same will almost certainly be true of other helminths. Although there is much to be learnt about the details of protein synthesis in para-sitic helminths, the similarity between parasitic helminths and their hosts makes it unlikely that protein synthesis will be a suitable target for chemotherapy. This may be one reason for the relative lack of interest in protein synthesis in helminths.

4.6. BIOSYNTHESIS OF NUCLEOTIDES AND NUCLEIC ACIDS

Nucleic acid synthesis, like protein synthesis, is a feature of all living organisms. Compared with the parasitic protozoa, there has been relatively little work on nucleotide synthesis in parasitic helminths. Helminths certainly have the ability to synthesise nucleic acids, but there is, as yet, little evidence that they synthesise purine bases *de novo* from simple precursors, and some species may be unable to synthesise pyrimidines as well. An exception is the insect parasitic nematode *N. glaseri* which, like the free-living nematode *C. briggsae*, does not seem to require an exogenous source of purines or pyrimidines[101]. The plant parasitic nematode *Aphelenchoides rutgersi* also seems to be able to synthesise both pyrimidines and purines *de novo*. If helminths do not synthesise purines, and in some cases pyrimidines, they must take up free bases or nucleosides (Section 4.1.10), and this would seem to be a potential site for chemotherapy.

Pyrimidine and purine synthesis is normally under strict metabolic control, and most animals show a considerable economy in the use of these bases. Purines and pyrimidines are not used as an energy source in organisms, and many tissues have 'salvage pathways' for the recovery of free bases resulting from the hydrolysis of nucleotides. These salvage pathways are particularly prominent in parasitic helminths. Virtually all the studies on purine and pyrimidine metabolism in helminths have been done on adults and there is very little information from larval and free-living stages.

4.6.1. Purine Nucleotide Synthesis

The biosynthesis of purine nucleotides starts with ribose-5-phosphate and involves a complex sequence of reactions, during which the purine ring is gradually built up (*Figure 4.15*). The initial product of purine nucleotide synthesis is inosinic acid (IMP). There is then another short series of reactions which can convert IMP to either AMP or GMP. The nucleoside monophosphates are phosphorylated to give the di- and triphosphates (ADP, GDP, ATP, GTP) by the action of nucleoside-

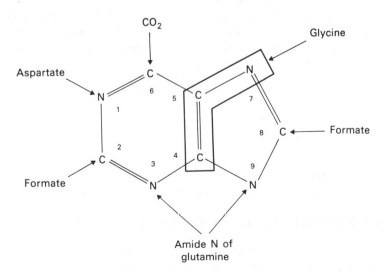

Figure 4.15 Precursors of the purine ring.

monophosphate kinase:

$$GMP + ATP \rightleftharpoons GDP + ADP$$

and nucleoside-diphosphate kinase:

$$GDP + ATP \rightleftharpoons GTP + ADP$$

Nucleoside-monophosphate kinase and nucleoside-diphosphate kinase have been found in *A. lumbricoides* and *S. mansoni* and are probably universally distributed. In addition to their role in nucleotide synthesis, these phosphate kinases are also involved in energy metabolism (Section 3.1.3).

Many helminths (cestodes, acanthocephalans, nematodes) have been shown to incorporate free purines (adenine) and purine nucleosides (adenosine) into nucleic acids. However, this is the result of salvage pathways. There is little evidence at present that helminths can synthesise IMP from simple precursors. The trematode *S. mansoni* is unable to synthesise IMP *de novo*[102]. However, there is evidence for purine synthesis in regenerating larval *M. corti* (tetrathyridia), although this is only very indirect[103]. And, finally, there are reports of purine synthesis in the nematode *A. cantonensis*[104].

Purine Salvage Pathways

These pathways convert free purines and purine nucleosides back to nucleotides, and so conserve the purine bases. There are two main mechanisms for this. The first involves adenine or guanine phosphoribosyl transferase:

$$adenine + 5\text{-phosphoribose-1-pyrophosphate} \rightleftharpoons AMP + PP_i$$

$$guanine + 5\text{-phosphoribose-1-pyrophosphate} \rightleftharpoons GMP + PP_i$$

The guanine phosphoribosyl transferase can also use hypoxanthine as a substrate and convert it to IMP. The second system involves two enzymes, purine nucleoside phosphorylase:

$$purine\ (adenine) + ribose\text{-1-P} \rightleftharpoons purine\ nucleoside\ (adenosine) + P_i$$

and a specific nucleoside kinase, such as adenosine kinase:

$$adenosine + ATP \rightleftharpoons AMP + ADP$$

The fact that helminths can incorporate free purines and purine nucleosides into nucleic acids indicates that these pathways must be present. Adenosine and guanosine kinases have been found in *A. lumbricoides*, but only in schistosomes have the purine salvage pathways been investigated[105].

Adenosine metabolism in *S. mansoni* is summarised in *Figure 4.16*. There are two, or possibly three, pathways for the synthesis of adenylic acid (AMP) from adenine or adenosine. Adenosine can be directly phosphorylated by adenosine kinase to give AMP. An alternative pathway is via adenosine deaminase to inosine and then via hypoxanthine to IMP. There is some evidence that schistosomes can convert IMP to AMP, and also to GMP. Adenine can be converted to adenosine by

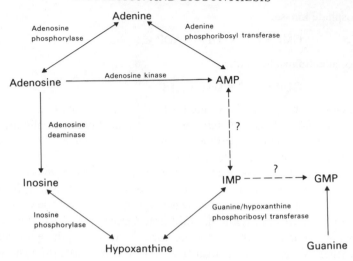

Figure 4.16 Purine salvage pathways in *S. mansoni*.

adenosine phosphorylase or directly to AMP by adenine phosphoribosyl transferase. Although it has not been demonstrated, the guanine/hypoxanthine phosphoribosyl transferase, which is responsible for the conversion of hypoxanthine to IMP, could also convert guanine to GMP.

The nematode *N. brasiliensis* can convert adenine to guanine and this presumably takes place via AMP and GMP.

Purine Nucleotide Cycle

This is a series of reactions involving some of the enzymes of purine metabolism:

$$AMP + H_2O \rightarrow IMP + NH_3$$

$$IMP + aspartate + GTP \rightarrow adenylosuccinate + GDP + P_i$$

$$adenylosuccinate \rightarrow AMP + fumarate$$

The net result of this cycle is the deamination of aspartate. AMP deaminase has been found in some nematodes (Section 3.5.2), but whether the purine nucleotide cycle is a significant source of ammonia in these nematodes is unknown. An alternative pathway is hydrolysis of AMP to adenosine, then via adenosine deaminase to inosine and resynthesis of AMP via hypoxanthine and IMP. All the enzymes for the latter pathway are present in *S. mansoni* (*Figure 4.16*).

4.6.2. Pyrimidine Nucleotide Synthesis

Pyrimidine synthesis follows a much simpler pathway than purine synthesis and is summarised in *Figure 4.17*. The first three enzymes of pyrimidine synthesis, aspartate transcarbamoylase, dihydro-orotase and orotate reductase, may be in a multi-

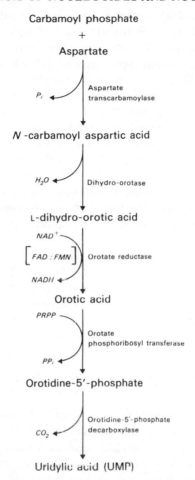

Figure 4.17 Pyrimidine synthesis: PRPP, 5-phosphoribose pyrophosphate; [FAD:FMN], flavin adenine dinucleotide:flavin adenine mononucleotide. Orotate reductase is a complex enzyme containing both FAD and FMN, as well as iron-sulphur centres.

functional complex. In contrast to purine synthesis, the D-ribose-5-P is not attached to the pyrimidine ring until after it has been formed. The initial product of pyrimidine synthesis is UMP, and this then acts as a precursor for the other nucleotides.

As with purine bases, helminths can incorporate exogenous pyrimidines (uracil) and pyrimidine nucleosides (uridine, thymidine) into nucleic acids, but again this involves the salvage pathways and not *de novo* synthesis. Exogenous thymidine is, however, said not to be incorporated into nucleic acids by *S. mansoni*.

Pyrimidine synthesis has been demonstrated in *Paragonimus ohirai*, and several of the enzymes involved have been shown to occur both in *P. ohirai* and *C. sinensis* (carbamoyl-phosphate synthetase, aspartate transcarbamoylase, dihydro-orotase, orotate phosphoribosyl transferase, orotidine-5-phosphate decarboxylase)[106]. There is indirect evidence that regenerating larval *M. corti* can synthesise pyrimidines *de novo*, and there are isolated reports that *F. hepatica* also synthesises pyrimidines[107,108]. The microfilariae of *D. immitis* can convert orotidine-5-phosphate to UMP (the last step in the pathway) and larval *M. corti* incorporate orotic acid into nucleic acids.

The larvae of *M. corti* will only incorporate orotate when the culture medium contains no free pyrimidines or pyrimidine nucleosides. The presence of free pyrimidines or pyrimidine nucleosides appears to prevent pyrimidine synthesis from orotate. This suggests that perhaps in *M. corti*, as in mammals, the *de novo* synthesis of purines and pyrimidines is under strict metabolic control. The apparent lack of *de novo* pyrimidine and purine synthesis in helminths might, therefore, be due not to the absence of the relevant pathways, but to their suppression by exogenous bases and nucleotides. In this context, it would be extremely interesting to know if the free-living stages of helminths synthesise these compounds from simple precursors. The possibility that regenerating larval *M. corti* synthesises pyrimidines and purines *de novo* could be explained by the relaxation of metabolic control in regenerating tissue.

Aspartate transcarbamoylase, the first enzyme in the pyrimidine pathway proper, has been demonstrated in several helminths (*F. hepatica, P. cervi, S. mansoni, M. benedeni, A. lumbricoides, A. cantonensis*) and dihydro-orotase has also been shown in *S. mansoni, A. lumbricoides* and *A. cantonensis*[87,109,110].

The key metabolite in pyrimidine synthesis is carbamoyl phosphate. The enzyme carbamoyl-phosphate synthetase catalyses the formation of carbamoyl phosphate from CO_2 and glutamine or ammonia:

$$2ATP + HCO_3^- + H_2O + \text{glutamine} \rightarrow$$
$$\text{carbamoyl phosphate} + \text{glutamate} + 2ADP + P_i$$

Three different carbamoyl-phosphate synthetases are known, a glutamine-dependent one, an ammonia-dependent one which requires N-acetylglutamate as an activator and, finally, a glutamine- and N-acetylglutamate-dependent enzyme. The ammonia-dependent enzyme, which in mammals is mitochondrial, functions in the urea cycle, the other variants are cytoplasmic and involved in pyrimidine or arginine synthesis. Until very recently, carbamoyl-phosphate synthetase seemed to be absent from all the helminths in which it had been looked for (*F. hepatica, P. cervi, E. granulosus, D. caninum, M. expansa, M. benedeni, M. dubius, A. lumbricoides, T. canis*). The absence of carbamoyl-phosphate synthetase in these helminths would be a block to pyrimidine synthesis. However, there have now been reports of low glutamine-dependent carbamoyl-phosphate synthetase activities in *A. lumbricoides, A. cantonensis, S. mansoni, P. ohirai* and *C. sinensis*[106,110]. The carbamoyl-phosphate synthetase from *A. lumbricoides* is inhibited by UDP and UTP and stimulated by 5-phosphoribosyl-1-pyrophosphate. The enzyme from *P. ohirai* and *C. sinensis* is similarly subject to feedback inhibition by end-products such as UDP, UTP, CDP, dUDP and dCDP and is again stimulated by 5-phosphoribosyl-1-pyrophosphate.

Carbamoyl-phosphate synthetase is an unstable enzyme and activity may be rapidly lost in homogenates. Also, the levels of carbamoyl-phosphate synthetase are normally fairly low in tissues, and the ratio of carbamoyl-phosphate synthetase to aspartate transcarbamoylase in vertebrate tissues is approximately 1:10.

Homogenates of *F. hepatica, P. cervi* and *M. benedeni* have been shown to be capable of synthesising carbamoyl phosphate[111], despite the apparent low, or non-existent, activity of carbamoyl-phosphate synthetase. The origin of the carbamoyl phosphate in these helminths is not certain. Ornithine transcarbamoylase seems to be absent in helminths[87,109], so carbamoyl phosphate cannot come from the cleavage of citrulline. There are, in micro-organisms, alternative sources of carbamoyl phosphate, such as the phosphorolytic cleavage of carbamoyl oxalate derived from the fermentation of allantoin. There is, however, no evidence that such pathways exist in metazoa.

Pyrimidine Salvage Pathways

The pyrimidine salvage pathways have been much less studied than the corresponding purine salvage pathways, but appear to involve analogous enzymes: pyrimidine phosphoribosyl transferases, pyrimidine nucleoside phosphorylases and specific pyrimidine nucleoside kinases. Since helminths incorporate exogenous pyrimidine bases and pyrimidine nucleosides into nucleic acids, these pathways must be presumed to be present. However, the only enzymes involved in pyrimidine salvage so far demonstrated in parasitic helminths are the pyrimidine nucleoside kinases: uridine and cytidine kinases in *A. lumbricoides*, uridine and thymidine kinases in *P. ohirai* and *C. sinensis*, and thymidine kinase in *H. diminuta* and *M. dubius*. Strangely, thymidine kinase was absent from the germinal tissue and developing eggs of *A. lumbricoides*[112]. Thymidine kinase activity does, however, show marked periodicity in many tissues, and this is probably related to the cell cycle.

4.6.3. Deoxyribonucleotide Synthesis

Deoxyribonucleotides (for DNA synthesis) are made not as might be expected, from 2-deoxyribose-5-phosphate, but by the reduction of the 2′ carbon of the corresponding ribonucleotide. This reduction is brought about by a complex multienzyme system, which in most cases requires thioredoxin as a cofactor. This system has not been studied in helminths, although several studies have indicated that ribonucleosides are incorporated into DNA in parasitic helminths. Most of this work has been histochemical and is open to question. However, Bolla and Roberts[113] have isolated labelled DNA after incubation of *H. diminuta* in labelled thymidine. This suggests that helminths can reduce the 2′ carbon, but the mechanism is unknown.

No studies seem to have been done to see if helminths can take up deoxyribonucleosides from the environment in the same way as they accumulate ribonucleosides (Section 4.1.10).

4.6.4. Nucleic Acid Synthesis

The incorporation studies referred to above demonstrate that helminths, like all other living organisms, can synthesise DNA and RNA, often at relatively high rates. However, there have been virtually no studies on the mechanisms of nucleic acid synthesis in parasitic helminths.

Ribonucleic Acid Synthesis

The synthesis of RNA requires nucleoside triphosphates and is catalysed by a DNA directed RNA polymerase:

$$NTP + (NMP)_n \rightleftharpoons (NMP)_{n+1} + PP_i$$

This enzyme requires a DNA template, it is ubiquitous in living organisms and so presumably occurs in helminths. Another polymerase, polynucleotide phosphorylase, which was thought to occur only in bacteria, has also been demonstrated in *A. lumbricoides*. This enzyme catalyses the synthesis of polynucleotides from dinucleotide phosphates:

$$NDP + (NMP)_n \rightleftharpoons (NMP)_{n+1} + P_i$$

Polynucleotide phosphorylase does not require a DNA primer and is almost certainly not involved in RNA synthesis. A possible function of this enzyme is in the degradation of *m*RNA. Nevertheless, polynucleotide phosphorylase is interesting, since it was the first enzyme discovered to be capable of synthesising long chain polynucleotides.

All forms of RNA, messenger RNA, transfer RNA and ribosomal RNA, are probably made by the same enzyme. The RNA formed by RNA polymerase then requires enzymatic modification (cleavage, chemical modification of bases, addition of polynucleotide sequences) before the functional finished products (*m*RNA, *t*RNA, *r*RNA) are released into the cytoplasm. The maturation of ribosomal RNA in eukaryotes is outlined in *Figure 4.18*. The sedimentation values for the different ribosomal RNA fractions vary somewhat from organism to organism, for example, 41s (37–42), 28s (24–30), 18s (16.8–20), as does the sedimentation value of the ribosomal particles, 60s (58–60) and 40s (37–40).

Experiments on *E. granulosus*[114] indicate that the formation of the different RNA fractions in helminths is probably the same as in other eukaryotes. There is evidence in *E. granulosus* for the involvement of 40–42.5s (equivalent to 41s) and 35s (equivalent to 32s) RNA in the formation of ribosomal RNA; 5s, 19.6s and 29.4s ribosomal RNA have been isolated together with transfer RNA. Pulse labelling of *E. granulosus* RNA has also demonstrated the presence of short-lived messenger RNA. Developing *A. lumbricoides* eggs have typical 80s eukaryote ribosomes with 60s and 40s sub-units, the sub-units containing 19s and 26s *r*RNA. In the free-living nematode *P. silusiae*[115], the formation of ribosomal RNA again seems to conform to the eukaryotic scheme in *Figure 4.18*. Inhibitors of RNA synthesis such as actinomycin D also inhibit RNA synthesis in helminths[113].

Ribonucleic Acid in Development

The different classes of RNA play an important role in embryogenesis, and some of the temporal aspects of RNA synthesis have been investigated during the development of *A. lumbricoides* eggs. In *A. lumbricoides* eggs, there is a burst of *r*RNA synthesis immediately after the penetration of the sperm. Most unusually, this synthesis occurs exclusively from the male genome (male pronucleus). Usually, in

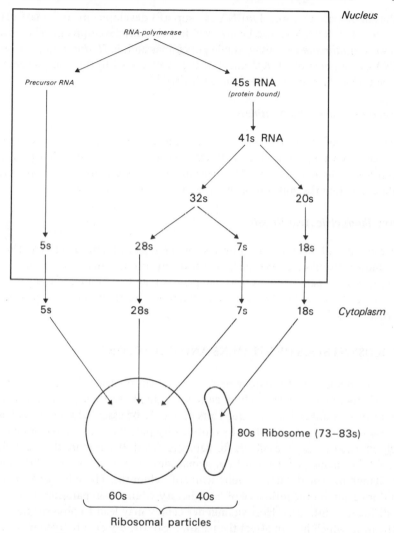

Figure 4.18 Formation of ribosomal RNA in eukaryotes.

developmental systems, the male genome does not have any influence until much later, normally around late blastula. In the later pronuclear stages of fertilisation of *A. lumbricoides* eggs, *r*RNA synthesis cannot be detected and synthesis does not start again until after the four-cell stage. The resumption of *r*RNA synthesis in *A. lumbricoides* eggs can be correlated with the reappearance of well defined nucleoli. There is strong evidence that the presence of nucleoli in cells is associated with *r*RNA synthesis. However, recently Kuhn and Tobler[116] found that the *r*RNA content of developing *A. lumbricoides* eggs increased steadily, with no post-fertilisation halt.

There is considerable evidence, from a variety of organisms, that the early stages of development depend on stable *m*RNA, synthesised and stored during oogenesis.

In the amphibian, preformed mRNA can support development to the late blastula stage. Stable mRNA may also be involved in helminth development. The fertilised eggs of *A. lumbricoides* contain stable polysomes and, in *H. diminuta*, preformed mRNA can support the development of the cysticercoid to the point where the genital primordia start to differentiate (day 6)[117].

Deoxyribonucleic Acid Synthesis

The synthesis of DNA utilises nucleoside triphosphates and requires a series of enzymes, DNA polymerase II and III, DNA ligase, together with RNA polymerase, to synthesise the RNA primer. The mechanism of DNA synthesis has not been studied in helminths, but is probably the same as in other eukaryotes.

Deoxyribonucleic Acid Repair

There are, in cells, enzymatic pathways for the repair of damaged DNA. The three best known systems are: enzymatic photoreactivation, which requires visible blue light; excision repair, which is light-independent; and recombination repair. The enzymatic photoreactivation system has been demonstrated in developing *A. lumbricoides* eggs[118].

4.7. BIOSYNTHESIS OF VITAMINS AND COFACTORS

The vitamin and cofactor requirements of an organism can only be determined by growth experiments using carefully defined media. Even then, the results may not be straightforward, since some nutrients may only be essential if others are lacking, and essential nutrients can often be replaced by precursors or related compounds. Such information is not available for parasitic helminths, nor are there any detailed data for free-living platyhelminths or nematodes. In general, we have little idea of the vitamin or growth factor requirements of helminths. There is a certain amount of information on the influence of host dietary vitamins on parasites, but the data are difficult to interpret. Host vitamin deficiency may lead to physiological changes in the host, which in turn affect the parasite. So, the effects observed in hosts on deficient diets may be direct, due to induced vitamin deficiency in the parasite, or they may be indirect, because of the effects on host metabolism. Vitamin deficiency in the host's diet does not necessarily mean that the parasite will be exposed to vitamin deficiency. Tissue parasites will be able to obtain their vitamins from the tissues (Section 4.1.11), whilst, in the gut, vitamins may be available from the exocrino-enteric circulation and from the gut flora.

Culture in precisely defined media has rarely been achieved in parasitic helminths. Vitamin supplements have been shown to be necessary for normal development, in culture, of *T. crassiceps, Diplostomum phoxini, N. brasiliensis, O. radiatum* and *C. punctata*. These species (and presumably all helminths) require vitamins, but these observations do not indicate which of the vitamins are important. Excess of the fat-soluble vitamins (A, D_3, E) were, however, toxic to cultured *H. microstoma*[119].

More precise data are available for the insect parasitic nematode *N. glaseri*, which has been shown to require folic acid (vitamin B_c) and biotin[101]; the plant parasitic nematode *Aphelenchoides rutgersi* also needs exogenous folic acid[120]; the free-living nematode *C. briggsae* requires thiamine, riboflavin, nicotinic acid, pyridoxine, folic acid and pantothenate. An alternative approach is to culture parasites in the presence of specific inhibitory vitamin analogues. The vitamin B_6 (pyridoxine) analogue 4-deoxypyridoxine and nicotinic acid analogues inhibit the growth of *H. diminuta* in culture, suggesting that pyridoxine and nicotinic acid are required by this tapeworm[121]. However, pantoyltaurine, a pantothenic acid analogue, had no effect on the culture of *H. diminuta*. No other studies with vitamin analogues appear to have been made with helminths. The absence of tryptophan oxidase in *S. mansoni* (Section 3.4.2) makes it likely that this parasite will also require nicotinic acid.

There have been a number of studies on the influence of host dietary vitamins on helminths. Dietary deficiency of the fat-soluble vitamins A, D and E do not appear to influence the growth of helminth parasites, although establishment may be affected. The trematode *S. mansoni* was also unaffected in vitamin C deficient hosts. However, for reasons stated above, it cannot be concluded that these vitamins are not required by helminths. Hosts on a vitamin A deficient diet are often more susceptible to parasitic infection.

In *H. diminuta*, host dietary deficiency of the B group vitamins, thiamine (B_1), riboflavin (B_2), choline, pantothenate and biotin, like A, D and E deficiency, had no effect on the parasite. In riboflavin deficient hosts, *H. diminuta* were larger than those from hosts on a full isocalorific diet. The reason for this riboflavin effect is not known. The only B group dietary deficiency which has been shown to affect *H. diminuta* is pyridoxine (B_6). The establishment, growth and development of *H. diminuta* were all affected in pyridoxine deficient hosts, and the worms showed reduced phosphorylase and transaminase activities. Phosphorylase and transaminases both require pyridoxal phosphate as a cofactor. The main form of B_6 in *H. diminuta* is pyridoxal, with small amounts of pyridoxamine and pyridoxine. Thus, in *H. diminuta*, a requirement has been demonstrated for nicotinic acid and pyridoxal, but it is almost certain that other vitamins and growth factors are needed.

The intermediary metabolism of vitamins by helminths is virtually unknown, the only data available being for vitamin A, vitamin B_{12} (cobalamin) and folic acid.

Vitamin A

In *A. lumbricoides*, the body wall and the intestine can convert carotene to vitamin A. This nematode can also absorb vitamin A directly.

Vitamin B_{12}

The physiologically active forms of B_{12} are adenosylcobalamin and methylcobalamin. In *S. mansonoides*, absorbed B_{12} is converted into adenosylcobalamin and hydroxycobalamin, but no methylcobalamin is detectable[122]. Hydroxycobalamin, an inactive form of the coenzyme, is a photolysis product of cobalamin, and it is unlikely to be an intermediate in adenosylcobalamin synthesis. Adenosylcobalamin has also been identified in *A. lumbricoides*, and both adenosylcobalamin and methylcobalamin have been found in *D. latum*. Adenosylcobalamin is the cofactor for methylmalonyl-CoA mutase, an enzyme that has been demonstrated in *S. mansonoides* (Section 3.1.4). Methylcobalamin, the coenzyme that could not be detected in *S. mansonoides*, is the methyl group carrier in methyl transferase reactions. Attempts to demonstrate methyl transferase activity in *S. mansonoides, M. corti* or *A. lumbricoides* have so far proved unsuccessful and is possibly correlated with the apparent absence of methylcobalamin. Methyl transferase activity has, however, been shown in the insect parasitic nematode *N. glaseri* and in the free-living nematode *C. briggsae*[101].

Folic Acid

The biologically active form of folic acid (*Figure 4.19*) is tetrahydrofolate (FH_4). In mammals, the conversion of folate to tetrahydrofolate involves two NADP-linked l reductases:

Folate ⟶ Dihydrofolate ⟶ Tetrahydrofolate

NADPH + H$^+$ NADP$^+$ NADPH + H$^+$ NADP$^+$

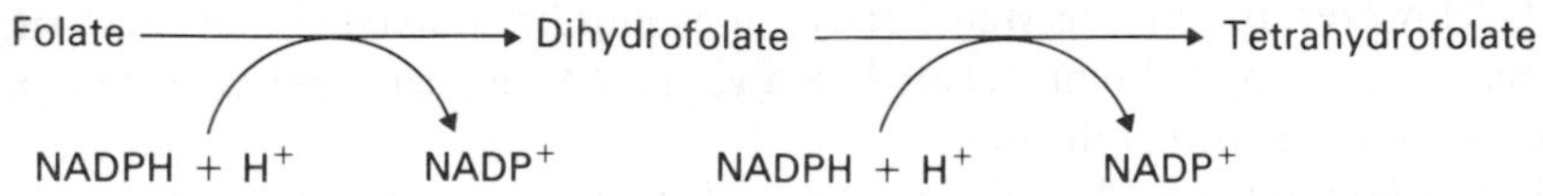

Folate metabolism is an important site for chemotherapy in bacteria and parasitic protozoa (sporozoans). These organisms are unable to metabolise folate, but instead synthesise dihydrofolate *de novo* and then reduce it to tetrahydrofolate. The synthesis of dihydrofolate can be blocked in bacteria and sporozoans by *para*-aminobenzoic acid analogues, such as the sulphonamides, and the dihydrofolate reductase of these organisms is much more sensitive to inhibition by 2,4-diaminopyrimidines and related heterocyclics than is the mammalian enzyme.

Despite its importance in the chemotherapy of bacterial and protozoan infections,

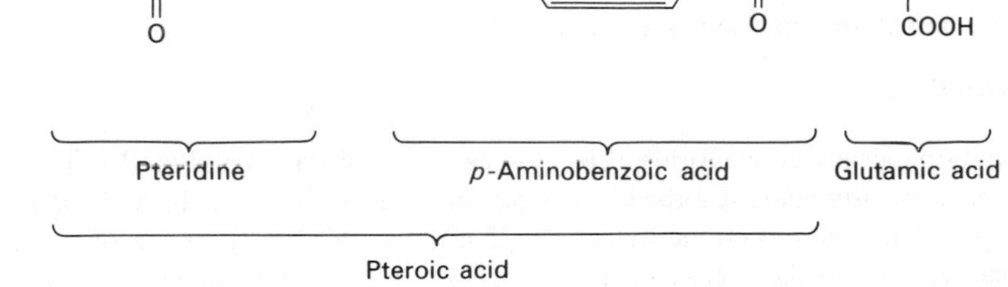

Pteridine   p-Aminobenzoic acid   Glutamic acid

Pteroic acid

Figure 4.19 Folic acid—the active form is 5,6,7,8-tetrahydrofolate.

folate metabolism has not been extensively investigated in parasitic helminths. It is, for example, uncertain if *N. brasiliensis* synthesises dihydrofolate *de novo*, or whether it requires folic acid[123]. Dihydrofolate reductase has been shown in *S. mansoni, N. brasiliensis*, in the filarial worms *D. immitis, L. carinii, D. viteae* and *Onchocercus volvulus* and in the plant parasitic nematode *A. avenae*[124,125]. In general, the dihydrofolate reductases of helminths are less sensitive, or only slightly more sensitive, to inhibition by heterocyclics than the mammalian enzyme. However, the drug suramin, which amongst other things inhibits dihydrofolate reductase, is an effective antifilarial compound.

The biochemical role of tetrahydrofolate is as an intermediate carrier of hydroxymethyl ($-CH_2OH$), formyl ($-CHO$) or methyl ($-CH_3$) groups in a variety of enzymatic reactions. Three of the enzymes involved in tetrahydrofolate metabolism have been found in parasitic nematodes. Serine hydroxymethyl transferase, which synthesis N^5,N^{10}-methylenetetrahydrofolate from tetrahydrofolate has been shown in *N. glaseri*; N^5,N^{10}-methylenetetrahydrofolate dehydrogenase, which is required for the synthesis of N^5,N^{10}-methenyltetrahydrofolate (a cofactor in purine synthesis), has been demonstrated in *N. brasiliensis* and *A. avenae*; finally N^{10}-formyltetrahydrofolate synthetase, which synthesises N^{10}-formyltetrahydrofolate from tetrahydrofolate and formate, has been found in *N. brasiliensis, N. glaseri* and *A. avenae*[101,124].

4.8. DETOXICATION REACTIONS

Animals have a number of ways of dealing with toxic metabolites or foreign chemicals. In mammals, in order to aid excretion, the solubility of toxic compounds is usually increased by conjugation with glycine or glucuronic acid, or by sulphonation. Conjugation with glutamine, ornithine or mercapturic acid (via glutathione) also occurs. Prior to conjugation, compounds may be partially detoxicated by oxidation, reduction, hydrolysis, hydroxylation or demethylation. In vertebrates, the reduction or hydroxylation of a wide range of compounds is brought about by the microsomal cytochrome systems.

The detoxication mechanisms of helminths have only recently started to be studied, despite their obvious relevance to chemotherapy and drug detoxication.

Microsomal Systems

There is no good evidence for microsomal cytochrome systems in helminths, and attempts to induce microsomal cytochromes in *A. lumbricoides* and *M. expansa* using 20-methylcholanthrene or 1,2-benzanthracene have proved unsuccessful[126]. The absence of cytochromes P_{450} and b_5 from *A. lumbricoides* and *M. expansa* may account for the inability of these two helminths to oxidise aldrin, aniline, biphenyl, *t*-butylbenzene or nitrobenzene, or to demethylate aminopyridine or 4-nitroanisole[127]. Nor can *A. lumbricoides* demethylate the insecticide Bidrin (dimethylamide), although this readily occurs in mammals and houseflies. Another microsomal-dependent reaction in mammals and insects is the conversion of precursor' organophosphates to more toxic metabolites. Insecticides such as phos-phorothionates (Parathion) and phosphorodithioates (Guthion) are converted by mammals and insects to the more toxic phosphate and phosphorothiolate analogues. These conversions do not, however, occur in *A. lumbricoides*[128].

The apparent absence of the microsomal systems in helminths would seem to restrict severely their ability to detoxicate drugs.

Nitro- and Azoreductases

Both *A. lumbricoides* and *M. expansa* show azo- and nitroreductase activity with a variety of substrates[126,129-131]. In these parasites, a single enzyme is probably responsible for both the nitro- and azoreductase activity, whereas in mammals these are separate enzymes. There are two types of nitro- and azoreductases in mammals, one microsomal requiring cytochrome P_{450} and the other non-microsomal, utilising NADPH. The helminth nitro- and azoreductases are, in contrast, NADH-linked.

Esterases

Parasites, in general, are well provided with esterases capable of hydrolysing foreign substrates such as *p*-aminobenzoyl, naphthyl and methylumbelliferyl esters (Section 4.1.1). Helminths can also hydrolyse aryl amides, such as β-naphthylamides and *p*-nitroanilides[132]. Parasitic helminths similarly have phosphatases capable of hydrolysing nitrophenyl phosphates (Section 4.1.1). The hydrolysis of organophosphates by *A. lumbricoides*, however, proceeds at a very low rate when compared with mammals and insects[128].

The helminths *M. expansa* and *A. lumbricoides* have been shown to possess aryl sulphatases as well as *N*- and *O*-deacetylases. The *N*-deacetylases of *A. lumbricoides* and *M. expansa* have been partially purified and characterised, and appear fairly similar[133-135]. These two helminths could not, however, hydrolyse β-glucuronides. The inability of *A. lumbricoides* to hydrolyse glucuronides would mean that the parasite could not hydrolyse the bilirubin diglucuronide found in the host intestine to free bilirubin (Section 4.4.2).

Rhodanese

Low levels of rhodanese, an enzyme that detoxicates cyanide, have been reported from nematodes, cestodes and trematodes (*A. lumbricoides, P. equorum, Anoplocephala magna, F. hepatica*):

$$CN^- + thiosulphate \rightarrow thiocyanate$$

Conjugation

Parasitic helminths have only a very limited ability to detoxicate compounds by conjugation. In both *A. lumbricoides* and *M. expansa*, there is no evidence of conjugation of phenolic compounds with phosphate, sulphate, β-glucuronide or β-glucoside; benzoic acid and aminobenzoate are similarly not conjugated with glycine, nor are amino compounds acetylated[127]. The liver fluke *F. hepatica* and the cestode *H. diminuta* also do not conjugate benzoic acid with ornithine or glycine, although there is a claim that *M. benedeni* can synthesise small quantities of hippuric acid (benzoic acid + glycine)[136].

However, glutathione aryl transferase activity has been detected in *A. lumbricoides* and *M. expansa*, and both of these parasites can conjugate glutathione with 1-chloro-2,4-dinitrobenzene[137]. Despite this, there is no evidence that these helminths conjugate halogenated anthelmintics with glutathione. Neither *M. expansa* nor *A. lumbricoides* possess measurable DDT dehydrochlorinase activity. This enzyme has an absolute requirement for glutathione and converts DDT to the less toxic DDE. On the other hand, there is some evidence that glutathione epoxide transferase activity may be present in helminths.

Significance of Detoxication Reactions

A knowledge of an organism's detoxication pathways is extremely useful in chemotherapy. The information can indicate which classes of compounds are likely to be rapidly catabolised and, secondly, the data can be used to design drugs that will give rise to active metabolites. Helminths have only a limited ability to detoxicate foreign compounds and really carry out only two types of detoxication reactions: the reduction of azo and nitro compounds and the hydrolysis of synthetic esters. Most anthelmintics will not, therefore, be rapidly destroyed by the parasite. The slow rate of hydrolysis of organophosphates by *A. lumbricoides* may in part explain this parasite's susceptibility to organophosphate anthelmintics. Conversely, helminths are unlikely to metabolise inactive precursors into toxic metabolites, although active groups could be masked by acetylation, since helminths possess active deacetylases.

4.9. NUTRITION OF PARASITIC HELMINTHS

Reliable information on the nutrition of parasitic helminths is extremely scarce and, with few exceptions, we really have very little idea of the kinds or quantities of amino acids, nucleosides, lipids or carbohydrates required. Nor do we know for certain which amino acids or vitamins are essential for parasite growth and development. How far the nutritional requirements of parasites determine their host specificity is again not known (Section 1.1.8).

Knowledge of the nutritional requirements of parasites comes from three sources: feeding experiments, *in vitro* culture, and biochemical studies. As discussed in Section 4.7, the effects of altering the host's diet are extremely difficult to interpret. Dietary modifications may influence the parasite directly or they can affect the host's physiology and this, in turn, affects the parasite. Intestinal helminths may also be able to obtain, directly from their hosts (via the exocrino-enteric circulation), requirements (such as vitamins) which are absent from the host's diet. The only vitamin requirement that has been demonstrated by feeding experiments is pyridoxine (B_6), which is necessary for *H. diminuta*. Protein-free diets do not affect the growth of *H. diminuta*, which is presumably able to get its amino acid requirements from the host. *In vivo*, roughage, bile and testosterone or progesterone are necessary for the normal growth and development of *H. diminuta*, although these factors are not needed in *in vitro* systems. Presumably *in vivo* these factors all act indirectly.

The *in vitro* culture of helminths should, in theory, give clear-cut results on the nutritional requirements of helminths. Unfortunately, it is not usually possible to grow helminth parasites in strictly defined media. Nevertheless, *in vitro* culture has shown that some helminths, at least, require a dietary source of sterols and porphyrins. An alternative approach is to use specific antimetabolites in the culture media, and in this way *H. diminuta* has been shown to have a specific requirement for pyridoxine (B_6) and nicotinic acid.

Biochemical studies indicate which compounds an organism can or cannot synthesise and the latter must presumably be obtained from its host. Even if a parasite can synthesise a particular compound, it may not be able to do so fast enough during periods of rapid growth or gamete production. Biochemical studies indicate that all parasitic helminths probably require a dietary source of sterols and a source of both saturated and unsaturated fatty acids. They may also all require an exogenous source of porphyrins, nicotinic acid, purines and possibly, in some cases, pyrimidines.

Crowding Effect

A phenomenon which may be related to nutrition is the crowding effect. Helminths from high-density infections are frequently stunted and produce less eggs per worm than parasites from low-density infections. Crowding effects have been described in nematodes, trematodes, acanthocephalans and cestodes, but have been most extensively studied in the rat tapeworm, *H. diminuta*.

If *H. diminuta* from low- and high-density infections (5 worms/rat and 50 worms/rat) are compared, there are striking morphological differences. Worms from high-density infections are shorter and reduced in weight (although the wet weight/dry weight ratio is unchanged). The numbers of immature proglottides in high- and low-density worms are similar, but in high-density worms the number of mature proglottides is reduced and the number of gravid proglottides severely reduced. The number of eggs/gravid proglottis is less in high-density infections, although the prepatent period is the same. This would suggest that in *H. diminuta* the production rate and the maturation rate of proglottides are independent of one another. It also indicates that the germinative region may be involved in the crowding effect. The germinative region is the area just behind the scolex where the proglottides begin their differentiation. The proglottides are budded off from the germinative region and do not themselves divide.

During development, the crowding effect is first noticeable at 5–7 days post-infection. This corresponds to the retardation phase of growth in *H. diminuta*, when the reproductive anlagen are starting to develop.

At the biochemical level, worms from high-density infections show a lower total percentage composition of carbohydrate and a consequent increase in the percentage composition of lipid and protein. However, although the crowding effect results in a lower carbohydrate concentration in the mature and gravid proglottides, the concentration of carbohydrate in the germinative and immature regions is not affected. The synthesis of DNA, RNA and protein are all reduced in worms from high-density infections, as is the uptake of precursors (amino acids and nucleosides). The reduced uptake of precursors is not, however, sufficient to account for the reduced rates of synthesis. The synthesis of DNA and RNA were most severely inhibited in the germinative, immature and mature regions and least in the gravid proglottides. Protein synthesis, on the other hand, was least affected in the germinative region.

The proportion of glycogen synthase I (Section 4.2.3) is higher in worms from high-density infections than low-density infections[138]. The levels of glycogen synthase I usually correlate well with the rate of glycogen synthesis. So, although worms from high-density infections contain less glycogen, their glycogen synthase system would appear to be more active.

Similar crowding effects have been found in mixed infections with *H. diminuta* and *H. citelli* and with *H. diminuta* and the acanthocephalan *M. dubius*. In the latter case, a crowding effect can be shown when the rat is the host, but not when hamsters are the host.

Several possibilities have been suggested to account for the crowding effect. It could be due to local immunity, to competition for nutrients or CO_2 or O_2, to actual physical crowding or to the inhibition of worm growth by secretory or excretory products. Rats can develop an immunity to *H. diminuta*, the response being dependent both on the strain of the rat and the size of the worm load. The crowding effect, however, is noticeable early in development, before any immune response is operative. No effect of oxygen on *in vitro* growth rate can be shown in *H. diminuta*, nor are there any reports of CO_2 having an effect. Cestodes and acanthocephalans do, however, all have an absolute requirement for carbohydrate.

Tapeworms from hosts kept on a low carbohydrate diet appear very similar to worms from high-density infections. Thus, *H. diminuta* from rats on a low starch diet are smaller, have less-mature and gravid proglottides and have fewer eggs per proglottis. Again, the number of immature proglottides and the maturation time (prepatent period) are not affected. Biochemically, *H. diminuta* from low starch hosts show a reduced percentage glycogen content and a consequent increased percentage of protein and lipid. Worms from low starch hosts are also said to have a higher rate of acid excretion and a higher rate of glucose uptake. In contrast, glucose uptake rates are not affected by worm density.

Low starch diets reduce the establishment of *H. diminuta* in their hosts and also cause regression of mature worms. In the fowl cestode *R. cesticillus*, destrobilisation occurs within 24 h of host starvation.

In *H. diminuta*, neither glucose nor sucrose are adequate replacements for starch in the diet. A possible reason for this is that starch is digested relatively slowly and so provides a higher glucose concentration in the intestine for a longer period of time. Alternatively, pure glucose or sucrose diets may adversely effect host intestinal flora.

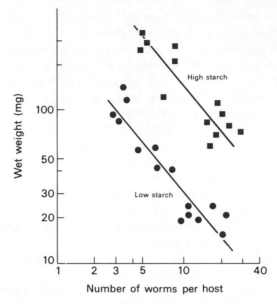

Figure 4.20 The effect of infection density and carbohydrate availability on the mean weight of individual *Hymenolepis diminuta.*

The effects on *H. diminuta* of high-density infections or low starch diets are very similar (*Figure 4.20*). This, however, does not necessarily mean that the same mechanism is involved in both cases. The maximum worm burden of *H. diminuta* in the rat is about 3 g, regardless of infection density. Mead and Roberts[139] have estimated that this weight of worms would use about 22% of the available carbohydrate in rats fed on a normal laboratory diet. So, competition for carbohydrate would seem to be a distinct possibility. The crowding effect seems to act primarily on the germinative region, and, if carbohydrate availability were the only factor involved, one might expect the glycogen content of the germinative region to be affected. However, this is not the case, although, of course, glycogen levels do not give any indication as to the actual rates of glycogen turnover. There have also been recent reports that in *in vitro* culture, conditioned media (media in which worms have already been grown) may mimic the crowding effect. This perhaps suggests that secretory or excretory products might be involved.

The effect of low carbohydrate diets on *H. diminuta* could be indirect, resulting from changes in intestinal flora and physiology. The presence of parasites also alters the physico-chemical and biotic conditions in the intestine (Section 1.1.8). The crowding effect (and possibly premunition) might also be the result of changes in intestinal conditions.

The rate of maturation of proglottides does not seem to be influenced by the crowding effect (the prepatent period is unaltered), only the number of proglottides produced changes. It is possible that there is some form of feedback mechanism involved between the mature region and the germinative region, such that the number of proglottides produced are integrated with the availability of nutrients.

The crowding effect is an example of a density-dependent regulatory factor, and perhaps one should look for its implications in terms of evolutionary stable strategies. The result of the crowding effect is to achieve the same total biomass of parasite, irrespective of initial infection density.

Energetics of Parasite Nutrition

There are two aspects to the energetics of parasite nutrition. First, how efficient are parasites at converting food to tissue? And, secondly, what is the loss of productivity to the host of parasitism?

The only comprehensive data on the efficiency of food conversion in parasites is for the plerocercoids of *S. solidus*, which occur in the body cavity of sticklebacks. These plerocercoids are unique in that they are the only case known in which the weight of the parasite can exceed the weight of the host. Growing plerocercoids place a tremendous metabolic strain on the fish and high incorporation rates by the parasite can give rise to a negative energy balance in the host. The plerocercoid appears to be more efficient at converting food into tissue than the host. Figures for gross efficiency (growth/food intake × 100) are 6 for unparasitised fish, 8 for parasitised fish, and 3.7 for parasitised fish minus parasite. However, gross efficiencies vary considerably throughout the life-cycle of animals. Very high efficiencies are often found in embryonic and growing stages (the plerocercoid is a growing stage), whilst adult animals tend to have low gross efficiencies unless they are producing gametes.

The loss of productivity to the host population as a whole, as a result of parasitism, is difficult to assess, but estimates have been made at around 10% or less. This is of the same order as estimates for the effects of predators on populations.

4.10. SUMMARY AND CONCLUSIONS

Quantitatively, synthetic pathways are well developed in parasitic helminths, but less well developed qualitatively. The range of compounds which parasitic helminths appear to be unable to synthesise *de novo* includes cholesterol, long chain fatty acids, unsaturated fatty acids, porphyrins, purines and possibly, in some cases, pyrimidines. The ability of helminths to synthesise and interconvert amino acids also seems relatively limited. Purines and pyrimidines are, of course, the basic building blocks of nucleic acids, and the fact that parasitic helminths may not be able to synthesise them seems particularly remarkable. However, this is not unique, and parasitic protozoa are also unable to synthesise purines *de novo*, although they can synthesise pyrimidines. The absence of porphyrin synthesis in helminths is again interesting. Iron porphyrins form the active centre of cytochromes, haemoglobins and a number of enzymes (catalase, peroxidases). Helminth eggs often contain appreciable amounts of porphyrins. In *A. lumbricoides*, the amount of haem in the total daily output of eggs is almost equal to the total haem content of the perienteric fluid. So, despite being unable to synthesise the porphyrin nucleus, helminths may still have a considerable haem requirement. Again, the absence of porphyrin synthesis is not restricted to parasitic helminths; the insect *Triatoma* and some parasitic protozoa (*Trypanosoma, Leishmania*) also require a dietary source of haem.

The reduced synthetic ability of helminths could be related to a number of factors: the low ATP production per mole of glucose catabolised in helminths; the free availability of nutrients in their environment; the lack of oxygen; the peculiarities of the different phyla; and 'epigenetic' loss of pathways.

In helminths, carbohydrate catabolism is relatively inefficient in terms of ATP produced per mole of glucose catabolised (Section 3.1.9). However, the rate of carbohydrate catabolism can be very high in helminths and the energy charge in helminth tissues is comparable with that of mammals. As a general principle, it is the rate of utilisation of ATP that determines the rate at which it is produced.

Catabolic pathways are primarily regulated by the energy charge or phosphorylation potential of the cell and to a lesser extent by the redox state (Section 5.1.2). The synthetic pathways leading to energy stores (carbohydrates and, in free-living stages, triacylglycerols) are also regulated by ATP, ADP or AMP. However, the synthesis of nucleotides, nucleic acids, complex lipids, amino acids and their derivatives is controlled by the concentrations of the end-products of biosynthesis. The products usually inhibit the initial step in the biosynthetic pathway. Parasitic helminths live in a nutrient-rich environment. Since synthetic pathways are under strict metabolic control, the presence of purines, pyrimidines, amino acids and so on in the environment may, in fact, suppress the helminth's synthetic pathways. There is some indirect evidence that this may be the case with purine and pyrimidine synthesis and possibly porphyrin synthesis as well. It would also explain such bizarre observations as the inability of *M. corti* and *S. mansoni* to synthesise serotonin, yet serotonin is a neurotransmitter in these parasites and so they must accumulate it from their environment.

Several of the syntheses that parasitic helminths are unable to perform have an absolute requirement for molecular oxygen: the desaturation of fatty acids; the cyclisation of squalene to give lanosterol; the conversion of coproporphyrinogen III to protoporphyrinogen IX. Many helminths live in an oxygen-poor environment. However, helminths can carry out at least one mono-oxygenase reaction, the conversion of proline to hydroxyproline, and traces of coproporphyrinogen oxidase have been found in *A. lumbricoides*. So, oxygen availability *per se* cannot account for the lack of oxidase and oxygenase reactions in helminths. Polyphenol oxidase, another oxygen-requiring enzyme, is involved in egg shell formation in a variety of helminths (Section 2.5.1). However, it is not certain whether polyphenol oxidase is active when the eggs are still in the parasite, or only after the eggs have been voided.

Microsomal mono-oxygenases, such as fatty acid mono-oxygenase and squalene oxido-cyclase, involve the microsomal cytochromes. Microsomal cytochromes appear to be absent from parasitic helminths and this also accounts for the relative inability of helminths to detoxify drugs. Proline-4-mono-oxygenase is not microsomal. Other microsomal enzymes such as glucose-6-phosphatase and 5'-nucleotidase also have rather low activities in parasitic helminths.

Some of the features of helminth syntheses are common to both free-living and parasitic members of the phyla and are not in any way related to parasitism. Steroid synthesis is absent in the majority of invertebrate groups, and both free-living and parasitic platyhelminths may be unable to synthesise polyunsaturated fatty acids. Porphyrin synthesis also seems to be lacking in free-living and parasitic nematodes.

Catabolic pathways, absent in adult parasitic helminths, are often present in the free-living stages. This has been called by Fairbairn 'epigenetic' loss of function. The adult parasite lacks a particular metabolic pathway, but nevertheless has the information for it, since the pathway is active in the free-living stages. Unfortunately, there have been very few studies on the synthetic capabilities of the free-living and intermediate stages of parasitic helminths. So we do not know if any of the synthetic pathways that are absent in the adult stage are, in fact, present in the free-living stages.

The synthetic pathways found in helminths are, in general, the same as those in mammals, although some enzymes originally thought only to occur in plants or micro-organisms have been found in helminths (isocitrate lyase, malate synthase, polynucleotide phosphorylase).

The reduced synthetic capabilities of parasitic helminths has led to the development of efficient uptake mechanisms. Parasites such as the rat tapeworm *H. diminuta* have been shown to possess at least 16 separate porters for low molecular weight compounds. The elaboration of transport mechanisms in parasitic helminths is in strong contrast to the general reduction of catabolic and synthetic pathways.

4.11. GENERAL READING

von Brand, T. (1973). *Biochemistry of Parasites*, 2nd edn. New York; Academic Press

Coles, G. C. (1973). 'The metabolism of Schistosomes: A review'. *Int. J. Biochem.*, **4**, 319–37

Coles, G. C. (1975). 'Fluke biochemistry—*Fasciola* and *Schistosoma*'. *Helminthol. Abstr.*, **A44**, 147–62

Davies, M. (1973). *Functions of Biological Membranes*. London; Chapman and Hall

Erasmus, D. A. (1972). *The Biology of Trematodes*. London; Arnold

Greichus, A. and Greichus, Y. A. (1975). 'Lipid metabolism in the hog roundworm *Ascaris lumbricoides suum*'. *Int. J. Biochem.*, **6**, 1–7

Lee, D. L. and Atkinson, H. J. (1977). *The Physiology of Nematodes*, 2nd edn. London; Macmillan

Pappas, P. W. and Read, C. P. (1975). 'Membrane transport in helminth parasites: A review'. *Exptl Parasitol.*, **37**, 469–530

Smyth, J. D. (1966). *The Physiology of Trematodes*. Edinburgh; Oliver and Boyd

Smyth, J. D. (1969). *The Physiology of Cestodes*. Edinburgh; Oliver and Boyd

4.12. REFERENCES

1. Fried, B., Gilbert, J. J. and Feese, R. C. (1976). *Int. J. Parasitol.*, **6**, 311–3
2. Castro, G. A. and Roy, S. A. (1974). *J. Parasitol.*, **60**, 887–9

3. Murthy, R. C. and Tayal, S. (1978). *Z. Parasitenkunde*, **56**, 63–8
4. Overturf, M. and Dryer, R. L. (1968). *Compar. Biochem. Physiol.*, **27**, 145–75
5. Dickinson, J. P. and Johnson, A. D. (1978). *Compar. Biochem. Physiol.*, **60B**, 277–9
6. Evans, A. A. F. (1971). *Int. J. Biochem.*, **2**, 262–4
7. Yeates, R. A. and Ogilvie, B. M. (1976). In *Biochemistry of Parasites and Host–Parasite Relationships*. Ed. H. Van den Bossche, pp. 307–10. Amsterdam; North-Holland
8. Reiner, E., Škrinjarić-Špoljar, M., Kralj, M. and Krvavica, S. (1978). *Compar. Biochem. Physiol.*, **60C**, 155–7
9. Butterworth, J. and Probert, A. J. (1970). *Exptl Parasitol.*, **28**, 557–65
10. Probert, A. J. and Lwin, T. (1974). *Exptl Parasitol.*, **35**, 253–61
11. Kwa, B. H. (1972). *Int. J. Parasitol.*, **2**, 29–33
12. Mead, R. W. and Roberts, L. S. (1972). *Compar. Biochem. Physiol.*, **41A**, 749–60
13. Dresden, M. H. and Lewis, J. C. (1977). *J. Parasitol.*, **63**, 941–3
14. Dresden, M. H. and Edlin, E. M. (1975). *J. Parasitol.*, **61**, 398–402
15. Moczoń, T. (1977). *Bull. Académie Polonaise des Sciences*, **25**, 479–81
16. Heath, D. D. (1971). *Int. J. Parasitol.*, **1**, 145–52
17. Barrett, J. (1976). *Parasitology*, **73**, 109–21
18. Rogers, W. P. and Brooks, F. (1977). *Int. J. Parasitol.*, **7**, 61–5
19. Rogers, W. P. and Brooks, F. (1976). *Int. J. Parasitol.*, **6**, 315–9
20. Tsang, V. C. W. and Damian, R. T. (1977). *Blood*, **49**, 619–33
21. Homandberg, G. A. and Peanasky, R. J. (1976). *J. Biol. Chem.*, **251**, 2226–33
22. Rhoads, M. L. and Romanowski, R. D. (1974). *Exptl Parasitol.*, **35**, 363–8
23. Byram, J. E. and Fisher, F. M. (1974). *Tissue and Cell*, **6**, 21–42
24. Podesta, R. B. (1977). *Exptl Parasitol.*, **43**, 12–24
25. Befus, A. D. and Podesta, R. B. (1976). In *Ecological Aspects of Parasitology*. Ed. C. R. Kennedy, pp. 303–25. Amsterdam; North-Holland
26. Podesta, R. B. (1977). *Exptl Parasitol.*, **42**, 289–99
27. Podesta, R. B., Stallard, H. E., Evans, W. S., Lussier, P. E., Jackson, D. J. and Mettrick, D. F. (1977). *Exptl Parasitol.*, **42**, 300–17
28. Dunkley, L. C. and Mettrick, D. F. (1977). *Exptl Parasitol.*, **41**, 213–28
29. Pappas, P. W. and Hansen, B. D. (1977). *J. Parasitol.*, **63**, 800–4
30. Love, R. D. and Uglem, G. L. (1978). *J. Parasitol.*, **64**, 426–30
31. Uglem, G. L. (1976). *Biochim. Biophys. Acta*, **443**, 126–36
32. Starling, J. A. (1975). *Trans. Am. Microsc. Soc.*, **94**, 508–23
33. Podesta, R. B., Evans, W. S. and Stallard, H. E. (1977). *Exptl Parasitol.*, **43**, 25–38
34. Henderson, D. (1977). *Parasitology*, **75**, 277–84
35. Podesta, R. B. and Mettrick, D. F. (1974). *Can. J. Physiol. Pharmacol.*, **52**, 183–97
36. Uglem, G. L., Love, R. D. and Eubank, J. H. (1978). *Exptl Parasitol.*, **45**, 88–92
37. Starling, J. A. and Fisher, F. M. (1975). *J. Parasitol.*, **61**, 977–90

38. Starling, J. A. and Fisher, F. M. (1978). *J. Compar. Physiol.*, **126**, 223–31
39. Al-Barwari, S. E. and Abdel-Fattah, R. F. (1974). *Bull. Endemic Dis.*, **15**, 105–11
40. Laurie, J. S. (1971). *Exptl Parasitol.*, **29**, 375–85
41. Schanbacher, L. M. and Beames, C. G. (1978). *J. Parasitol.*, **64**, 89–92
42. Hurstead, S. T. and Williams, J. F. (1977). *J. Parasitol.*, **63**, 314–21
43. Chappell, L. H. and Read, C. P. (1973). *Parasitology*, **67**, 289–305
44. Isseroff, H., Ertel, J. C. and Levy, M. G. (1976). *Compar. Biochem. Physiol.*, **54B**, 125–33
45. Asch, H. L. and Read, C. P. (1975). *Exptl Parasitol.*, **38**, 123–35
46. Halton, D. W. (1978). *Parasitology*, **76**, 29–37
47. Rutherford, T. A., Webster, J. M. and Barlow, J. S. (1977). *Can. J. Zool.*, **55**, 1773–81
48. Surgan, M. H. and Roberts, L. S. (1976). *J. Parasitol.*, **62**, 78–86, 87–93
49. King, J. W. and Lumsden, R. D. (1969). *J. Parasitol.*, **55**, 250–60
50. Hammond, R. A. (1968). *J. Exptl Biol.*, **48**, 217–25
51. Pappas, P. W., Uglem, G. L. and Read, C. P. (1973). *Parasitology*, **66**, 525–38
52. McCracken, R. O., Lumsden, R. D. and Page, C. R. (1975). *J. Parasitol.*, **61**, 999–1005
53. Page, C. R. and MacInnis, A. J. (1975). *J. Parasitol.*, **61**, 281–90
54. Page, C. R., MacInnis, A. J. and Griffith, L. M. (1977). *J. Parasitol.*, **63**, 91–5
55. Levy, M. G. and Read, C. P. (1975). *J. Parasitol.*, **61**, 627–32, 648–56
56. Tkachuck, R. D., Weinstein, P. P. and Mueller, J. F. (1976). *J. Parasitol.*, **62**, 94–101
57. Hariri, M. (1975). *J. Parasitol.*, **61**, 440–8
58. Bennett, J. L. and Bueding, E. (1973). *Molec. Pharmacol.*, **9**, 311–9
59. Podesta, R. B. and Mettrick, D. F. (1975). *Exptl Parasitol.*, **37**, 1–14
60. Podesta, R. B. (1978). *Can. J. Zool.*, **56**, 2344–54
61. Podesta, R. B. (1977). *Exptl Parasitol.*, **43**, 295–306
62. Rotunno, C. A., Kammerer, W. S., Esandi, M. V. P. and Cereijido, M. (1974). *J. Parasitol.*, **60**, 613–20
63. Harpur, R. P. and Popkin, J. S. (1973). *Can. J. Physiol. Pharmacol.*, **51**, 79–90
64. Ridley, R. K., Slonka, G. F. and Leland, S. E. (1977). *J. Parasitol.*, **63**, 348–56
65. Rubin, H. and Trelease, R. N. (1975). *J. Parasitol.*, **61**, 577–88
66. Rubin, H. and Trelease, R. N. (1976). *J. Cell Biol.*, **70**, 374–83
67. Dendinger, J. E. and Roberts, L. S. (1977). *Compar. Biochem. Physiol.*, **58B**, 215–9
68. Dendinger, J. E. and Roberts, L. S. (1977). *Compar. Biochem. Physiol.*, **58B**, 231–6
69. Lumsden, R. D. (1975). *Exptl Parasitol.*, **37**, 267–339
70. Trimble, J. J. and Lumsden, R. D. (1975). *J. Parasitol.*, **61**, 665–76
71. Rumjanek, F. D., Broomfield, K. E. and Smithers, S. R. (1979). *Exptl Parasitol.*, **47**, 24–35

72. Fripp, P. J., Williams, G. and Crawford, M. A. (1976). *Compar. Biochem. Physiol.,* **53B**, 505-7

73. Meyer, H., Mueller, J. and Meyer, F. (1978). *Biochem. Biophys. Res. Commun.,* **82**, 834-9

74. Meyer, F., Meyer, H. and Bueding, E. (1970). *Biochim. Biophys. Acta,* **210**, 257-66

75. Sasi, P. K. and Raj, R. K. (1978). *Experientia,* **34**, 1156-7

76. Fioravanti, C. F. and MacInnis, A. J. (1977). *Compar. Biochem. Physiol.,* **57B**, 227-33

77. Willett, J. D. and Downey, W. L. (1974). *Biochem. J.,* **138**, 233-7

78. Davey, K. G. (1976). In *Biochemistry of Parasites and Host-Parasite Relationships.* Ed. H. Van den Bossche, pp. 359-72. Amsterdam; North-Holland

79. Dennis, R. D. W. (1977). *Int. J. Parasitol.,* **7**, 171-9, 181-8

80. Rogers, W. P. (1978). *Compar. Biochem. Physiol.,* **61A**, 187-90

81. Fioravanti, C. F. and MacInnis, A. J. (1976). *J. Parasitol.,* **62**, 749-55

82. Tarr, G. E. and Fairbairn, D. (1973). *J. Parasitol.,* **59**, 428-33

83. Barrett, J. (1976). *Parasitology,* **73**, 109-21

84. Oldenborg, V., Van Vugt, F. and Van Golde, L. M. G. (1975). *Biochim. Biophys. Acta,* **398**, 101-10

85. Webb, R. A. and Mettrick, D. F. (1973). *Int. J. Parasitol.,* **3**, 47-58

86. Bishop, S. H. (1975). *J. Parasitol.,* **61**, 79-88

87. Kurelec, B. (1972). *Compar. Biochem. Physiol.,* **43B**, 769-80

88. Langer, B. W., Smith, W. J. and Theodorides, V. J. (1971). *J. Parasitol.,* **57**, 836-9

89. Cain, G. D. and Fairbairn, D. (1971). *Compar. Biochem. Physiol.,* **40B**, 165-79

90. Kurelec, B. and Rijavec, M. (1976). In *Biochemistry of Parasites and Host-Parasite Relationships.* Ed. H. Van den Bossche, pp. 101-7. Amsterdam; North-Holland

91. Hopkins, F. G. and Morgan, E. J. (1945). *Biochem. J.,* **39**, 320-4

92. Bolla, R. I., Weinstein, P. P. and Lou, C. (1972). *Compar. Biochem. Physiol.,* **43B**, 487-501

93. Cain, G. D. (1976). *Exptl Parasitol.,* **40**, 112-5

94. Cain, G. D. and Bassow, F. (1976). *Int. J. Parasitol.,* **6**, 79-82

95. Cain, G. D. and Welshman, I. R. (1973). *Int. J. Parasitol.,* **3**, 623-30

96. Parker, R. D. and MacInnis, A. J. (1977). *Exptl Parasitol.,* **41**, 2-16

97. Naquira, C., Paulin, J. and Agosin, M. (1977). *Exptl Parasitol.,* **41**, 359-69

98. Agosin, M. and Naquira, C. (1978). *Compar. Biochem. Physiol.,* **60B**, 183-7

99. Noble, S., Leushner, J. and Pasternak, J. (1978). *Biochim. Biophys. Acta,* **520**, 219-28

100. Harpur, R. P. and Jackson, D. M. (1975). *J. Parasitol.,* **61**, 808-14

101. Jackson, G. J. and Platzer, E. G. (1974). *J. Parasitol.,* **60**, 453-7

102. Senft, A. W., Miech, R. P., Brown, P. R. and Senft, D. G. (1972). *Int. J. Parasitol.,* **2**, 249-60

103. Heath, R. L. and Hart, J. L. (1970). *J. Parasitol.,* **56**, 340-5

104. Wong, P. C. L. and Ko, R. C. (1979). *Compar. Biochem. Physiol.*, **62B**, 129–32

105. Senft, A. W., Senft, D. G. and Miech, R. P. (1973). *Biochem. Pharmacol.*, **22**, 437–47

106. Kobayashi, M., Yokogawa, M., Mori, M. and Tatibana, M. (1978). *Int. J. Parasitol.*, **8**, 471–7

107. Togan, I. and Gülen, S. (1974). *Proc. Third Int. Congr. of Parasitology (Munich)* 3, p. 1492

108. Türkoğlu, C., Buğra, K. Tremblay, G. C. and Gülen, S. (1978). *Proc. Fourth Int. Congr. of Parasitology (Warsaw)* F, p. 55

109. Kurelec, B. (1973). *J. Parasitol.*, **59**, 1006–11

110. Aoki, T. and Aoki, H. (1978). *Proc. Fourth Int. Congr. of Parasitology (Warsaw)* F, p. 74

111. Kurelec, B. (1974). *Compar. Biochem. Physiol.*, **47B**, 33–40

112. Farland, W. H. and MacInnis, A. J. (1978). *J. Parasitol.*, **64**, 564–5

113. Bolla, R. I. and Roberts, L. S. (1970). *J. Parasitol.*, **56**, 1151–8

114. Agosin, M., Repetto, Y. and Dicowsky, L. (1971). *Exptl Parasitol.*, **30**, 233–43

115. Scott Noble, J. and Pasternak, J. (1975). *Biochim. Biophys. Acta*, **402**, 51–61

116. Kuhn, O. and Tobler, H. (1978). *Biochim. Biophys. Acta*, **521**, 251–266

117. Bolla, R. I. and Roberts, L. S. (1971). *Compar. Biochem. Physiol.*, **40B**, 885–92

118. MacInnis, A. J. Unpublished results

119. Chowdhury, N. (1978). *Z. Parasitenkunde*, **56**, 29–38

120. Thirugnanam, M. and Myers, R. F. (1974). *Exptl Parasitol.*, **36**, 202–9

121. Roberts, L. S. and Mong, F. N. (1973). *J. Parasitol.*, **59**, 101–4

122. Tkachuck, R. D., Weinstein, P. P. and Mueller, J. F. (1977). *J. Parasitol.*, **63**, 694–700

123. Gutteridge, W. E., Ogilvie, B. M. and Dunnett, S. J. (1970). *Int. J. Biochem.*, **1**, 230–4

124. Platzer, E. G. (1974). *Compar. Biochem. Physiol.*, **49B**, 3–13

125. Jaffe, J. J., McCormack, J. J. and Meymarian, E. (1972). *Biochem. Pharmacol.*, **21**, 719–31

126. Douch, P. G. C. (1976). *Xenobiotica*, **6**, 531–6

127. Douch, P. G. C. and Blair, S. S. B. (1975). *Xenobiotica*, **5**, 279–92

128. Knowles, C. O. and Casida, J. E. (1966). *J. Agric. Food Chem.*, **14**, 566–72

129. Douch, P. G. C. (1975). *Xenobiotica*, **5**, 293–302, 401–6, 657–63, 773–80

130. Douch, P. G. C. (1976). *Xenobiotica*, **6**, 399–404

131. Douch, P. G. C. and Gahagan, H. M. (1977). *Xenobiotica*, **7**, 301–7

132. Douch, P. G. C. (1978). *Compar. Biochem. Physiol.*, **60B**, 63–6

133. Douch, P. G. C. and Gahagan, H. M. (1976). *Xenobiotica*, **6**, 769–73

134. Douch, P. G. C. and Gahagan, H. M. (1977). *Xenobiotica*, **7**, 309–14

135. Douch, P. G. C. (1978). *Xenobiotica*, **8**, 177–82

136. Kurelec, B. (1971). *Int. J. Biochem.*, **2**, 245–8

137. Douch, P. G. C. and Buchanan, L. L. (1978). *Xenobiotica*, **8**, 171–6

138. Dendinger, J. E. and Roberts, L. S. (1977). *Compar. Biochem. Physiol.*, **58B**, 215–9
139. Mead, R. W. and Roberts, L. S. (1972). *Compar. Biochem. Physiol.*, **41A**, 749–60
140. Pappas, P. W. and Gamble, H. R. (1978). *Exptl Parasitol.*, **79**, 256–61
141. Matthews, B. E. (1977). *Symp. Br. Soc. Parasitol.*, **15**, 93–119
142. Rogers, W. P. and Brooks, F. (1978). *Int. J. Parasitol.*, **8**, 449–52
143. Chen, S. and Howells, R. E. (1979). *Parasitology*, **78**, 343–54
144. Meyer, H., Nevaldine, B. and Meyer, F. (1978). *Biochemistry*, **17**, 1822–7, 1828–33
145. Briggs, M. H. (1972). *Biochim. Biophys. Acta*, **280**, 481–5
146. Krusberg, L. R. (1971). In *Plant Parasitic Nematodes*, vol. 2. Eds B. M. Zuckerman, W. F. Mai and R. A. Rohde, pp. 213–34. New York; Academic Press.
147. Lusier, P. E., Podesta, R. B. and Mettrick, D. F. (1978). *J. Parasitol.*, **64**, 1139–40
148. Brockelman, C. R. and Jackson, G. J. (1978). *J. Parasitol.*, **64**, 803–9
149. Moczoń, T. (1977). *Acta Parasitol. Polonica*, **24**, 275–82
150. Davey, K. G. (1971). *Int. J. Parasitol.*, **1**, 61–6; (1979). *ibid*, **9**, 121–5
151. Mansour, T. E., Lago, A. D. and Hawkins, J. L. (1957). *Federation Proc.*, **16**, 319
152. Guerra, A. (1968). *Federation Proc.*, **27**, 472

5 Metabolic Regulation

There are two separate aspects to metabolic control in parasitic helminths. First, there is regulation at the cellular level and, secondly, there is the regulation of metabolic changes that occur during the life-cycle of the parasite. In many ways, these are two rather different processes, although they both involve feedback mechanisms, in the one case allosteric, and in the other environmental and genetic.

Regulation of metabolic pathways at the cellular level is, of course, necessary for maximum economy. The rate of energy production must be closely matched to energy utilisation, so that the ATP/ADP ratio stays relatively constant, and the flux through the synthetic pathways has to be related to synthetic requirements. During their life-cycle, many helminths occupy widely differing environments, ranging from the free-living situation to the tissues of invertebrates and warm- and cold-blooded vertebrates (Chapter 1). The different life-cycle stages of helminths frequently show major differences in metabolism. The metabolic changes that occur during the life-cycle of helminths, and the environmental and genetic factors that control them, constitute what may be referred to as 'developmental' regulation.

5.1. CELLULAR REGULATION

Regulation at the cellular level comprises the ways in which the fluxes through the different metabolic pathways are controlled and also the mechanisms by which the activities of the different pathways, both catabolic and anabolic, are integrated.

5.1.1. General Theory

Metabolic regulation can be exerted at three different levels: first, at the level of each individual enzymatic step; secondly, at the level of the specialised regulatory enzymes; and, thirdly, by changes in the rate of enzyme synthesis. All enzymes respond to changes in pH, and the rates of reaction depend on the concentrations of the substrates and products and on the availability of cofactors. So, in a way, the activities of all the enzymes in a metabolic pathway are regulated. When the flux through the pathway alters, the actual activities of all of the enzymes involved change (i.e. their turnover numbers alter). However, certain enzymes are responsible for initiating the changes in the flux rate. These are the regulatory enzymes and, by responding to factors other than substrate concentration, they bring about the integration of metabolic pathways. There are two types of regulatory enzyme, allosteric enzymes and covalently modulated enzymes. In allosteric enzymes, the catalytic activity is modulated by specific metabolites which become bound, noncovalently, to sites on the enzyme distinct from the catalytic site. It is a feature of allosteric enzymes that they are polymeric and show sigmoidal kinetics. Covalently modulated enzymes exist in active and inactive forms and are interconverted by the action of other enzymes. Many covalently modulated enzymes are also allosteric.

Allosteric and covalently modulated enzymes can respond rapidly to metabolic changes in the cell, allosteric enzymes within seconds, and covalently modulated enzymes within minutes. In contrast, enzyme synthesis as a method of control may require hours or days and, as a consequence, regulation by enzyme synthesis is usually related to nutritional change.

A feature of metabolic regulation is biochemical homeostasis, that is, the intracellular metabolites are maintained at nearly constant levels, despite large changes in the flux rate. If the regulation of metabolic pathways depended solely on the availability of substrates or the removal of products, changes in the flux rate would be accompanied by large changes in metabolite levels. Instead, the regulatory enzymes, by responding to relatively small changes in specific metabolite levels, bring about large changes in flux rate without major changes in metabolite pool sizes. In general, the intracellular levels of metabolites are such that the catalytic and allosteric sites of enzymes are not saturated (metabolite concentrations being of the same order as K_m). So, altering metabolite levels brings about variations in catalytic activity and modulation of K_m is a more efficient method of regulation than altering V_{max}. In contrast, the intracellular concentrations of cofactors (ATP, NAD) are sufficiently high to saturate their binding sites (the concentrations being well in excess of K_m), so in this case it is not changes in cofactor levels which are important in modulation, but alterations in cofactor ratios (ATP/ADP, NAD/NADH).

Identification of Regulatory Points

Enzymes can be divided into two types, those that catalyse reactions in the cell which are close to their thermodynamic equilibrium and those that catalyse reactions which are far displaced from their equilibrium (non-equilibrium enzymes). The equilibrium constant for the reaction:

$$A + B \rightleftharpoons C + D$$

is defined as:

$$K' = \frac{[C]\ [D]}{[A]\ [B]}$$

The thermodynamic equilibrium constant (K_{eq}) is obtained if the concentrations of substrates and products approach infinite dilution or if thermodynamic activities are used in the equation instead of concentrations. Since the equilibrium constant is usually calculated from experiments where the reactants are not at infinite dilution, the constant is referred to as the apparent equilibrium constant (K'). If an enzyme has a high activity relative to the flux through the pathway, the ratio of products/substrates will approximate to K' of that reaction, that is, it will be a near-equilibrium enzyme. The reaction cannot, of course, be at equilibrium, since at equilibrium there would be no net flux through the system. On the other hand, if an enzyme has a low catalytic activity relative to the capacity of the rest of the enzymes in the sequence, the reaction it catalyses will be displaced from equilibrium. This arises because the enzyme does not have sufficient activity to bring substrates and products into equilibrium. Such non-equilibrium enzymes restrict the flux through the pathway and, as such, are potential control points.

A near-equilibrium enzyme may have a catalytic capacity one thousand times greater than the flux through the pathway. In order for such an enzyme to reduce the flux by half, its own activity would have to be reduced 2000 fold. On the other hand, any alteration in the catalytic capacity of a non-equilibrium enzyme, since it is rate-limiting, will immediately be reflected in changes in the flux rate. Non-equilibrium reactions thus constitute potential control points. There are two main experimental methods which have been used to identify the non-equilibrium reactions in metabolic pathways; comparison of the mass action ratio with the equilibrium constant and the measurement of maximal enzyme activities.

The steady-state contents of the substrates and products of a reaction can be measured in freeze clamped tissue and the mass action ratio (Γ) calculated. If the value of the mass action ratio is similar to that of the apparent equilibrium constant, it can be concluded that the reaction is near equilibrium in the cell. If, however, the mass action ratio is much smaller than the apparent equilibrium constant $(\Gamma/K' < 0.2)$, the reaction is far displaced from equilibrium in the cell and the enzyme is catalysing a non-equilibrium reaction.

Since non-equilibrium enzymes catalyse the rate-limiting steps in a metabolic sequence, they can also be identified from measurement of maximal enzyme activities. If the activities of all of the enzymes in a metabolic sequence are measured *in vitro*, the enzymes can then be classified into low- and high-activity groups. Enzymes of the low-activity group are then considered to be catalysing non-equilibrium reactions. In general, the difference in activities between these two groups of enzymes is 10 to 1000 fold. To use this approach, the enzymes must, of course, be assayed under optimal conditions. An enzyme with a high activity, however, need not necessarily catalyse a near-equilibrium reaction *in vivo*, because in the cell its activity may be greatly inhibited. So, enzyme activity data should, where possible, be compared with mass action ratio results, since the mass action ratio reflects more accurately the conditions *in vivo*. The actual rate-limiting enzyme in a pathway may, of course, change under different conditions. In glycolysis, for example, hexokinase may be the rate-limiting enzyme under certain conditions, phosphofructokinase under others. Both hexokinase and phosphofructokinase are regulatory enzymes, but by definition there can only be one rate-limiting enzyme in a pathway at any one time.

Mass action ratios and maximal enzyme activities have been used extensively to identify the potential control points in metabolic pathways. Potential control points can also be identified by supplementation and isotope equilibrium experiments. For example, in a pathway:

$$A \rightleftharpoons B \rightarrow C \rightleftharpoons D$$

if $B \rightarrow C$ is the regulatory step, D will be more readily synthesised from C than from A or B. Using isotopically labelled A, the specific activity of B will rise rapidly to that of A since this is a near-equilibrium enzyme. However, with non-equilibrium reactions the product is slow in reaching isotopic equilibrium with the substrate, and so C will only gradually reach isotopic equilibrium. By following the changes in specific activity of metabolites with time, the non-equilibrium steps can be identified. Experimentally, supplementation and isotope equilibrium experiments are difficult to interpret because cells may be differentially permeable to intermediates, and added compounds may be metabolised by more than one pathway.

Finally, it is possible to speculate on which reactions would be suitable regulatory points on the basis of their location in the pathway. The most likely control points are at the start of a sequence or immediately after a branch point in the pathway. In this way, long stretches of uncontrolled metabolism are avoided. Enzymes which catalyse reactions with large free-energy changes are also often, but not necessarily, non-equilibrium.

The non-equilibrium enzymes in a pathway have so far been referred to as potential regulatory enzymes or potential regulatory sites. To prove that such enzymes are indeed regulatory, the flux through the pathway must be altered and the changes in the steady-state concentrations of the substrates of the non-equilibrium enzymes measured. If the substrate concentration changes in the opposite direction to the flux (substrate concentration decreases whilst flux increases or vice versa), this indicates that the enzyme is regulatory. A change in substrate concentration in the opposite direction to the catalytic activity occurs because the enzyme is being modified by factors other than just substrate concentration. In order to do this, the flux through the pathway must be perturbed and, for pathways such as carbohydrate breakdown, this can be done by comparing active and resting tissue or by using aerobic and anaerobic conditions. This approach can, of course, only show that an enzyme is regulatory—it cannot be used to show that an enzyme is not regulatory.

The use of changes in flux and steady-state levels of intermediates to identify control points is extensively used in the study of electron transport and has led to the development by Chance and co-workers of the cross-over theorem. This states that, if a pathway is inhibited at a specific enzyme, the substrate content will increase, whilst the products decrease, so a 'cross-over' will occur. The cross-over theorem assumes conservation of intermediates, which occurs in the cytochrome chain where the components alter their oxidation/reduction states but not their concentrations. The cross-over theorem is not valid when applied to non-conserved reactions (i.e. when the levels of intermediates change) and so, in the case of regulatory enzymes in a metabolic sequence, changes in product content are irrelevant. All that is necessary to identify regulatory enzymes is to establish the non-equilibrium character of the reaction and show that the substrate content and flux rate change in opposite directions.

Once the regulatory enzymes have been identified, the effects of possible modulators can be tested on isolated enzymes and a control theory formulated. Unfortunately, the effects of modulators are often investigated without it first being established that the enzyme is in fact regulatory. A difficulty in this approach is to extrapolate the properties of isolated enzymes *in vitro* to the conditions in the cell. It is assumed that factors that influence activity *in vitro* are equally important *in vivo*. In most cases, studies *in vitro* involve enzyme concentrations of the order of 1 μg/ml. In the cell, enzyme concentrations can be as high as 1 mg/ml and this may constitute a major difference. Testing modulators can also be fraught with problems. If a coupled enzyme assay is being used, care must be taken to ensure that the modulators are not inhibiting the coupling enzymes, and the effects of activators and inhibitors are often dependent on the pH and on the nature of the activating metal ions. A further complication with some enzymes is that, whilst some compounds are activators, others are de-inhibitors, i.e. their effects are only noticeable when the enzyme is inhibited.

When a control theory has finally been formulated, it must then be tested; this is done by perturbing the system and seeing if the metabolite levels change in the predicted manner.

Compartmentation

A major problem in studying metabolic control is compartmentation within the cells of both enzymes and metabolites. Compartmentation itself is a control mechanism, pathways are kept separate and metabolites may be present in several independent pools. Differential centrifugation can give information on the intracellular distribution of enzymes, but determining the intracellular distribution of metabolites is much more difficult. Most methods of metabolite measurement give the total metabolite content and do not take into account the differential distribution between cytoplasm and mitochondria. The error in the measurement of metabolites which are primarily cytoplasmic, such as the glycolytic intermediates, is not large as the mitochondrial volume is relatively small (5–10% of the total cell volume). Attempts have been made to estimate the intramitochondrial levels of metabolites by making use of enzyme equilibria data. Recent rapid separation techniques have now made possible the direct measurement of intramitochondrial metabolite levels and these indicate large mitochondrial/cytoplasmic differences. In the cytoplasm, the ATP/ADP ratio is usually high, in the range 2–6, whilst in the mitochondrion the ratio is low, 0.5 or less, and the tricarboxylic acid cycle intermediates are present in much higher concentrations in the mitochondria than in the cytoplasm.

Isoenzymes

Many enzymes occur in multiple molecular forms, or isoenzymes, and these isoenzymes frequently differ in their kinetic and allosteric properties. Different tissues often contain different isoenzymes and, if the same enzyme occurs in separate cellular compartments of the same cell, it is usually present as different isoenzymes.

In many cases, the properties of the different isoenzymes can be related to their different metabolic functions in different tissues. When enzymes are investigated using whole homogenates or whole animal extracts, as is often the case with helminths, the different properties of the separate isoenzymes are masked.

Isoenzymes have been described in helminths for a number of enzymes, lactate dehydrogenase, malate dehydrogenase, glutamate dehydrogenase, pyruvate kinase, phosphoenolpyruvate carboxykinase and hexokinase, and certainly many more exist. In helminths, in addition to different isoenzymes being found in different cellular compartments and in different tissues, isoenzyme patterns also change during the course of the life-cycle (Section 5.2.1).

5.1.2. Control of Carbohydrate Catabolism in Helminths

In mammals, the regulatory enzymes have been identified and their properties investigated for most of the major catabolic and anabolic pathways. Control mechanisms in helminths have only recently begun to be investigated, although they are of great potential interest in chemotherapy. Studies on metabolic control in parasitic helminths have concentrated almost entirely on carbohydrate catabolism. With the exception of glycogen synthesis (Section 4.2.3), the control of synthetic pathways has not been investigated in helminths. This is despite the fact that the reduced synthetic capabilities of parasites could be due not so much to the absence of synthetic pathways but to inhibition of the pathways by exogenous nutrients (Section 4.10).

In some ways, the control mechanisms of helminths are simpler than those of mammals, as carbohydrate is the sole energy source in adult helminths and there is no appreciable lipid or amino acid catabolism. On the other hand, the pathways of carbohydrate breakdown in helminths are different from those in mammals and this presents new regulatory problems. In particular, many helminths have a branch point at phosphoenolpyruvate and the partial reverse tricarboxylic acid cycle has no counterpart in mammalian systems.

The regulation of carbohydrate catabolism in helminths can be considered in a number of separate units; glycolysis, the phosphoenolpyruvate branch point, the malate branch point and the tricarboxylic acid cycle.

5.1.3. Glycolysis

Measurements of the intracellular levels of the glycolytic intermediates have been made in *A. lumbricoides*[1], *F. hepatica*[2,3] and *M. expansa*[4] and the mass action ratios for the glycolytic enzymes in these helminths calculated. A comparison of the mass action ratios with the apparent equilibrium constants for the glycolytic enzymes in these parasites shows that the reactions catalysed by hexokinase, phosphofructokinase and pyruvate kinase are all displaced from equilibrium. The reactions catalysed by phosphoglucomutase, glucose-phosphate isomerase, aldolase, triose-phosphate isomerase, phosphoglyceromutase and phosphopyruvate hydratase,

Table 5.1 The mass action ratios of glycolytic enzymes in parasitic helminths

Enzyme	Apparent equilibrium constant	Mass action ratio		
		A. lumbricoides[1]	F. hepatica[2,3]	M. expansa[4]
Hexokinase	5.5×10^3	—	0.4	0.02
Phosphogluco-mutase	5.5×10^{-2}	7×10^{-2}	—	--
Glucose-phosphate isomerase	0.47	0.16	0.20	0.44
Phosphofructo-kinase	1.2×10^3	0.11	0.16	0.48
Aldolase	6.8×10^{-5} M	8.5×10^{-5} M	3.7×10^{-6} M	3.3×10^{-6} M
Triose-phosphate isomerase	4×10^{-2}	4.7×10^{-2}	2.9×10^{-1}	3.1×10^{-1}
Phosphoglycero-mutase	0.1	0.09	0.11	0.16
Phosphopyruvate hydratase	4.6	2.6	3.3	1.22
Phosphoglycero-mutase + phospho-pyruvate hydratase	0.5	0.46	0.36	0.20
Pyruvate kinase	15×10^3	7.0	1.35	1.66

Superscripts are to references at end of this chapter.

on the other hand, are all near equilibrium (*Table 5.1*). In *M. expansa* and *F. hepatica*, the aldolase reaction appears to be slightly displaced from equilibrium, but the combined aldolase/triose-phosphate isomerase reaction is near equilibrium. A similar situation has been found in mammalian tissues, and the apparent non-equilibrium position of aldolase is thought to be due to technical problems in the assays. Glyceraldehyde-3-phosphate dehydrogenase has a relatively high activity in helminths. For this reason, it is assumed to catalyse a near-equilibrium reaction and the glyceraldehyde-3-phosphate dehydrogenase equilibrium has been used to estimate the cytoplasmic free $[NAD^+]/[NADH]$ ratio in *A. lumbricoides* muscle[5]. In mammals, glyceraldehyde-3-phosphate dehydrogenase is also thought to catalyse a near-equilibrium reaction, although the mammalian enzyme is allosterically modulated by NAD. The significance, if any, of this modulation in the control of glycolysis is not known.

The non-equilibrium enzymes of glycolysis in *A. lumbricoides, F. hepatica* and *M. expansa* are thus hexokinase, phosphofructokinase and pyruvate kinase, and these are, therefore, potential regulatory sites. Measurement of maximal activities of the glycolytic enzymes in a variety of helminths again indicates that phosphory-lase, hexokinase and phosphofructokinase are the rate-limiting enzymes as they are in all other glycolytic systems which have been studied in detail. A relationship frequently found in helminths (and other animals) is that the sum of the maximal activities of hexokinase and phosphorylase in the tissues is equal to the maximal activity of phosphofructokinase.

Hexokinase controls the activation of glucose, not only for entry into glycolysis but also for catabolism via the pentose phosphate pathway and for synthetic reactions (the formation of glycogen and complex polysaccharides). Phosphorylase similarly controls the activation of glycogen for catabolism via glycolysis or the pentose phosphate pathway and for synthetic reactions. The control of glycolysis from glucose involves hexokinase and phosphofructokinase, and the control of glycolysis from glycogen uses phosphorylase and phosphofructokinase.

The key regulatory role of phosphofructokinase in glycolysis has been confirmed in *M. expansa* by showing that, when the glycolytic flux rate was increased by the addition of glucose to the incubation medium, the levels of fructose-6-phosphate decreased, i.e. the substrate level and the flux rate changed in opposite directions[4]. Phosphofructokinase has also been shown to be the rate-limiting enzyme in *S. mansoni* by supplementation experiments.

The regulatory properties of hexokinase, phosphorylase and phosphofructokinase have been looked at in several helminths.

Hexokinase

In mammals, hexokinase is inhibited by its product, glucose-6-phosphate; inhibition of phosphofructokinase leads to an increase in fructose-6-phosphate and glucose-6-phosphate and so the phosphorylation of glucose is inhibited. The hexokinases of *A. lumbricoides*[6], *D. immitis*[7] and *H. diminuta*[8] are all inhibited by glucose-6-phosphate, as are the glucokinase and mannokinase enzymes of *S. mansoni*. In *E. granulosus* scoleces, the glucokinase, fructokinase and mannokinase enzymes are inhibited by glucose-6-phosphate, whilst mannose-6-phosphate inhibits mannokinase and galactokinase.

Product inhibition of hexokinase limits the conversion of glucose to glycogen. In mammalian liver, this problem is overcome by having another enzyme, glucokinase, which has a lower affinity for glucose, but is not inhibited by glucose-6-phosphate. Glucokinases proper have not been described in helminths, but K_i of helminth hexokinase for glucose-6-phosphate is an order of magnitude larger than that of the mammalian enzyme. So, the hexokinases of *A. lumbricoides*[6], *D. immitis*[7] and *H. diminuta*[8] are much less sensitive to glucose-6-phosphate inhibition than is the mammalian enzyme, and this may overcome the potential bottleneck in glycogen synthesis. A glucose-6-phosphate insensitive glucokinase has, however, recently been described from the nematode *A. cantonensis*[61].

Both mammalian and *A. lumbricoides* hexokinase and the glucokinase of *S. mansoni* are inhibited by high levels of ADP, but this is not thought to be physiologically significant. In mammals, hexokinase exists as a number of isoenzymes. Mammalian hexokinase also occurs both in the cytoplasm and bound to the endoplasmic reticulum. Three isoenzymes of hexokinase have been reported in *D. immitis*[7], and the hexokinase of *A. lumbricoides*, like the mammalian enzyme, occurs in both soluble and membrane-bound forms[9]. It has been suggested that the reversible binding of hexokinase and other glycolytic enzymes to cell membranes may be involved in regulation, but this has not been established.

Phosphorylase

The regulation of phosphorylase in mammalian tissues involves the enzymatic inter-conversion of a high-activity form, phosphorylase *a*, and a low-activity form, phosphorylase *b*. The conversion of phosphorylase *b* to phosphorylase *a* is regulated by phosphorylase *b* kinase, which itself is controlled by a 3′,5′-cyclic-AMP dependent protein kinase. In addition, phosphorylase *b* is modulated by ATP, inorganic phosphate, glucose-6-phosphate and AMP. The control of mammalian phosphoryl-ase is summarised in *Figure 5.1*. Despite the fact that glycogen is the major, and

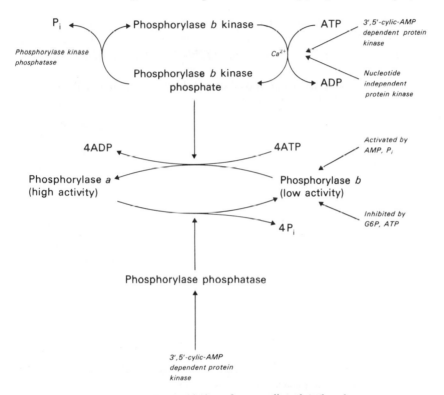

Figure 5.1 The regulation of mammalian phosphorylase.

probably the sole, energy reserve in helminths, the regulation of glycogen phos-phorylase has received relatively little attention. In *S. mansoni*, phosphorylase exists in active and inactive forms, and there is evidence for the interconversion of these forms via a phosphorylase kinase and a fluoride-sensitive phosphatase[10]. The glycogen phosphorylase of *S. mansoni* is also stimulated by AMP. The anthelmintic niridazole causes glycogen depletion in *S. mansoni* and this is the result of inhibition of phosphorylase phosphatase. In niridazole-treated worms, the glycogen phosphory-lase remains permanently active so the schistosome catabolises all its glycogen reserves. Niridazole also inhibits mammalian phosphorylase phosphatase, but to a much lesser extent[10]. The glycogen phosphorylase of *F. hepatica* exists in active and inactive forms; activation is stimulated by 3′,5′-cyclic-AMP and the activity of the enzyme is increased by AMP[63,67]. In adult *H. diminuta*, the phosphorylase is also stimulated by AMP. The cysticercoids of *H. diminuta* have *a* and *b* forms of phosphorylase and their interconversion is regulated by a 3′,5′-cyclic-AMP dependent protein kinase and a phosphorylase phosphatase[11]. So, most of the features of the control mechanism of mammalian phosphorylase seem to occur in helminth systems.

Phosphofructokinase

The key regulatory enzyme in glycolysis is undoubtedly phosphofructokinase and, to date, some 27 different compounds have been described as modulators for this enzyme in mammalian and bacterial systems (*Table 5.2*). These modulators can be

Table 5.2   Modulators of phosphofructokinase from mammalian and bacterial sources

Inhibitors	Activators*	De-inhibitors†
ATP	5′-AMP	5′-AMP
Citrate	3′,5′-cyclic-AMP	3′,5′-cyclic-AMP
Isocitrate	ADP	ADP
Succinate	NH_4^+	NH_4^+
Malate	K^+	SO_4^{2-}
Mg^{2+}	Inorganic phosphate	Inorganic phosphate
Ca^{2+}	Fructose-1,6-bisP	Fructose-6-P
Pyrophosphate	Aspartate	Fructose-1,6-bisP
Phosphocreatine		Glucose-1,6-bisP
3-P-glycerate		Mannose-1,6-bisP
2-P-glycerate		
2,3-bisP-glycerate		
Phosphoenolpyruvate		
6-P-gluconate		
3′,5′-cyclic-GMP		
Oleate		

*Activators increase activity at non-inhibitory levels of ATP.
†De-inhibitors increase activity at inhibitory levels of ATP.

grouped into inhibitors, activators (compounds which increase activity at non-inhibitory ATP levels) and de-inhibitors (which increase activity at inhibitory ATP levels). Some compounds can act both as activators of phosphofructokinase and as de-inhibitors. Different modulators are effective in different organisms, and modulation can depend on the pH and on the type of buffer system. However, with the exception of some micro-organisms such as *Entamoeba histolytica*, which have unregulated phosphofructokinases, the main regulatory features that appear common to all phosphofructokinases are as follows:

(1) Inhibition by high ATP levels; this is accompanied by a decreased affinity for fructose-6-phosphate.

(2) At inhibitory ATP levels, citrate inhibits.

(3) The ATP and citrate inhibition is relieved by AMP, fructose-1,6-bisphosphate and 3',5'-cyclic-AMP.

(4) At inhibitory levels of ATP, increasing the concentration of fructose-6-phosphate has a cooperative effect on the enzyme.

In parasitic helminths, the regulatory properties of phosphofructokinase have been investigated in some detail in three species, *S. mansoni*, *F. hepatica* and *M. expansa*. In *S. mansoni*, the enzyme is inhibited by ATP and this is increased by citrate. The ATP inhibition is relieved by fructose-6-phosphate, ADP, AMP, 3',5'-cyclic-AMP, inorganic phosphate, NH_4^+ and SO_4^{2-}, but these modulators did not, however, activate the enzyme at non-inhibitory ATP levels. In mammalian systems, ADP, inorganic phosphate, AMP, 3',5'-cyclic-AMP and NH_4^+ are all potent activators of phosphofructokinase, as well as being de-inhibitors. Relatively high levels of citrate are required to inhibit *S. mansoni* phosphofructokinase and this apparent inhibition could be due to chelation of Mg^{2+} ions by citrate. High concentrations of ADP, AMP and 3',5'-cyclic-AMP inhibit *S. mansoni* phosphofructokinase, but a similar inhibition of mammalian phosphofructokinase by these nucleotides has not been reported. Some plant phosphofructokinases are, however, inhibited by high levels of ADP and to a lesser extent by AMP. The phosphofructokinase of *S. mansoni* is some 60 to 80 times more sensitive to inhibition by trivalent organic antimonial compounds than is the enzyme from mammalian tissues. This may form the basis for the use of antimony compounds in the treatment of schistosomiasis. The effect of trivalent antimonials on *S. mansoni* phosphofructokinase is reversible and probably involves interaction with a fructose-6-phosphate site on the enzyme. The phosphofructokinases from *D. viteae*, *B. pahangi* and *L. carinii* show a similar high sensitivity to antimony, and the enzymes from *A. lumbricoides* and *H. diminuta* are only slightly less sensitive[12].

The phosphofructokinase of *M. expansa*[13] is inhibited by ATP, and this inhibition is relieved by fructose-6-phosphate, AMP and NH_4^+. The enzyme is also inhibited by Ca^{2+} and activated by NH_4^+ and AMP. Both ITP and GTP can act as substrates for *M. expansa* phosphofructokinase (as they can for the mammalian enzyme) and, unlike ATP, high levels of these two triphosphates are not inhibitory either to mammalian or *M. expansa* phosphofructokinase.

In *F. hepatica*, the phosphofructokinase is again inhibited by ATP, and this inhibition is relieved by AMP and fructose-6-phosphate. The enzyme is also activated by 3',5'-cyclic-AMP. The phosphofructokinase of *F. hepatica* can be extracted in active and inactive forms. The inactive enzyme is converted to the active form by incubation with 3',5'-cyclic-AMP, which also modulates the active enzyme[14]. Activation of the enzyme can be reversed by dialysis and this is accompanied by dissociation of the enzyme into sub-units. The activation and deactivation of the phosphofructokinase from *F. hepatica* does not, therefore, involve phosphorylation of the enzyme (since it is reversible by dialysis) and so is not protein kinase dependent. Phosphofructokinase from mammalian sources can also be isolated in active and inactive forms, and inactivation of the mammalian enzyme is again accompanied by dissociation into sub-units. This inactivation can be prevented or reversed by a variety of compounds including ATP and sulphydryl protecting agents. The activation of the inactive mammalian phosphofructokinase, like the *F. hepatica* enzyme, does not involve phosphorylation of the enzyme and it is not thought to be of physiological significance. There is some evidence, though, that the phosphofructokinase of yeast may exist in interconvertible phosphorylated and dephosphorylated *a* and *b* forms.

Apart from *M. expansa*, *F. hepatica* and *S. mansoni*, little work has been done on other helminth phosphofructokinases. The enzyme from *D. dendriticum* is inhibited by ATP and this inhibition is relieved by AMP[15]. The phosphofructokinases of *A. lumbricoides* and *T. pisiformis* are activated by 3',5'-cyclic-AMP, and the enzyme from *A. lumbricoides*[16] is also activated by K^+ and NH_4^+.

In general, the phosphofructokinases of parasitic helminths show the main regulatory features found in other phosphofructokinases, namely, inhibition by ATP and relief of this inhibition by fructose-6-phosphate, AMP and 3',5'-cyclic-AMP. In addition, K^+, NH_4^+ and ADP have all been found to be activators in different helminth systems.

In mammals, modulation of phosphofructokinase by citrate coordinates the glycolytic and tricarboxylic acid cycle fluxes. The phosphofructokinase from *S. mansoni* is inhibited by citrate, and this is of interest since the tricarboxylic acid cycle is of little importance in this parasite. Whether or not helminth phosphofructokinases are also modulated by metabolites such as phosphoenolpyruvate, malate or succinate, as they are in some other organisms, has not yet been investigated. Control of phosphofructokinase by succinate or malate could serve to integrate glycolysis with the reverse tricarboxylic acid cycle, in the same way that citrate integrates the classical tricarboxylic acid cycle with glycolysis. Similarly, control via phosphoenolpyruvate could be of significance in helminths where phosphoenolpyruvate forms a branch point in catabolism. The ability of ITP and GTP to replace ATP as a substrate for *M. expansa* phosphofructokinase is interesting in view of the fact that the phosphoenolpyruvate carboxykinase reaction is one of the major energy-producing steps in this and many other gastrointestinal helminths (Section 3.1.4). The phosphoenolpyruvate carboxykinase reaction results, of course, in the formation of ITP or GTP and not ATP.

Fructose-1,6-bisphosphatase

The phosphofructokinase step is essentially irreversible; the enzyme fructose-1,6-bisphosphatase catalyses the reaction:

$$\text{fructose-1,6-bisphosphate} \rightarrow \text{fructose-6-phosphate} + P_i$$

In gluconeogenic tissues, this reaction bypasses the energy barrier of the phosphofructokinase reaction. Fructose-1,6-bisphosphatase also occurs in muscle tissue, where it may form a substrate cycle with phosphofructokinase (Section 4.2.1). In mammals, fructose-1,6-bisphosphatase is inhibited by AMP; phosphofructokinase, on the other hand, is activated by AMP. By having a substrate cycle, the sensitivity of the system to AMP is thereby greatly increased.

Fructose-1,6-bisphosphatase is found in parasitic helminths (*A. lumbricoides, D. dendriticum, F. hepatica, S. solidus*), and the enzyme from *D. dendriticum, F. hepatica* and *A. lumbricoides* eggs has been shown to be inhibited by AMP. High levels of fructose-1,6-bisphosphate also inhibit the enzyme from *D. dendriticum* and *F. hepatica*, and the fructose-1,6-bisphosphatase of mammals is similarly inhibited by substrate. In addition, the mammalian enzyme is said to be modulated by citrate and 3-phosphoglycerate, as well as being under endocrinal control. It has also been suggested that both phosphofructokinase and fructose-1,6-bisphosphatase might be regulated by a phosphorylation–dephosphorylation cycle.

5.1.4. Pyruvate Kinase/Phosphoenolpyruvate Carboxykinase Branch Point

In many helminths, phosphoenolpyruvate is an important branch point, leading either via pyruvate kinase to pyruvate, or else via phosphoenolpyruvate carboxykinase to oxaloacetate and the reverse tricarboxylic acid cycle. Alterations in the incubation conditions of parasitic helminths *in vitro*, in particular varying the amount of oxygen, usually leads to changes in the nature of the end-products from carbohydrate catabolism. The changes in end-products can be correlated with changes in the relative flux rates through pyruvate kinase and phosphoenolpyruvate carboxykinase.

Pyruvate Kinase

As discussed above, pyruvate kinase appears to catalyse a non-equilibrium reaction and is, therefore, a potential regulatory enzyme. The position of pyruvate kinase, immediately after a branch point, would again suggest that it should be a regulatory site. The next enzyme in the sequence, lactate dehydrogenase, catalyses a near-equilibrium reaction and is not involved in controlling the flux through the pathway[17] (fructose-1,6-bisphosphate activated lactate dehydrogenases have, however, been found in micro-organisms). In *H. diminuta*, the major lactate dehydrogenase isoenzyme is inhibited by excess pyruvate[18] (heart-type LDH), and this presumably prevents the accumulation of excessive amounts of lactate. The specificity of lactate dehydrogenase for L(+)- or D(−)-lactate differs in different groups of invertebrates. The lactate dehydrogenases from *A. lumbricoides, H. contortus, H. diminuta* and *F. hepatica* are specific for L(+)-lactate, the enzyme from *M. dubius* for D(−)-lactate.

Measurement of the maximal activities of helminth pyruvate kinases does not put them clearly into the low-activity group, as would be expected for a rate-limiting enzyme. In mammalian tissues, pyruvate kinase also shows this anomalous behaviour in having a relatively high activity and yet catalysing a non-equilibrium reaction. This may be related to the occurrence of multiple kinetic forms (isoenzymes) of pyruvate kinase in tissues.

Possible modulators of helminth pyruvate kinase have been extensively investigated, particularly in *F. hepatica, H. diminuta* and *M. expansa*, and the results are summarised in *Table 5.3*. One problem is that the effects of modulators on pyruvate kinase (and phosphoenolpyruvate carboxykinase) are strongly dependent on pH and

Table 5.3 Modulators of helminth pyruvate kinases

Species	Activators	Inhibitors	No effect
Hymenolepis diminuta[21,22]			
Isoenzyme I (restricted to adult)	–	HCO_3^-, lactate	FBP, G6P, ATP, alanine, citrate, succinate, malate, glutamate, proline
Isoenzymes II, III, IV, V	FBP	ATP, Ca^{2+}	Alanine
Moniezia expansa[13,23]			
Isoenzyme I	–	–	FBP
Isoenzyme II	FBP	ATP, malate	Succinate, oxaloacetate, fumarate, alanine, lactate
Ligula intestinalis[28] (plerocercoid)	FBP	ATP, malate	Alanine
Fasciola hepatica[24]	FBP	ATP, malate	Alanine, fumarate, succinate, HCO_3^-
Dicrocoelium dendriticum[25]	FBP	ATP, malate	–
Schistosoma mansoni[26]	–	–	FBP, ATP
Microphallus similis[20] (sporocyst)	FBP	ATP, alanine	–
Haemonchus contortus[27]	FBP	Malate	–
Litomosoides carinii[26]	FBP	ATP	–
Dirofilaria immitis[26]	FBP	ATP	–

Superscripts are to references at end of this chapter.

metal ions. So, the effects depend both on the metal ion used and the buffer system; which cation is active *in vivo* (Mg^{2+}, Mn^{2+} or Zn^{2+}) is not known. Mammalian and helminth pyruvate kinases both require K^+ for maximal activity.

In mammals, there are two types of pyruvate kinase; the isoenzyme from muscle is inhibited by ATP, whilst the isoenzyme from liver and from the muscles of diving mammals is activated by fructose-1,6-bisphosphate and inhibited by alanine and ATP. The modulation of liver pyruvate kinase by fructose-1,6-bisphosphate, alanine and ATP is related to the control of glyconeogenesis from lactate or other metabolic intermediates. The modulation of muscle pyruvate kinase by fructose-1,6-bisphosphate and alanine in diving mammals is related to regulation during anaerobic conditions. The pyruvate kinases from muscles of free-living invertebrates appear to be similar to the pyruvate kinase of diving mammals, although not all of them are inhibited by alanine[19].

In parasites, the major precursor of glycogen is absorbed glucose, and glyconeogenesis from amino acids or other metabolic intermediates is probably less important. The modulation of pyruvate kinase in helminths is concerned primarily with the regulation of metabolic end-products rather than glyconeogenesis. In this context, it is interesting that alanine, an important glyconeogenic substrate in mammals, is a powerful inhibitor of the mammalian liver enzyme. But, with the exception of the sporocysts of *M. similis*[20], alanine is not a modulator in helminth systems.

Both fructose-1,6-bisphosphate sensitive and fructose-1,6-bisphosphate insensitive isoenzymes of pyruvate kinase are found in *H. diminuta* and *M. expansa*. The fructose-1,6-bisphosphate insensitive enzymes of these helminths differ from the mammalian muscle isoenzyme in being insensitive to ATP as well. The pyruvate kinase of *S. mansoni* is also fructose-1,6-bisphosphate and ATP insensitive; this helminth is a homolactic fermenter and so may not need to modulate its pyruvate kinase. All of the other helminths so far investigated have pyruvate kinases which are activated by fructose-1,6-bisphosphate and inhibited by ATP. Isoenzymes of pyruvate kinase have not, however, been investigated in helminths other than *H. diminuta* and *M. expansa*; and so parasites which have fructose-1,6-bisphosphate sensitive pyruvate kinases may also have fructose-1,6-bisphosphate insensitive isoenzymes as well.

In addition to fructose-1,6-bisphosphate and ATP, lactate, malate, alanine, calcium and bicarbonate have all been described as modulators of pyruvate kinase from different helminths (*Table 5.3*). There is, however, no consistent pattern. Malate inhibits pyruvate kinase from *M. expansa, L. intestinalis, F. hepatica, D. dendriticum* and *H. contortus* but has no effect in *H. diminuta*; lactate and bicarbonate inhibit the pyruvate kinase from *H. diminuta* but are without effect in *M. expansa* or *F. hepatica*. Mammalian pyruvate kinase is also inhibited by excess magnesium, ADP and phosphoenolpyruvate.

Phosphoenolpyruvate Carboxykinase

The equilibrium position of the phosphoenolpyruvate carboxykinase reaction is not clear. In mammalian tissues, phosphoenolpyruvate carboxykinase is thought to be the rate-limiting enzyme in glyconeogenesis. However, its non-equilibrium nature has not been established and no physiological modulators of the enzyme are known. In the mammal, phosphoenolpyruvate carboxykinase activity is controlled primarily by synthesis, although there are reports of a possible protein regulator.

In parasitic helminths, phosphoenolpyruvate carboxykinase catalyses the reverse reaction, that is, oxaloacetate formation, rather than phosphoenolpyruvate formation as in mammals. The only helminth systems so far investigated are *A. lumbricoides* and *F. hepatica* and, in both, phosphoenolpyruvate carboxykinase appears to be catalysing a non-equilibrium reaction[3,5]. Determination of the mass action ratio of phosphoenolpyruvate carboxykinase requires the measurement of tissue oxaloacetate levels and a knowledge of the pCO_2. Both of these can be subject to considerable error, and so the non-equilibrium nature of the phosphoenolpyruvate carboxykinase reaction in helminths is still open to question.

Phosphoenolpyruvate carboxykinase might be expected to be a regulatory enzyme on theoretical grounds, since it is situated immediately after a branch point. The next enzyme in the sequence, malate dehydrogenase, catalyses a near-equilibrium reaction and is not involved in controlling the flux through the branch[17].

Like pyruvate kinase, phosphoenolpyruvate carboxykinase does not fall into the low-activity group as would be expected for a regulatory enzyme. Again, this may be related to the presence of isoenzymes. Phosphoenolpyruvate occurs in both the cytoplasm and mitochondria and there is considerable species variation in the relative intracellular distribution of the enzyme. In parasitic helminths, phospho-enolpyruvate carboxykinase tends to be predominantly cytoplasmic and, in *M. ex-pansa*, the cytoplasmic and mitochondrial isoenzymes appear to have similar properties[29].

Table 5.4   Modulators of helminth phosphoenolpyruvate carboxykinases

Species	Activators	Inhibitors	No effect
Hymenolepis diminuta[21]	HCO_3^-	Lactate	G6P, FBP, citrate, suc-cinate, alanine, malate, glutamate, proline
Moniezia expansa[13] Isoenzymes I, II	–	ATP, ITP	AMP, ADP, FBP, NH_4^+, pyruvate, fumarate, suc-cinate, malate
Fasciola hepatica[24]	NADH	ATP, ITP, citrate (in the presence of Zn^{2+})	AMP, $3',5'$-AMP, fum-arate, succinate, pyruvate
Haemonchus contortus[27]	NADH, malate	–	–

Superscripts are to references at end of this chapter.

In contrast to pyruvate kinase, very few modulators of phosphoenolpyruvate carboxykinase have been described in helminths (*Table 5.4*) but again there is no consistent pattern. Bicarbonate ions activate the phosphoenolpyruvate carboxy-kinase of *H. diminuta*, whilst NADH activates the enzyme from *F. hepatica* and *H. contortus*. Amongst possible modulators of the enzyme from various helminths are lactate, citrate, ATP and ITP. The phosphoenolpyruvate carboxykinases of free-living invertebrates (molluscs and coelenterates) are also inhibited by ITP but, in many cases, this inhibition is relieved by alanine[30]. In micro-organisms, a whole range of activators for phosphoenolpyruvate carboxykinase have been described (fructose-1, 6-bisphosphate, acetyl-CoA, fatty acids, fatty acyl-CoA, aspartate).

Control of the Branch Point

On the basis of the known modulators of pyruvate kinase and phosphoenolpyruvate carboxykinase in helminths, no overall scheme for the control of the phosphoenol-pyruvate branch point can be formalised. Different metabolites act as modulators in different helminths, although, as the tables show, the list of effectors which have been tried on the different species is not comprehensive. It is, nevertheless, possible in one or two species to postulate control mechanisms for the branch point. In *M. expansa*, anaerobiosis leads to an increase in lactate production, and this is accom-panied by a fall in the intracellular levels of malate[31]. Malate is an inhibitor of pyruvate kinase in *M. expansa*, so the fall in malate levels would result in an increase in pyruvate kinase activity leading to a rise in lactate production. Malate is also a modulator in *D. dendriticum* and *H. contortus*. In *H. contortus*, malate may have a dual role, activating phosphoenolpyruvate carboxykinase and inhibiting pyruvate kinase. Unfortunately, there is no information on the changes in the intracellular malate pool in *H. contortus* under aerobic and anaerobic conditions. The phosphoenolpyruvate carboxykinase from *H. contortus* is also activated by NADH, as is the enzyme from *F. hepatica*. So, in these two helminths, the fall in the NAD/NADH ratio, which accompanies anaerobiosis, will stimulate carbon dioxide fixation. Finally, in *H. diminuta*, bicarbonate has a reciprocal effect, inhibiting pyruvate kinase and activating phosphoenolpyruvate carboxykinase. The phosphoenolpyruvate branch point in this parasite may be regulated by the concentration of carbon dioxide[21]. The pyruvate kinase/phosphoenolpyruvate carboxykinase switch would, therefore, appear to be controlled by different effectors in different helminths and, interestingly, the same conclusion seems to apply to molluscs, where again phosphoenolpyruvate is an important branch point.

In molluscs, pyruvate kinase and phosphoenolpyruvate carboxykinase have essentially non-overlapping pH profiles, pyruvate kinase having an optimum in the range pH 7.5–8.5, phosphoenolpyruvate carboxykinase in the region pH 5.5–6.5 (the pH optimum for both enzymes depending on the metal ion). It has been proposed in molluscs that pH is, in fact, the key regulator of the phosphoenolpyruvate branch point. When molluscs become anaerobic, acidic end-products accumulate, the tissue pH falls and so there is a decrease in pyruvate kinase activity and an increase in phosphoenolpyruvate carboxykinase activity. In parasitic helminths, the pH profiles of pyruvate kinase and phosphoenolpyruvate carboxykinase do not show such a clear separation and in *H. diminuta* it has been concluded that pH changes, within the physiological range, would not lead to any appreciable change in the relative activities of the two enzymes[21].

In helminths, pyruvate kinase has a higher affinity for phosphoenolpyruvate than does phosphoenolpyruvate carboxykinase, and there is usually a four- to fivefold difference in $K_{m \ PEP}$ between the two enzymes. So, under normal conditions, pyruvate kinase may be saturated with phosphoenolpyruvate and the flux through pyruvate kinase controlled by effectors (in particular, fructose-1,6-bisphosphate and ATP). Phosphoenolpyruvate carboxykinase, on the other hand, may not be saturated with phosphoenolpyruvate, the intracellular levels of phosphoenolpyruvate being of the same order as K_m. The flux through phosphoenolpyruvate carboxykinase and phosphoenolpyruvate carboxykinase may be modified by a phosphorylation–dephosphorylation mechanism similar to the phosphorylase kinase system. enolpyruvate carboxykinase.

In mammalian liver, there is some evidence that the activity of both pyruvate kinase and phosphoenolpyruvate carboxykinase may be modified by a phosphorylation–dephosphorylation mechanism similar to the phosphorylase kinase system. Whether the phosphoenolpyruvate branch point of helminths could similarly be regulated by a protein kinase dependent phosphorylation of pyruvate kinase and phosphoenolpyruvate carboxykinase has yet to be investigated.

5.1.5. Malate Branch Point

In helminths such as *A. lumbricoides* and *H. diminuta*, malate is another important branch point in catabolism, being either oxidised via the malic enzyme to pyruvate or else, via its equilibrium with fumarate, reduced to succinate (Section 3.1.3).

On theoretical grounds, one would expect the malic enzyme and either fumarase or fumarate reductase to be regulatory enzymes, since they are situated immediately after a branch point. However, in *A. lumbricoides*, the activity of all three enzymes is relatively high, so they do not appear to be rate-limiting. There are no known modulators of fumarase and it almost certainly catalyses a near-equilibrium reaction. Similarly, no modulators have been described for fumarate reductase. The reduction of fumarate to succinate is, however, coupled to the phosphorylation of ADP and so may be regulated by the availability of ADP and P_i. The malic enzyme also appears to be a near-equilibrium enzyme in *A. lumbricoides* and has been used to estimate the mitochondrial free $[NAD^+]/[NADH]$ ratio[5].

The malic enzyme from *A. lumbricoides* is, however, activated by fumarate and inhibited by pyruvate, oxaloacetate and volatile fatty acids (2-methylbutyrate, 2-methylvalerate and tiglate), but it was not affected by ATP nor NADH[32,33]. So, if volatile fatty acids accumulate, the pathway will be inhibited. In contrast, the NAD-linked malic enzyme of mammalian mitochondria is inhibited by ATP, as is the enzyme from insects and molluscs. Some molluscan malic enzymes are also inhibited by alanine and NADPH. Although there is no evidence that the malic enzyme from *A. lumbricoides* is displaced from equilibrium, it is modulated in an apparently adaptive manner. However, it is not sensitive to either the energy level or the redox state of the cell (i.e. it is not modulated by NADH or ATP).

In helminths, the dismutation of malate involves the transport across the inner mitochondrial membrane of malate, reducing equivalents (NADH) and also probably fumarate. So, it is possible that the control of the malate branch point may take place at the level of these transport mechanisms.

5.1.6. The Tricarboxylic Acid Cycle

The entry of carbohydrate into the tricarboxylic acid cycle is controlled by the pyruvate dehydrogenase complex and, in mammals, this enzyme exists in active and inactive forms. The active form is inactivated by a protein kinase dependent phosphorylation, and the inactive phosphorylated enzyme activated via a phosphatase. Interconversion of the active and inactive forms of mammalian pyruvate dehydrogenase is regulated by the ratios of acetyl-CoA/CoA, NAD/NADH and ATP/ADP, as well as the concentrations of pyruvate, thiamine pyrophosphate and metal ions. The active form of pyruvate dehydrogenase is also inhibited by NADH, acetoin and acetyl-CoA. A pyruvate dehydrogenase complex has been demonstrated in a number of parasitic helminths (*H. diminuta, S. solidus, F. hepatica, A. lumbricoides*). The classical tricarboxylic acid cycle is not, however, important in these helminths, and the main function of pyruvate dehydrogenase in parasites is probably in the formation of acetate. Modulation of the pyruvate dehydrogenase complex may, therefore, be involved together with pyruvate kinase and phosphoenolpyruvate carboxykinase in controlling the nature of the end-products from carbohydrate breakdown.

Regulation of the pyruvate dehydrogenase complex has not been investigated in helminths, although there is evidence that the pyruvate dehydrogenase of *A. lumbricoides* does exist in active and inactive forms[34].

In the tricarboxylic acid cycle of mammals, at least four enzymes are under regulatory control: citrate synthase, NAD-linked isocitrate dehydrogenase, 2-oxoglutarate decarboxylase and succinate dehydrogenase. The equilibrium nature of these four reactions has, however, not been established. In mammals, citrate synthase is inhibited by ATP, NADH, fatty acyl-CoA and citrate (the inhibition by ATP may be non-physiological); NAD-linked isocitrate dehydrogenase is activated by ADP and inhibited by ATP and NADH (and by Ca^{2+} in muscle); 2-oxoglutarate decarboxylase is inhibited by high NAD/NADH ratios and high succinyl-CoA/CoA ratios; and succinate dehydrogenase is strongly inhibited by oxaloacetate. In helminths, modulators of citrate synthase and 2-oxoglutarate decarboxylase have not been studied. The modulators of bacterial citrate synthase can be correlated with the metabolic fate of citrate. Modulators of the bacterial enzyme from different sources include acetyl-CoA, 2-oxoglutarate, oxaloacetate and AMP, in addition to ATP, NADH, citrate and fatty acyl-CoA. In parasitic helminths, the tricarboxylic acid cycle has a low activity, and a study of the regulatory properties of citrate synthase might give some indication as to the metabolic fate of citrate.

Isocitrate Dehydrogenase

The NAD-linked isocitrate dehydrogenases of helminths (*A. lumbricoides, H. contortus*) are, like the mammalian enzyme, activated by ADP. In general, helminths contain very little NAD-linked isocitrate dehydrogenase, most of the isocitrate dehydrogenase being NADP-linked. There is, however, growing evidence that, in invertebrates generally, part of the tricarboxylic acid cycle flux may go via the NADP-linked enzyme. No modulators of helminth (or any other invertebrate) NADP-linked isocitrate dehydrogenase have been described, but allosteric NADP-linked isocitrate dehydrogenases do exist in bacteria.

Succinate Dehydrogenase

The succinate dehydrogenase of mammals is inactivated by oxaloacetate. The inactive mammalian enzyme can be activated by incubation with compounds which bind to the active site (succinate, fumarate, malonate) and by incubation with a variety of anions, nucleotides and reducing agents. The significance of the active and inactive forms of succinate dehydrogenase in the regulation of the mammalian tricarboxylic acid cycle is not clear. The succinate dehydrogenase of *F. hepatica* is, like the mammalian enzyme, inhibited by oxaloacetate and activated by incubation with anions, nucleotides and compounds which bind to the active site[35]. Fumarate reductase activity, on the other hand, is not activated by incubation with substrates or anions and is not inhibited by oxaloacetate. The regulatory properties of *F. hepatica* succinate dehydrogenase could be important in the control of the tricarboxylic acid cycle in this parasite. The major pathway of carbohydrate breakdown in *F. hepatica* involves carbon dioxide fixation into phosphoenolpyruvate to give oxaloacetate, which is converted to succinate by a partial, reversed tricarboxylic acid cycle, the classical tricarboxylic acid cycle being of minor importance. Oxaloacetate formation would inhibit succinate oxidation and hence the classical tricarboxylic acid cycle. Fumarate reductase activity, on the other hand, is not inhibited by oxaloacetate, so the reverse tricarboxylic acid cycle would be unaffected. The succinate dehydrogenase of *A. lumbricoides* is also inhibited by oxaloacetate.

5.1.7. Hormones and 3′,5′-cyclic-AMP

The hormonal control of metabolism in invertebrates has received relatively little attention and mammalian hormones rarely have an effect in invertebrate systems. It would, in fact, seem advantageous for parasitic helminths not to have their metabolism influenced by host hormone changes. In *F. hepatica*, for example, thyroxine, histamine, adrenalin, noradrenalin, progesterone, testosterone and hydrocortisone have no effect on metabolism. There are, however, isolated reports that insulin stimulates metabolism in *T. crassiceps* and *Schistosomatium douthitti* (insulin is also said to affect the metabolism of molluscs) and thyroxine is said to speed the growth of *D. latum* and to stimulate oxygen uptake in several parasites (adults and cercariae of *S. douthitti, Haematoloechus* sp.)[62].

A number of hormones that affect mammalian metabolism, such as adrenalin and noradrenalin, have been found in helminths (*Table 4.11*), and, in the infective larvae of *H. contortus*, exsheathing is accompanied by changes in noradrenalin levels[36]. Serotonin (5-hydroxytryptamine) is also widely distributed in parasites[37] and a 5-hydroxytryptamine like compound occurs in *F. hepatica*. However, the compound in *F. hepatica* appears to differ from serotonin both in its absorption spectrum and its chromatographic properties and is possibly dopamine[38]. With one exception, none of these amines have been shown to affect the metabolism of the parasite that they are found in and so they are probably primarily neurotransmitters. The exception is serotonin; this stimulates glycolysis in *F. hepatica*, increases metabolism in schistosomes and decreases propionate production in *T. colubriformis*. In *F. hepatica*, serotonin activates adenyl cyclase and this leads to a rise in intracellular 3′,5′-cyclic-AMP levels[39]. A whole variety of mammalian hormones, including glucagon and the catecholamines, use 3′,5′-cyclic-AMP as a 'second messenger'. These hormones bind to specific receptors on the cell surface and this activates the adenyl cyclase which is on the inner face of the membrane. Cyclic-3′,5′-AMP can modulate enzymes directly, as in the case of phosphofructokinase, or it can exert its effects via 3′,5′-cyclic-AMP dependent protein kinases. In the mammalian cell, protein kinase (kinase kinase) exists in active and inactive forms, the inactive form being a combination of two sub-units, one regulatory and one catalytic. The cyclic nucleotide combines with the regulatory sub-unit, the sub-units dissociate and the catalytic unit is unmasked. Among the enzymes regulated by protein kinases are triacylgly-

cerol lipase, cholesterol esterase, phosphorylase b kinase, phosphorylase phosphatase, pyruvate dehydrogenase, glycogen synthase and possibly pyruvate kinase,
phosphoenolpyruvate carboxykinase and fructose-1,6-bisphosphatase. Not all
protein kinases are, of course, cyclic-AMP dependent.

In the cell, 3',5'-cyclic-AMP is destroyed by a cyclic-AMP phosphodiesterase, and
this enzyme is a potential mechanism for regulating 3',5'-cyclic-AMP levels. A number of modulators have been described for mammalian phosphodiesterase and the
enzyme may also be regulated by a protein activator as well as being inducible.

The essential features of the 3',5'-cyclic-AMP dependent protein kinase system
have been found in parasitic helminths[63]. In $S.$ $mansoni$, there is an adenyl cyclase,
a cyclic-AMP phosphodiesterase and a 3',5'-cyclic-AMP dependent protein kinase[40].
Phosphodiesterase has also been demonstrated in $S.$ $japonicum$. The adenyl cyclase
of $S.$ $mansoni$ is stimulated by serotonin, glucagon and prostaglandins. The adenyl
cyclase of $F.$ $hepatica$ is similarly stimulated by serotonin, and there is also a
phosphodiesterase present and a 3',5'-cyclic-AMP dependent protein kinase[39,41,64].
In $F.$ $hepatica$, both the adenyl cyclase and the 3',5'-cyclic-AMP dependent protein
kinase are concentrated at the anterior end. This may explain why, if liver fluke are
cut in half, only the anterior end will synthesise new glycogen, whilst in intact
worms glycogen is synthesised equally in both halves[42]. In $F.$ $hepatica$, the phosphodiesterase was found to be inhibited by dopamine and activated by imidazole,
whilst serotonin, prostaglandins and theophylline were ineffective[43]. The lack of
inhibition by theophylline made $F.$ $hepatica$ phosphodiesterase appear more similar
to the enzyme of certain bacteria than to the mammalian one. However, more
recently, the phosphodiesterase of $F.$ $hepatica$ has been shown to be theophylline-
sensitive and also to be inhibited by caffeine, D-lysergic acid and papaverine[44].

Adenyl cyclase, phosphodiesterase and 3',5'-cyclic-AMP have been demonstrated
in adult $A.$ $lumbricoides$ muscle[45], whilst adenyl cyclase has also been found in the
tegument of $H.$ $microstoma$[65].

5.1.8. Energy Charge

In addition to being substrates for energy-yielding and energy-utilising reactions, the
adenylate nucleotides, ATP, ADP and AMP, are also important enzyme modulators.
Atkinson[46] has proposed that the energy status of the cell can be expressed as the
energy charge (adenylate charge):

$$\text{energy charge} = \tfrac{1}{2} \; \frac{[ADP] + 2[ATP]}{[AMP] + [ADP] + [ATP]}$$

The energy charge integrates the pathways which produce and utilise high-energy
phosphate. The mid-point for control by the energy charge is 0.85, this being the
adenylate ratio at which ATP production in the cell equals energy utilisation. In
tissues, the energy charge normally lies between 0.75 to 0.95, and parasitic helminths are no exception (*Table 5.5*). Use has been made of the energy charge to
assess the metabolic integrity of helminths in *in vitro* culture and to monitor the
effects of anthelmintics[3,47,48,49].

The enzyme myokinase (adenylate kinase) has been found in helminths (*A. lumbricoides, F. hepatica, H. diminuta*), this enzyme catalysing the reaction:

$$ATP + AMP \rightleftharpoons 2ADP$$

In all of the helminths so far studied (*Table 5.5*), the mass action ratio for myokinase [ATP] [AMP]/[ADP]^2 is approximately equal to the apparent equilibrium constant for the reaction, which is 0.44. This indicates that myokinase is active in

Table 5.5   Adenylate charge, phosphorylation potential and myokinase equilibrium in parasitic helminths

Species	Adenylate charge	Phosphorylation potential (M^{-1})	$\dfrac{[ATP][AMP]}{[ADP]^2}$
Ascaris lumbricoides[50]	0.86	946	0.52
Globodera rostochiensis[66] (hatched juveniles)*	0.77	–	0.22
Nematodirus battus[52]	0.69	–	0.39
Nippostrongylus brasiliensis[48,52]	0.78	–	0.36
Fasciola hepatica[47,50]	0.66	325	0.47
Hymenolepis diminuta[50]	0.71	571	0.35
Moniezia expansa[4,49]	0.8	–	0.37
Schistocephalus solidus[45] (plerocercoid)	0.71	108	0.47

*Plant parasite.
Superscripts are to references at end of this chapter.

these helminths and is catalysing a near-equilibrium reaction. One function of myokinase in tissues may be to amplify changes in the ATP/ADP ratio. The [ADP]^2 function in the mass action ratio of myokinase means that small changes in the ATP/ADP ratio will lead to relatively large changes in the AMP levels.

In many tissues, a decline in the energy charge is accompanied by a decrease in the total adenylate pool. The drop in energy charge activates AMP deaminase, this removes AMP, and ATP is formed at the expense of ADP via the myokinase reaction. This gives a temporary increase in the energy charge, but, if the ATP levels drop too far, AMP deaminase is inhibited in order to conserve adenylate nucleotides. High levels of AMP deaminase are found in vertebrate muscles, but, in invertebrates, AMP deaminase is often low or absent, and this seems to be the case in parasitic helminths (Section 3.5.2). Some bacteria may use AMP nucleosidase as an alternative to AMP deaminase. In *F. hepatica*, the decline in energy charge as a result of anthelmintic treatment was not always accompanied by a fall in the total adenylate nucleotide pool[47,51]. In contrast, the decrease in energy charge brought about by anthelmintics in *M. expansa* was accompanied by a significant drop in the total nucleotide content[49].

5.1.9. Phosphorylation Potential

An alternative way of expressing the energy status of the cell is by the phosphorylation potential:

$$\text{phosphorylation potential} = \frac{[ATP]}{[ADP]\,[P_i]}$$

If there is no energy input, the phosphorylation potential is low, $5\ \mu M^{-1}$. The extent to which this value is exceeded by the observed ratio is a measure of the potential of the cell to do work, and in most tissues it usually varies from 200 to $800\ M^{-1}$. Again, helminths are no exception and fall into this general range (*Table 5.5*), the higher the phosphorylation potential the more 'energised' is the cell. This would seem to be a more sensitive guide than the adenylate charge which tends to vary very little from the mid control point ratio of 0.85.

5.1.10. Phosphagens

Muscle tissue of both vertebrates and invertebrates usually contains a reserve of high-energy phosphate in the form of phosphagens. The phosphagen bases are all guanidines and they react reversibly with ATP:

guanidine + ATP ⇌ phosphagen + ADP   (*phosphagen phosphotransferase*)

Some seven or eight different guanidines have been found as phosphagens in nature, although the major ones are arginine and creatine. Creatine is the sole phosphagen in vertebrates, whilst arginine is the only phosphagen in the majority of invertebrates. A few invertebrates also have creatine, and annelids have all seven phosphagens (individual species never have more than two or, in the case of annelids, three different phosphagens). Muscle tissue usually has enough ATP to sustain contraction for only a fraction of a second. When there is a sudden energy demand, ATP is split to ADP and inorganic phosphate and the ATP is immediately rephosphorylated via the phosphotransferase reaction. The ATP levels are maintained at the expense of the phosphagen until metabolism can be accelerated to meet the new energy demand. It is not usually possible to detect any differences in the ATP/ADP ratio between resting and active muscle, unless both glycolysis and the phosphotransferase reaction are blocked.

A number of parasitic helminths are extremely unusual in that they possess no detectable phosphagens. At the most, only traces of phosphagen occur in adult *F. hepatica, M. expansa, H. diminuta* and in adults and eggs of *A. lumbricoides*, nor are there significant levels of phosphotransferase activity in these parasites[45]. In adult *A. lumbricoides* muscle and in the eggs, traces of arginine phosphotransferase activity have been detected using isotopic assays, but the activity is so low (less than $1\ \mu mole/min/g$) that it is difficult to see how it could be of physiological importance. An unusual phosphorus compound 1,2-propanediol-2-phosphate has been isolated from *A. lumbricoides* muscle, but there is no evidence that this compound is involved in energy metabolism. The more usual metabolite of 1,2-propanediol is in fact the 1-phosphate. Phosphate compounds like 1,2-propanediol phosphate can act as modulators of haemoglobin (Section 2.5.2).

There has been no systematic survey of the distribution of phosphagens in helminths, but arginine phosphate has been reported from adults and larvae of *S. ratti* and from adult *T. vulpis*. There are also unconfirmed reports of creatine phosphate in adult *A. caninum* and *Wuchereria bancrofti*. A taurocyamine phosphotransferase seems to be present in the plerocercoids of *S. solidus* but not in the plerocercoids of *L. intestinalis*. However, no phosphagens have been detected in either species[45]. Free-living nematodes and platyhelminths appear to have arginine phosphate, but phosphagens may be absent from some free-living platyhelminths.

The absence of phosphagens from several of the larger parasitic helminths has interesting implications for the control of metabolism in these parasites. If there is no reserve of high-energy phosphate, a sudden energy demand should lead to a transient drop in the ATP/ADP ratio. Possibly, parasitic helminths are living in a sheltered environment and are not subject to sudden energy demands, or they may be able to accelerate glycolysis sufficiently quickly that a reserve of high-energy phosphate is not necessary. Alternatively, these helminths may have some other method of maintaining their ATP/ADP ratios; the myokinase reaction, for example, might provide a means of restoring ATP levels, at least temporarily, by catalysing the rephosphorylation of part of the ADP.

5.2. DEVELOPMENTAL REGULATION

The metabolic changes that take place during the life-cycle of a parasite can be studied by comparing the metabolism of the adult parasite with that of the free-living and intermediate stages. However, whilst there is a wealth of information about the metabolism of adult helminths, relatively little is known about the metabolism of the larval stages.

5.2.1. Metabolic Changes During the Life-cycle

The metabolism of adult and larval helminths is discussed in detail in Sections 3.1, 3.2 and 3.3. In general, the free-living stages of nematodes and trematodes (miracidia and cercariae) are aerobic. They have a normal glycolytic sequence and tricarboxylic acid cycle, a mammalian-type cytochrome chain and can catabolise fatty acids by β-oxidation. In contrast, the energy metabolism of adult parasitic nematodes and trematodes is essentially anaerobic. The adults either fix carbon dioxide and have a partial reversed tricarboxylic acid cycle or they rely on glycolysis alone. Many adult nematodes and trematodes have branched cytochrome chains, and none of them appear to be able to catabolise lipids by β-oxidation. The intramolluscan stages of trematodes (sporocysts and rediae) are facultative anaerobes and resemble the adult more than the free-living stages. However, unlike adult trematodes, sporocysts and rediae may be able to catabolise amino acids and lipids as well as carbohydrate.

Adult cestodes and acanthocephalans also have specialised pathways of anaerobic carbohydrate breakdown, branched cytochrome chains are common and none of them have an active β-oxidation sequence. Of the larval stages of cestodes, the cysti-cercoids of cyclophyllidean tapeworms, which are found in the haemocoel of arthropods, and the free-swimming pseudophyllidean coracidia appear to be largely aerobic. The acanthocephalan cystacanth (also from the haemocoel of arthropods) is again probably aerobic, although neither cystacanths nor cysticercoids can metabolise fatty acids by β-oxidation. The metabolism of larval cestodes from vertebrate intermediate hosts (plerocercoids, tetrathyridia, cysticerci) is similar to that of the adult cestode and, like the adult, they excrete reduced organic acids (mostly succinate, lactate and acetate) as end-products of carbohydrate catabolism. Despite this, the metabolism of the adults and larvae of such cestodes are not identical. There are, for example, quantitative differences in the organic acids excreted by adult and larval stages and, in *Diphyllobothrium latum*, there are differences in K_m and the specific activities of the NADH oxidase and succinoxidase systems between the adult and plerocercoid.

In parasitic helminths, the transition from one stage of the life-cycle to the next is accompanied by major metabolic changes. In *A. lumbricoides*, for example, invasion of the final host involves modification of the tricarboxylic acid cycle and glycolytic pathway, the β-oxidation sequence and the glyoxylate cycle cease to function and there are changes in the nature of the terminal oxidases. These changes all occur in reverse when the free-living eggs leave the host. In trematodes, there may be two metabolic switches in the life-cycle, one when the miracidia infect their molluscan host and the second when the cercariae enter the final vertebrate host.

The metabolic changes during the life-cycle of a parasite may include alterations in the intracellular distribution of enzymes, and there is evidence that different iso-enzymes are functioning in the adult and larval stages. For example, in *A. lumbricoides*, different isoenzymes of malate, lactate and glutamate dehydrogenase are present in the free-living and parasitic stages. The process of invasion of a host by infective stages may not then simply just involve the switching-on and switching-off of certain key enzymes. At infection, all of the enzymes of the free-living phase may be replaced by isoenzymes adapted for the parasitic stage, and the converse happens when free-living stages are shed from the host. Changes in synthetic pathways during the life-cycle of parasitic helminths have not been studied, although there are indications in cestodes that the pathways of pyrimidine and purine synthesis, which appear to be absent in the adult, may function in the larvae (Section 4.6).

The life-cycle of a parasite is accompanied by cyclic changes in metabolic pathways and isoenzyme patterns. The reason for this is twofold. First, the metabolism of the free-living and parasitic stages are orientated towards different ends. The free-living stages are adapted for growth and survival, whilst the metabolism of the adult parasite is geared towards reproduction. This might explain the heavy dependence on lipid catabolism in the free-living stages of many parasites. Secondly, the physical environment of the different stages can be very different and this necessitates different metabolic adaptations (Chapter 1). From the metabolic point of view, the main environmental factors are the availability of oxygen and carbon dioxide and the temperature.

5.2.2. The Role of Oxygen and Carbon Dioxide

Oxygen and carbon dioxide tensions in different parasitic environments have been summarised in Sections 1.1.1 and 1.1.2. In many parasitic sites, the oxygen tension is low. Pathways such as the tricarboxylic acid cycle and the β-oxidation sequence produce large amounts of reduced cofactors which have to be reoxidised via aerobic oxidase systems. Metabolic schemes which would allow β-oxidation or the tricarboxylic acid cycle to function anaerobically are theoretically possible, but do not occur in helminths (Sections 3.3.2 and 3.4.4). So, it is not surprising that helminths, which live in oxygen-poor environments, should have an essentially anaerobic energy metabolism, their specialised cytochrome chains using what little oxygen is available. Why parasites which live in aerobic sites in the body, such as the tissues and bloodstream, should also have a basically anaerobic energy metabolism requires alternative explanations (Section 3.2.9).

The carbon dioxide tension in parasitic environments can often be very high, up to 700 mmHg in the intestines of ruminants. The K_{m_a} of phosphoenolpyruvate carboxykinase for bicarbonate is also high (25 mM), so high levels of carbon dioxide will favour carbon dioxide fixation. It has been suggested that the anaerobic pathways of carbohydrate breakdown found in intestinal helminths are an adaptation to the high environmental pCO_2 rather than to the low pO_2. High environmental carbon dioxide concentrations are not, however, essential for carbon dioxide fixation. Larval cestodes found in fish (the plerocercoids of *S. solidus* and *L. intestinalis*) fix carbon dioxide, although the pCO_2 in aquatic vertebrates is only 2–10 mmHg, and many free-living invertebrates also fix carbon dioxide under anaerobic conditions (Section 3.1.4). Interestingly, altering the pCO_2 does not seem to affect the metabolic end-products produced by helminths[53].

Carbon dioxide fixation also has a number of advantages for parasitic helminths. It increases the ATP yield per mole of glucose catabolised and it leads to the retention of at least part of the tricarboxylic acid cycle (Section 3.1.9).

5.2.3. The Role of Temperature

When an infective stage invades a mammalian or avian host, there is a sudden rise in ambient temperature to 37–43 °C, and this has a number of very important physiological consequences.

Raising the temperature increases the rate of reaction of a chemical process, although the actual extent to which a reaction is speeded up depends on the energy of activation. A rise in temperature also increases the rate of protein denaturation. Thus, the so-called 'temperature optimum' for an enzyme is the result of the combination of two different processes, one due to the kinetic effect of temperature on reaction rates, the other related to enzyme stability. In addition to rate of reaction, several other enzyme parameters are affected by temperature. The affinity of an enzyme for its substrate can be temperature-dependent, as can its pH optimum. The effects of modulators may also vary with temperature. Cellular pH is temperature-dependent, decreasing by approximately 0.015–0.02 pH units/°C rise. The equilibrium constant of a reaction varies with temperature, so, in the case of near-equilibrium enzymes, altering the temperature may lead to a change in metabolite pool sizes. The extent by which the equilibrium constant is altered for a given rise in temperature depends on the standard change in enthalpy of the reaction. The effect of altering the temperature on the activity of individual enzymes and on the overall activity of metabolic pathways can be very complex and cannot be readily predicted. The increase in rate of reaction brought about by an increase in temperature may be offset by a decrease in the affinity of the enzyme for its substrate. Or the effects of modulators may alter such that, at high temperatures, the activators are less effective and the inhibitors more effective. These sorts of processes may form the biochemical basis of metabolic temperature compensation[54].

There is considerable evidence that there is a close relationship between the various temperature-dependent parameters of enzyme activity and an organism's normal environmental temperature range. Correlations have been described between environmental temperature and K_{m_a} and between environmental temperature and thermostability of enzymes from a variety of sources. Some thermodynamic aspects of enzyme activity (the energy, entropy and enthalpy of activation) have also been correlated with environmental temperature. During infection, all of the enzymes of the free-living stage of a parasite may, therefore, have to be replaced by isoenzymes with temperature characteristics adapted to the higher temperature of the final host.

The properties of membrane-bound enzymes (such as succinate dehydrogenase) and membrane transport systems are dependent on the physical state of the membrane. Changing the temperature alters the physical properties of membrane lipids and this is reflected in changes in the rate of reaction and allosteric properties of membrane-bound enzymes. Frequently, membrane lipids undergo sharp phase changes at critical temperatures and there are corresponding sudden changes in the properties of the membrane-bound enzymes. For mammalian and avian membrane-bound enzymes, Arrhenius plots frequently show two breaks, one at around 30 °C, the other at 10 °C. The membrane-bound enzymes of ectotherms usually show one low-temperature break, often about 5 °C. Again, there is a correlation between the breaks in the Arrhenius plots and the animal's normal body temperature range Exactly what the two breaks in the mammalian system represent is not clear. They may reflect the start and finish of a phase change, or two separate phase changes or, possibly, they may be the result of the two lipid faces of the membrane having different transition temperatures. Infection of an endothermic host must then be accompanied by changes in the parasite's membranes, such that the physical state of the membrane, and hence the properties of the membrane-bound enzymes, are retained at the new environmental temperature. Changes in membrane composition with changes in environmental temperature have been found in acclimatising fish, hibernating mammals and in micro-organisms. The sorts of changes that take place are alterations in the fatty acid composition of the membranes (chain length and saturation) and changes in the relative proportions of the different phospholipid and steroid classes. There is some evidence in the nematode *S. ratti* that infection is accompanied by changes in lipid composition and this is dealt with in detail in Sections 4.3.1 and 2.3.1. The physical state of an animal's depot fat will also vary with temperature and must be similarly regulated.

5.2.4. Other Environmental Factors

In helminths, temperature and the availability of oxygen and carbon dioxide play a major part in determining the metabolism of the different life-cycle stages. Other environmental factors which may influence metabolism during the life-cycle include osmotic pressure, redox potential, availability of nutrients and ions, viscosity of the media and hydrostatic pressure.

The osmotic pressure of the environment determines the amount of osmotic work an organism has to perform. The different ionic compositions of different environments may also act as developmental triggers. A drop in osmotic pressure, for example, triggers hatching in schistosome eggs (Section 1.1.5) and sodium ions are necessary for the excystment of tapeworm cyticercoids.

The redox potential is a complex parameter (Section 1.1.3). Low redox conditions are often an important hatching trigger for nematodes and trematodes, and the redox conditions may affect the functioning of cytochrome chains.

Most parasitic stages have available to them an ample supply of low molecular weight nutrients. This may, in part, be responsible for the suppression of synthetic pathways in adult parasites. The relative absence of gluconeogenic pathways in adult helminths may similarly be correlated with the availability of hexoses in parasitic sites.

It has often been suggested that the invading stages of parasites may require a specific nutrient or factor from their hosts[55]. This compound would then initiate the next phase of the life-cycle. The specific metabolite could act by replacing a missing factor in the parasite's system. Suitable sites for such an interaction might be the parasite's endocrine system or the cytochrome chain. This is a very attractive model for the regulation of parasite development by host substances. The initiating metabolite would presumably have to be a macromolecule in order to have the required degree of specificity. Unfortunately, there is no evidence at all for this type of interaction between host molecules and parasite systems.

Viscosity and hydrostatic pressure are known to affect parasite establishment, movement and reproduction, but it is not known if they have any physiological effects.

5.2.5. Timing of the Metabolic Changes

The differences in metabolic pathways and enzyme properties between the free-living and parasitic stages of helminths can, to a large extent, be related to the differences between the free-living and parasitic environments. The actual process of infection of, or egression from, a host is rapid and there is no gradual acclimatisation. So when, during infection, for example, do the different metabolic changes actually take place and do they all happen simultaneously or are they spread out over a period of time? The enzymes for the parasitic phase could be preformed but inactive in the infective stage or the enzymes could be synthesised *de novo* at infection, *m*RNA being transcribed from DNA, or stable *m*RNA might be involved.

The infective stages of helminths usually possess at least some of the enzyme systems characteristic of the adult. Phosphoenolpyruvate carboxykinase and fumarate reductase activity have been demonstrated in several infective nematode larvae (Section 3.1.14), and infective *A. lumbricoides* eggs contain adult-type malic dehydrogenase isoenzymes. Larval trematodes may be similarly 'pre-adapted' for their vertebrate host. Using two species of trematode, one parasitic in fish (*Zoogonus rubellus*), the other parasitic in gulls (*Himasthla quissetenis*), Vernberg[56] found that there was a correlation between the Q_{10} of the larval trematode and the body temperature of the final host.

So, at least some of the enzymes of the adult stage may be preformed in infective nematode and trematode larvae. However, whether or not the enzymes of the adult pathways function to any extent in the infective larva or whether they remain inactive until after infection is not clear. In some cases, it seems that, although the infective larvae contain the enzymes of adult-type pathways, one of the key enzymes in the sequence is either absent, or has only a very low activity. The infective eggs of *A. lumbricoides*, for example, have significant levels of phosphoenolpyruvate carboxykinase and fumarate reductase, but the malic enzyme is hardly detectable[9]. Activation of the adult pathway would require an increase in malic enzyme activity and this could be initiated by the environmental change. Similarly, eggs developing in the adult parasite, before they are shed from the host, contain enzyme systems characteristic of the free-living phase. Unembryonated *A. lumbricoides* eggs, from the uterus of the female, have a complete sequence of tricarboxylic and β-oxidation enzymes, but again, in each case, one of the enzymes (NAD-linked isocitrate dehydrogenase and 3-(OH)-acyl-CoA dehydrogenase) appears to be absent or is only just detectable.

Most of the metabolic changes associated with the transition from the free-living to the parasitic environment may then have already occurred by the time the infective stage is formed. In the same way, eggs developing in the parasitic female contain many of the enzyme systems characteristic of the free-living stage. Following infection or egression, an increase in activity of one or a few key enzymes initiates the metabolic change.

In nematodes, metabolic switches often coincide with a moult. Another morphological event which accompanies metabolic changes is the loss of the tail by penetrating cercariae. When the cercariae of *S. mansoni* penetrate a host, there is a rapid change from the aerobic metabolism of the cercaria to the predominantly lactic acid producing schistosomule. It has been suggested that it is the loss of the tail which initiates the switch[57]. Within 15–30 min of infection, the schistosomules are no longer able to survive in water like the cercariae, and there is also a reduction in the rate of pyruvate uptake. Penetrating schistosome cercariae lose their glycoprotein coat and this may account for the permeability changes.

Most of the post-infection metabolic changes in helminths tend to involve the loss or reduction of enzyme systems, rather than the acquisition of new pathways. In invading *A. lumbricoides* larvae, part of the tricarboxylic acid cycle, the β-oxidation sequence and the glyoxylate cycle are all lost. The little evidence available suggests that the post-infection changes are also spread out over a period of time. In the developing and infective *A. lumbricoides* egg, the terminal oxidase is cytochrome oxidase, and cytochrome oxidase is still present in third-stage larvae recovered from the lungs, but disappears in fourth-stage larvae. Whether the suppression of metabolic pathways in helminths also involves sudden changes in key enzymes and slower changes in the rest (as postulated for the activation of pathways) is not known.

During the course of the metabolic switches, the various pathways must remain under tight metabolic control. The part played by allosteric and covalently modulated enzymes in controlling the change from one phase of the life-cycle to the next has not been studied.

5.2.6. Dormancy and Delayed Development

The infective stages of many helminth parasites are dormant, so infection also involves the activation of a dormant stage. In *A. lumbricoides*, the onset of dormancy in the infective egg and its subsequent reactivation during hatching are not accompanied by any significant changes in the activities of the catabolic enzymes (glycolysis, tricarboxylic acid cycle, β-oxidation sequence). It can, however, be correlated with changes in the steady-state levels of metabolic intermediates and, in particular, the [ATP]/[ADP] ratio. The dormant, infective *A. lumbricoides* egg is characterised by a high [ATP]/[ADP] ratio and a low cytoplasmic free [NAD$^+$]/[NADH] ratio. Following activation, the [ATP]/[ADP] ratio falls and the free [NAD$^+$]/[NADH] ratio rises. In the dormant egg, the key regulatory enzymes of carbohydrate breakdown (phosphorylase, hexokinase, phosphofructokinase, pyruvate kinase) are all inhibited. The inhibition and activation of the regulatory enzymes in *A. lumbricoides* eggs can be accounted for by changes in the steady-state levels of the intracellular metabolites. There is no evidence in the dormant eggs for any sort of specific inhibitory metabolite, although specific metabolic inhibitors such as guanosine-5'-diphosphate-2'-diphosphate (ppGpp) have been found to regulate metabolism in some micro-organisms. However, it is not known how the changes in metabolite levels are controlled in *A. lumbricoides* eggs. One possibility is that, in the dormant egg, the cytoplasmic/mitochondrial NADH shuttle (Section 3.2.4) is not operating and so the cytoplasm becomes reduced. Another way in which dormancy could be initiated in infective larvae is if, in preparation for the parasitic phase, the enzymes of the free-living stage were replaced by isoenzymes adapted to function at the higher temperatures of the final host. The infective eggs of *A. lumbricoides* have been found to show a rather modified form of temperature adaptation[58] which may support this idea.

The stage in a parasitic life-cycle which makes the transition from one environment to the next appears, almost invariably, to be non-feeding (miracidia, cercariae, infective nematode larvae). Perhaps such stages cannot cope both with feeding and with the environmental changes. In some species of nematode, there are, however, reports that, after invasion, the infective larvae increase in size and may possibly feed.

A phenomenon found in parasitic nematodes, which may be related to dormancy, is delayed development[59]. After invasion of the host, the infective larvae, instead of developing directly into the adult, may enter a diapause-like state for varying lengths of time. This temporary cessation of growth occurs at a precise point in development, usually the early L_4 stage, but occasionally the L_3 or L_5. Frequently, only a proportion of the invading larvae become arrested, but in some species it may be an obligatory part of the life-cycle. Arrested development has been well documented in at least ten species of parasitic nematode, but has been most extensively studied in *H. contortus*. Whether or not an invading larva becomes arrested depends on the interaction of a whole range of host, parasite and environmental factors. The proportion of larvae becoming arrested can depend on the strain of the parasite, the density of infection, the age, sex and strain of the host as well as the host's immunological and endocrine status. The main environmental stimulus in initiating delayed development is temperature, or possibly the change in temperature, to which the infective larvae have been exposed prior to infection. Photoperiod may also have an influence.

Arrested larvae are often extremely resistant to anthelmintic treatment. There may be several reasons for this. First, the arrested larvae occur in the tissues, not the gut lumen, and so anthelmintics may not reach them. Secondly, arrested larvae have a low metabolic rate and may not be so susceptible as the adults, or the metabolism of the arrested larva and the adult may be rather different. There is, at the moment, no information on the biochemistry of arrested stages. The phenomenon may be under hormonal control and in arrested *Ostertagia ostertagia* larvae, neurosecretory material has been shown to accumulate in the anal ganglion. The only other biochemical observation on arrested larvae is the formation of crystalloids in the intestine of arrested *H. contortus* larvae (Section 2.1).

5.2.7. Environmental and Genetic Control

During the course of a parasite's life-cycle, metabolic pathways are lost, new ones appear and enzymes are replaced by isoenzymes adapted to the different environmental conditions. These processes are under both genetic and environmental control. Enzymes for the parasitic phase may be present in infective stages and are activated during infection. A similar process occurs when eggs or larvae are shed from the host into the free-living environment. Activation of pathways may involve the synthesis of one or a few key enzymes, or the switch may be controlled by cellular feedback mechanisms.

Temperature change seems to be one of the important stimuli in initiating metabolic change during the infection of mammalian or avian hosts. The respiratory rates of the infective larvae of *N. brasiliensis* and *N. americanus* show a break in the Arrhenius plot above 30 °C, indicating a change in metabolism above this temperature, whilst the incubation of infective larvae of *S. ratti* at 37 °C brings about an irreversible decrease in QO_2. A similar temperature-dependent metabolic switch has been suggested in the plerocercoids of *S. solidus*. Above about 30 °C the plerocercoids cease to synthesise somatic tissue and change over to an adult type of metabolism geared towards genital development. It has been postulated that there are two enzyme systems in these plerocercoids, one concerned with somatic growth, with a temperature optimum at 23 °C, and the adult system with an optimum at 40 °C. For other helminth stages, it may be a decrease in temperature which is the stimulus. When arthropod vectors take up microfilariae with their mammalian blood meal, the drop in temperature triggers the development in the invertebrate host.

As well as temperature, the osmotic pressure, pH, rH, pCO_2 and pO_2 all change during infection, and invading stages are exposed to a variety of host metabolites, some of which have a physiological role during infection (Section 1.1). Many of these stimuli have been shown to be involved in initiating hatching and exsheathment, but it has yet to be shown if the same stimuli are also responsible for controlling the switches in metabolic pathways. So far, only temperature change has been found to have a direct effect on metabolism. It would seem very unlikely that there is only a single stimulus involved in initiating development and it probably involves the interaction of a variety of factors. Certainly, things other than change in temperature must be involved in the infection of ectothermal hosts.

Another problem that has not been resolved is whether environmental stimuli, such as increase in temperature, influence infective stages via sense organs and hormonal systems (triggering effect) or whether they exert their influence by acting directly on the metabolic pathways (long-lasting effect). Alteration in temperature, for example, might modify the behaviour of membrane-bound enzymes and activate enzymes with different temperature characteristics. Increased carbon dioxide concentrations could provide substrate for carboxylating reactions and affect intracellular pH. Of course, there is no reason why a particular stimulus, such as temperature or pCO_2, should not act both directly and as a trigger.

A specific carbon dioxide receptor has been found in the infective larvae of some trichostrongyles and in some plant parasitic nematodes[60]. The proposed model involves two free sulphydryl groups which react with carbon dioxide to form a carbon bridge:

$$-S-\overset{|}{\underset{|}{C}}-S-$$

The requirement for a low redox potential in the exsheathment of infective larvae might be related to the need to keep the receptor sulphydryl groups reduced. This model, if it is correct, is totally different from the way in which vertebrates monitor carbon dioxide tension. Vertebrates respond to pH change caused by alteration in the bicarbonate buffer system.

If a stimulus is acting as a trigger for a metabolic switch, this implies that, after exposure to the stimulus for a critical period, the changes will then proceed in its absence. This possibility has not really been studied in parasites. Nor is it known if different aspects of the metabolic changes, such as the loss of the β-oxidation sequence and the development of branched cytochrome chains, respond to different environmental cues.

We are only just beginning to get an idea of the extent of the metabolic changes which take place during the life-cycles of parasites, and we really know even less of how these changes are controlled.

5.3. SUMMARY AND CONCLUSIONS

Metabolism is controlled by a series of hierarchical mechanisms ranging from behavioural to molecular. These controls enable an organism efficiently to divide its energy input between different processes (growth, reproduction, locomotion, osmoregulation and so on) and between different pathways. The basis of metabolic control is, therefore, energy partition.

Developmental regulation attempts to look at the ways in which the relative importance of different processes changes during the life-cycle of the parasite. Cellular regulation, on the other hand, is concerned with the control of flux rates though individual pathways.

A feature of cellular regulation is that the control mechanisms are symmetrical; mechanisms for accelerating a particular step are balanced by mechanisms for inhibiting it.

The metabolic pathways found in parasitic helminths are often different from those found in mammals and might be expected to pose new regulatory problems. The only pathways in which control has been looked at in detail in helminths are those involved in carbohydrate catabolism. The same enzymes appear to be regulatory in both helminths and mammals. No new regulatory enzymes have yet been discovered in parasitic helminths, and both helminth and mammalian regulatory enzymes appear to be modulated by similar metabolites. Nevertheless, there are differences in detail between the properties of the regulatory enzymes of mammals and those of helminths, and these differences can be exploited by chemotherapy.

During its life-cycle, a parasite may occupy a series of differing environments and there are corresponding alterations in metabolism. These metabolic switches reflect the changes in the physico-chemical properties of the environment and the changing roles of the different parasitic stages. The free-living and intermediate stages are specialised for growth and survival, the adult stages for reproduction. There is little direct evidence on the ways in which the metabolic switches that occur during the life-cycle of parasites are controlled, and much of this section is largely speculative. The developmental switches appear to be under both genetic and environmental control. In some cases, it has been shown that enzymes are synthesised prior to infection, but activation of the pathways depends upon environmental factors. The latter may have a direct (long-lasting) effect on metabolism or they may act as triggers (indirect).

5.4. GENERAL READING

Barrett, J. (1976). 'Energy metabolism in nematodes'. In *The Organisation of Nematodes*. Ed. N. A. Croll, pp. 11–70. London; Academic Press

Barrett, J. (1977). 'Energy metabolism and infection in helminths'. *Symp. Br. Soc. Parasitol.*, **15**, 121–44

von Brand, T. (1973). *Biochemistry of Parasites*. 2nd edn. London; Academic Press

Bryant, C. (1975). 'Carbon dioxide utilisation and the regulation of respiratory metabolic pathways in parasitic helminths.' *Adv. Parasitol.*, **13**, 139–65

Bryant, C. (1978). 'The regulation of respiratory metabolism in parasitic helminths'. *Adv. Parasitol.*, **16**, 311–31

Denton, R. M. and Pogson, C. I. (1976). *Metabolic Regulation*. London; Chapman and Hall

Fairbairn, D. (1970). 'Biochemical adaptation and loss of genetic capacity in helminth parasites'. *Biol. Rev.*, **45**, 29–72

Newsholme, E. A. and Start, C. (1973). *Regulation in Metabolism*. London; Wiley

Rogers, W. P. (1962). *The Nature of Parasitism*. London; Academic Press

5.5. REFERENCES

1. Barrett, J. and Beis, I. (1973). *Compar. Biochem. Physiol.*, **44B**, 751–61
2. Cornish, R. A. and Bryant, C. (1976). *Int. J. Parasitol.*, **6**, 387–92
3. Prichard, R. K. (1978). *Parasitology*, **76**, 277–88
4. Behm, C. A. and Bryant, C. (1975). *Int. J. Parasitol.*, **5**, 209–17
5. Barrett, J. and Beis, I. (1973). *Compar. Biochem. Physiol.*, **44A**, 331–40
6. Supowit, S. C. and Harris, B. G. (1976). *Biochim. Biophys. Acta*, **422**, 48–59
7. Hutchison, W. F., Turner, A. C. and Oelshlegel, F. J. (1977). *Compar. Biochem. Physiol.*, **58B**, 131–4
8. Komuniecki, R. W. and Roberts, L. S. (1977). *Compar. Biochem. Physiol.*, **57B**, 45–9
9. Barrett, J. (1976). In *Biochemistry of Parasites and Host-Parasite Relationships*. Ed. H. Van den Bossche, pp. 117–23. Amsterdam; North-Holland
10. Bueding, E. and Fisher, J. (1970). *Molec. Pharmacol.*, **6**, 532–9
11. Moczoń, T. (1977). *Acta Parasitol. Polonica*, **27**, 275–82
12. Saz, H. J. and Dunbar, G. A. (1975). *J. Parasitol.*, **61**, 794–801
13. Behm, C. A. and Bryant, C. (1975). *Int. J. Parasitol.*, **5**, 339–46
14. Mansour, T. E. (1967). *Federation Proc.*, **26**, 1179–85
15. Köhler, P. and Hanselmann, K. (1973). *Compar. Biochem. Physiol.*, **45B**, 825–45
16. Sugden, P. H. and Newsholme, E. A. (1975). *Biochem. J.*, **150**, 113–22
17. Moon, T. W., Hulbert, W. C., Mustafa, T. and Mettrick, D. F. (1977). *Compar. Biochem. Physiol.*, **56B**, 249–54
18. Logan, J., Ubelaker, J. E. and Vrijenhoek, R. C. (1977). *Compar. Biochem. Physiol.*, **57B**, 51–3

19. Zammit, V. A., Beis, I. and Newsholme, E. A. (1978). *Biochem. J.*, **174**, 989–99

20. McManus, D. P. and James, B. L. (1975). *Compar. Biochem. Physiol.*, **51B**, 299–306

21. Moon, T. W., Mustafa, T., Hulbert, W. C., Podesta, R. B. and Mettrick, D. F. (1977). *J. Exptl Zool.*, **200**, 325–36

22. Carter, C. E. and Fairbairn, D. (1975). *J. Exptl Zool.*, **194**, 439–48

23. Bryant, C. (1972). *Int. J. Parasitol.*, **2**, 333–40

24. Prichard, R. K. (1976). *Int. J. Parasitol.*, **6**, 227–33

25. Köhler, P. (1974). *Compar. Biochem. Physiol.*, **49B**, 335–44

26. Brazier, J. B. and Jaffe, J. J. (1973). *Compar. Biochem. Physiol.*, **44B**, 145–55

27. Prichard, R. K. (1974). *Proc. Third Int. Congr. of Parasitology (Munich)* 3, pp. 1446–7

28. McManus, D. P. (1975). *Int. J. Biochem.*, **6**, 79–84

29. Behm, C. A. and Bryant, C. (1975). *Int. J. Parasitol.*, **5**, 347–54

30. Zammit, V. A. and Newsholme, E. A. (1978). *Biochem. J.*, **174**, 979–87

31. Bryant, C. and Behm, C. A. (1976). In *Biochemistry of Parasites and Host-Parasite Relationships*. Ed. H. Van den Bossche, pp. 89–94. Amsterdam; North-Holland

32. Landsperger, W. J. and Harris, B. G. (1976). *J. Biol. Chem.*, **251**, 3599–602

33. Landsperger, W. J., Fodge, D. W. and Harris, B. G. (1978). *J. Biol. Chem.*, **253**, 1868–73

34. Barrett, J. (1978). *Z. Parasitenkunde*, **55**, 223–7

35. Barrett, J. (1978). *Parasitology*, **76**, 269–75

36. Rogers, W. P. and Head, R. (1972). *Compar. Gen. Pharmacol.*, **3**, 6–10

37. Tomosky-Sykes, T. K., Mueller, J. F. and Bueding, E. (1977). *J. Parasitol.*, **63**, 492–4

38. Gianutsos, G. and Bennett, J. L. (1977). *Compar. Biochem. Physiol.*, **58C**, 157–9

39. Abrahams, S. L., Northup, J. K. and Mansour, T. E. (1976). *Molec. Pharmacol.*, **12**, 49–58

40. Higashi, G. I., Kreiner, P. W., Keirns, J. J. and Bitensky, M. W. (1973). *Life Sci.*, **13**, 1211–20

41. Gentleman, S., Abrahams, S. L. and Mansour, T. E. (1976). *Molec. Pharmacol.*, **12**, 59–68

42. Ehrlich, I. (1966). *Proc. First Int. Congr. of Parasitology (Rome)* 1, pp. 64–5

43. Simonic, T., Sartorelli, P. and Locatelli, A. (1975). *Ann. Parasitol.*, **4**, 461–8

44. Mansour, T. E. and Mansour, J. M. (1977). *Biochem. Pharmacol.*, **26**, 2325–30

45. Barrett, J. (1977). Unpublished results

46. Atkinson, D. E. and Walton, G. M. (1967). *J. Biol. Chem.*, **242**, 3239–41

47. Cornish, R. A. and Bryant, C. (1976). *Int. J. Parasitol.*, **6**, 393–8

48. Richards, A. J., Bryant, C., Kelly, J. D., Windon, R. G. and Dineen, J. K. (1977). *Int. J. Parasitol.*, **7**, 153–8

49. Rahman, M. S. and Bryant, C. (1977). *Int. J. Parasitol.*, **7**, 403–9

50. Barrett, J. and Beis, I. (1973). *Int. J. Parasitol.*, **3**, 271–3

51. Metzger, H. and Düwel, D. (1973). *Int. J. Biochem.*, **4**, 133–43
52. Ballantyne, A. J., Sharpe, M. J. and Lee, D. L. (1978). *Parasitology*, **76**, 211–20
53. Ward, P. F. V. and Huskisson, N. S. (1978). *Parasitology*, **77**, 255–71
54. Hochachka, P. W. and Somero, G. N. (1968). *Compar. Biochem. Physiol.*, **27**, 659–68
55. Rogers, W. P. and Sommerville, R. I. (1968). *Adv. Parasitol.*, **6**, 327–48
56. Vernberg, W. B. and Vernberg, F. J. (1968). *Exptl Parasitol.*, **23**, 347–54
57. Von Kruger, W. M. A., Gazzinelli, G., Figueiredo, E. A. and Pellegrino, J. (1978). *Compar. Biochem. Physiol.*, **60B**, 41–6
58. Wilson, P. A. G. (1967). *Nature*, **213**, 715–7
59. Schad, G. A. (1977). In *Regulation of Parasite Populations*. Ed. G. W. Esch, pp. 111–67. New York; Academic Press
60. Croll, N. A. and Viglierchio, D. R. (1969). *J. Parasitol.*, **55**, 895–6
61. Oguchi, M., Kanda, T. and Akamatsu, N. (1979). *Compar. Biochem. Physiol.*, **63B**, 335–40
62. Cornford, E. M. (1974). *Exptl Parasitol.*, **36**, 210–21
63. Mansour, T. E. (1979). *Science*, **205**, 462–9
64. Northup, J. K. and Mansour, T. E. (1978). *Molec. Pharmacol.*, **14**, 804–19, 820–33
65. Conway-Jones, P. B. and Rothman, A. H. (1978). *Exptl Parasitol.*, **46**, 152–6
66. Atkinson, H. J. and Ballantyne, A. J. (1977). *Ann. Appl. Zool.*, **87**, 167–74
67. Simonic, T. and Locatelli, A. (1978). *Arch. Veterin. Ital.*, **29**, 101–3

6 General Summary

Parasitism is essentially an ecological problem, i.e. the relationship of an organism to its environment, only in this case the environment is the body of another animal. What we have been trying to investigate is the metabolism of a parasite within its host. However, the metabolism of an infected host is not the same as an uninfected host, and the metabolism of a parasite *in vivo* is different from that of a parasite *in vitro*. There is a dynamic equilibrium between a parasite and its host and this steady state is easily disturbed by experimentation. Ideally, the host–parasite complex should be considered as a whole and not each part in isolation. Experimentally, this has not often proved feasible.

Parasites are usually highly specific with regards to their site of parasitism and also to the range of host species that they can invade. So, is there anything unique about the physics or chemistry of the parasites' environment which can account for this specificity? In general, it seems to be the overall pattern of physico-chemical parameters which delineate the different parasitic habitats, rather than requirements for specific factors or nutrients. What the host does provide for the parasite is a stable environment, and parasites can be thought of as exploiting the homeostatic mechanisms of their hosts. The presence of parasites, however, frequently leads to physiological changes in the host which may modify the parasites' environment. Some of these changes could be of adaptive value to the parasite.

The metabolism of metazoan parasites is not coupled to that of the host as it is, in say, viruses. However, compared with free-living animals, parasitic helminths show considerable reductions in both catabolic and anabolic pathways, though it might have been argued that a parasite with an efficient metabolism would make less demands on its host. The reduction of metabolic pathways found in parasitic helminths should be considered not as a degenerate condition but as a form of biochemical economy. Although the parasitic stages of helminths lack many of the catabolic and anabolic pathways found in free-living organisms, these pathways are often present in the free-living and intermediate stages of the life-cycle. So, the parasitic stages still possess the information necessary to synthesise these pathways, since they occur at other stages of the life-cycle.

The biochemical (and morphological) adaptations found in parasitic helminths are all adaptations to different features of the parasites' environment. These features are also present in free-living environments and few, if any, parasitic adaptations are wholly restricted to parasites. Anaerobic pathways of carbohydrate breakdown involving carbon dioxide fixation, for example, are found in a number of free-living invertebrates, whilst the ability to take up nutrients through the body surface occurs in many marine organisms. Even the extensive metabolic switches which take place during the life-cycle of parasites have parallels in the metamorphoses of insects and amphibians.

There is no single metabolic adaptation which distinguishes parasites from their free-living relatives, rather it is the combination of adaptations which gives them their unique character.

7 Appendixes

APPENDIX 7.1. POSSIBLE MODE OF ACTION OF SOME ANTHELMINTICS

The actual biochemical mode of action of few anthelmintics are known with any certainty and most anthelmintics seem to have multiple effects. Many of the apparent differences in response to anthelmintics by different species of parasite may reflect differences in the pharmokinetic behaviour of the anthelmintics rather than differences in biochemical action.

Compound	Mode of action
Antimonial drugs (stibophen, stibocaptate, antimony potassium tartrate)	Inhibit phosphofructokinase (Section 5.1.3), also cause selective tissue damage.
Avermectins	May interfere with 4-aminobutyric acid metabolism.
Benzimidazoles	A variety of effects. Thiabendazole and cambendazole inhibit the fumarate reductase of nematodes, thiabendazole also inhibits the fumarate reductase of *H. diminuta* and *F. hepatica*. In *A lumbricoides*, the site of fumarate reductase inhibition by thiabendazole appears to be at the level of the reduction of rhodoquinone by flavoprotein 1, although there may be a second site of inhibition between succinate dehydrogenase and the terminal oxidase. At high concentrations, benzimidazoles are uncouplers of oxidative phosphorylation and, in *F. hepatica* and *M. expansa*, mebendazole and cambendazole cause a drop in ATP levels. The structure of benzimidazoles would suggest that they might act as purine analogues. Mebendazole inhibits glucose uptake in nematodes and some trematodes and cestodes. Recently, benzimidazoles have been shown to bind to tubulin and prevent microtubule formation. Thiophanate, although not a benzimidazole,

Compound	Mode of action
	probably cyclises to a benzimidazole *in vivo*. In nematodes, benzimidazole resistance is becoming an increasing agricultural problem.
Bephenium	Acetylcholine mimic. Vertebrate tissue is, however, relatively insensitive to the bephenium ion.
Bisaminomethylphenoxyalkanes (bunamidine, diamphenethide)	Disrupt the tegument of schistosomes, resulting in reduced glucose uptake and inhibition of alkaline phosphatase.
Cyanine dyes (cyanine 863, dithiazanine)	Inhibit oxygen uptake in several species of parasite. It is claimed that cyanine dyes inhibit aldolase and oxidative phosphorylation. Also inhibit glucose uptake in *T. vulpis*.
Diethylcarbamazine	Causes contraction and spontaneous activity in *A. lumbricoides* muscle preparations.
Diflubenzuron	Inhibits chitin synthesis in plant parasitic nematodes.
Hycanthone	Blocks acetylcholine receptors in schistosomes and, to a lesser extent, inhibits acetylcholine esterase.
Levamisole	At high concentrations, inhibits the fumarate reductase of nematodes and trematodes, but not cestodes. In *A. lumbricoides*, the site of fumarate reductase inhibition seems to be at the level of the reduction of rhodoquinone by flavoprotein 1. Levamisole causes rapid, sustained contraction of nematode muscle and acts as a ganglionic stimulant in nematode and mammalian tissue. It also stimulates the mammalian immune system.
Niridazole	Inhibits glycogen phosphorylase phosphatase in schistosomes (Section 5.1.3).
Organophosphorus compounds (haloxon, trichlorphon, dichlorvos, naphthalophos, crufomate)	Inhibit acetylcholine esterase; the enzyme from helminths is ten times more sensitive to inhibition by these compounds than mammalian acetylcholine esterase. Also, inhibition of the mammalian enzyme is reversible, that of the helminth enzyme is not. The acetylcholine esterases of insects and birds are, again, much more sensitive to inhibition by organophosphorus compounds than the mammalian enzyme.

Compound	Mode of action
Pyrantel	Pyrantel, and its analogue morantel, cause depolarisation and contraction of *A. lumbricoides* muscle. Methydridine may have a similar mode of action. Pyrantel is a hundred times more potent than acetylcholine in causing contraction of *A. lumbricoides* muscle. Morantel also inhibits fumarate reductase.
Piperazine	Causes hyperpolarisation of *A. lumbricoides* muscle by increasing the permeability to chloride ions. This results in reversible, flaccid paralysis. Piperazine may mimic the inhibitory neurotransmitter of nematodes.
Praziquantel	Increases Ca^{2+} permeability of schistosome muscle.
p-Rosaniline	Acetylcholine mimic and, to a lesser extent, inhibits acetylcholine esterase.
Salicylanilides	Multiple effects. All of them are potent uncouplers of oxidative phosphorylation, and may prevent the site 1 phosphorylation of ADP associated with the reduction of fumarate to succinate (Section 3.2.3). The ATP levels in *F. hepatica* and *H. diminuta* fall after treatment with salicylanilides. Several salicylanilides have been reported to inhibit succinic dehydrogenase and to inhibit propionate production in liver fluke. Oxyclozanide is reported to inhibit malic dehydrogenase in *F. hepatica*.

There are a whole group of anthelmintics which are substituted phenols and bear a structural relationship to 2,4-dinitrophenol (bithionol, bromophenophos, desaspidin, dichlorophen, disophenol, hetol, hexachlorophene, niclofolan, nitroxynil). Like the salicylanilides, these are all potent uncouplers of phosphorylation. In addition, disophenol inhibits nematode fumarate reductase and nitroxynil induces an irreversible, tonic paralysis in nematodes. Substituted phenols may also act as feeding repellents in *F. hepatica*.

In the blood of the host, the substituted phenols are detoxicated by being bound to the plasma proteins.

286 APPENDIXES

Compound	Mode of action
Tetramisole	A racemic mixture of levamisole and much less active R(+) isomer, dexamisole.
Thiosinamine (1-allylthiourea)	Inhibits phenolase in the vitellaria of *S. mansoni.*

References
Coles, G. C. (1977). *Pest. Sci.,* 8, 536–43
Coles, G. C. (1977). In *Perspectives in the Control of Parasitic Disease of Animals in Europe.* Ed. D. W. Jolly and J. M. Sommerville, pp. 53–63. London; Royal College of Physicians
Köhler, P. and Bachmann, R. (1978). *Molec. Pharmacol.,* 14, 155–63
Sanderson, B. E. (1973). *Symp. Br. Soc. Parasitol.,* 11, 53–82
Van den Bossche, H. (1976). In *Biochemistry of Parasites and Host-Parasite Relationships.* Ed. H. Van den Bossche, pp. 553–72. Amsterdam; North-Holland

APPENDIX 7.2. LIST OF ABBREVIATED NAMES

Acanthocephala
E. gadi–Echinorhynchus gadi
M. dubius–Moniliformis dubius
M. hirudinaceus–Macracanthorhynchus hirudinaceus
P. minutus–Polymorphus minutus

Cestoda
A. magna–Anoplocephala magna
B. gowkongensis–Bothriocephalus gowkongensis
C. verticillatum–Calliobothrium verticillatum
D. caninum–Dipylidium caninum
D. latum–Diphyllobothrium latum
E. granulosus–Echinococcus granulosus
E. multilocularis–Echinococcus multilocularis
H. citelli–Hymenolepis citelli
H. diminuta–Hymenolepis diminuta
H. microstoma–Hymenolepis microstoma
H. nana–Hymenolepis nana
K. sinensis–Khawia sinensis
L. intestinalis–Ligula intestinalis
L. tenuis–Lacistorhynchus tenuis
M. benedeni–Moniezia benedeni
M. corti–Mesocestoides corti
M. expansa–Moniezia expansa
P. lintoni–Pterobothrium lintoni
R. cesticillus–Raillietina cesticillus
S. erinacei–Spirometra erinacei
S. mansonoides–Spirometra mansonoides

S. solidus—Schistocephalus solidus
T. crassiceps—Taenia crassiceps
T. crassus—Triaenophorus crassus
T. hydatigena—Taenia hydatigena
T. nodulosus—Triaenophorus nodulosus
T. pisiformis—Taenia pisiformis
T. saginata—Taenia saginata
T. solium—Taenia solium
T. taeniaeformis—Taenia taeniaeformis

Nematoda
A. avenae—Aphelenchus avenae
A. caninum—Ancylostoma caninum
A. cantonensis—Angiostrongylus cantonensis
A. columnaris—Ascaris columnaris
A. dissimilis—Ascaridia dissimilis
A. duodenale—Ancylostoma duodenale
A. galli—Ascaridia galli
A. lumbricoides—Ascaris lumbricoides
A. tetraptera—Aspiculuris tetraptera
B. pahangi—Brugia pahangi
B. trigonocephalum—Bunostomum trigonocephalum
*C. briggsae—Caenorhabditis briggsae**
C. elegans—Caenorhabditis elegans
C. hawkingi—Chandlerella hawkingi
C. punctata—Cooperia punctata
C. trispinosus—Camallanus trispinosus
D. filaria—Dictyocaulus filaria
D. immitis—Dirofilaria immitis
D. uniformis—Dirofilaria uniformis
D. viteae—Dipetalonema viteae (=witei)
D. viviparus—Dictyocaulus viviparus
E. ignotus—Eustrongylides ignotus
E. vermicularis—Enterobius vermicularis
G. rostochiensis—Globodera rostochiensis (=Heterodera)
G. strigosum—Graphidium strigosum
H. contortus—Haemonchus contortus
H. gallinae—Heterakis gallinae
H. rubidus—Hyostrongylus rubidus
H. schachtii—Heterodera schachtii
L. appendiculata—Leidynema appendiculata
L. carinii—Litomosoides carinii
M. apri—Metastrongylus apri
M. elongatus—Metastrongylus elongatus
M. nigrescens—Mermis nigrescens
N. americanus—Necator americanus

N. battus—Nematodirus battus
N. brasiliensis—Nippostrongylus brasiliensis
N. glaseri—Neoaplectana glaseri
O. cuniculi—Obeliscoides cuniculi
O. equi—Oxyuris equi
O. ostertagia—Ostertagia ostertagia
O. radiatum—Oesophagostomum radiatum
O. volvulus—Onchocercus volvulus
P. decipiens—Porrocaecum decipiens
P. equorum—Parascaris equorum
P. redivivus—Panagrellus redivivus*
R. anomala—Rhabditis anomala
R. bufonis—Rhabdias bufonis
R. maupasi—Rhabditis maupasi
S. brevicaudata—Strongyluris brevicaudata
S. cervi—Setaria cervi
S. dentatus—Stephanurus dentatus
S. edentatus—Strongylus edentatus
S. equinus—Strongylus equinus
S. muris—Syphacia muris
S. papillosus—Strongyloides papillosus
S. ratti—Strongyloides ratti
S. simiae—Strongyloides simiae
S. trachea—Syngamus trachea
T. aceti—Turbatrix aceti*
T. axei—Trichostrongylus axei
T. canis—Toxocara canis
T. cati—Toxocara cati (=mystax?)
T. colubriformis—Trichostrongylus colubriformis
T. confusa—Tetrameres confusa
T. decipiens—Terranova decipiens
T. muris—Trichuris muris
T. mystax—Toxocara mystax
T. retortaeformis—Trichostrongylus retortaeformis
T. spiralis—Trichinella spiralis
T. suis—Trichuris suis
T. vulpis—Trichuris vulpis
W. bancrofti—Wuchereria bancrofti

Trematoda
C. emasculans—Cercaria emasculans
C. lingua—Cryptocotyle lingua
C. sinensis—Clonorchis sinensis
D. dendriticum—Dicrocoelium dendriticum
D. merlangi—Diclidophora merlangi

D. phoxini–Diplostomum phoxini
E. liei–Echinostoma liei
E. revolutum–Echinostoma revolutum
F. buski–Fasciolopsis buski
F. gigantica–Fasciola gigantica
F. hepatica–Fasciola hepatica
F. magna–Fascioloides magna
G. fimbriata–Gyrocotyle fimbriata
G. parvispinosa–Gyrocotyle parvispinosa
H. cylindracea–Haplometra cylindracea
H. medioplexus–Haematoloechus medioplexus
L. constantiae–Leucochloridiomorpha constantiae
M. monodi–Mesocoelium monodi
M. pygmaeus–Microphallus pygmaeus
M. similis–Microphallus similis
M. temperatus–Megalodiscus temperatus
P. cervi–Paramphistomum cervi
P. megalurus–Philophthalmus megalurus
P. microbothrium–Paramphistomum microbothrium
P. ohirai Paragonimus ohirai
P. westermani–Paragonimus westermani
S. douthitti–Schistosomatium douthitti
S. japonicum–Schistosoma japonicum
S. mansoni –Schistosoma mansoni
S. rodhaini–Schistosoma rodhaini

*Free-living species.

APPENDIX 7.3. LIST OF OTHER ABBREVIATIONS

ACP–acyl carrier protein
ADH–antidiuretic hormone
ATP, ADP, AMP–adenosine-5′-tri-, di- and monophosphate
CoA–coenzyme A
CoQ–coenzyme Q
CTP, CDP, CMP–cytidine-5′-tri-, di- and monophosphate
Δ–depression of freezing point
dCDP–deoxycytidine-5′-diphosphate
dUDP–deoxyuridine-5′-diphosphate
DDE–dichlorodiphenyldichloroethylene
DDT–dichlorodiphenyltrichloroethane
DNA–deoxyribonucleic acid
E_h–redox potential (mV)
FAD–flavin adenine dinucleotide

FBP—fructose-1,6-bisphosphate
FBPase—fructose-1,6-bisphosphatase
FH_2—dihydrofolate
FH_4—tetrahydrofolate
FMN—flavin mononucleotide
FP—flavoprotein
GH—growth hormone
G6Pase—glucose-6-phosphatase
GTP, GDP, GMP—guanosine-5'-tri-, di- and monophosphate
ITP, IDP, IMP—inosine-5'-tri, di- and monophosphate
K'—apparent equilibrium constant
K_a—dissociation constant (acid)
K_{eq}—thermodynamic equilibrium constant
K_i—inhibitor constant
K_m—Michaelis constant
K_{m_a}—apparent Michaelis constant
K_t—transport constant
L_3, L_4, L_5—third-, fourth- and fifth-stage larvae (nematodes)
NAD(H)—β-nicotinamide adenine dinucleotide (reduced)
NADP(H)—β-nicotinamide adenine dinucleotide phosphate (reduced)
NHI—non-haem iron
NTP, NDP, NMP—nucleoside tri-, di- and monophosphate
pCO_2—partial pressure of carbon dioxide (mmHg)
pO_2—partial pressure of oxygen (mmHg)
PFK—phosphofructokinase
pH—hydrogen ion concentration
P_i—inorganic phosphate
PP_i—pyrophosphate
ppGpp—guanosine-5'-diphosphate-2'-diphosphate
PRPP—5-phosphoribose pyrophosphate
P : O—phosphorylation : oxygen uptake ratio
Q—quinone
Q_{10}—temperature coefficient
QCO_2—μl CO_2 used/mg dry weight/h
QO_2—μl O_2 used/mg dry weight/h
RNA—ribonucleic acid
mRNA, rRNA, tRNA—messenger, ribosomal and transport RNA
RQ—respiratory quotient
RQ_9—rhodoquinone-9
SGF—sparganum growth factor
UQ—ubiquinone
UTP, UDP, UMP—uridine-5'-tri-, di- and monophosphate
V_m—maximum absorption rate
V_{max}—maximum enzyme activity

Systematic Index

The numbers in italics refer to figures or tables. This index should be used in conjunction with the table of contents and/or the subject index.

Subject Index

The numbers in italics refer to figures or tables.